# HOW to GROW a BABY

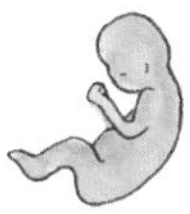

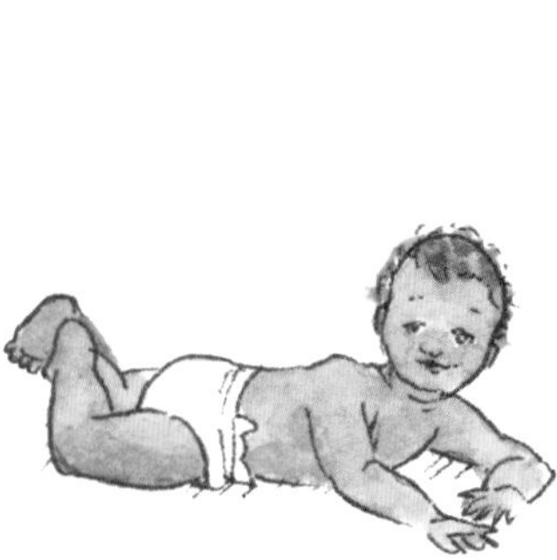

# HOW *to* GROW *a* BABY

A Science-Based Guide to Nurturing New Life, from Pregnancy to Childbirth and Beyond

Amy J. Hammer, RN

*Illustrated by* Michelle Lassaline

RB

ROOST BOOKS

**ROOST BOOKS**
An imprint of Shambhala Publications, Inc.
2129 13th Street
Boulder, Colorado 80302
roostbooks.com



The information presented in this book is for educational purposes only and is not intended to diagnose or treat any health conditions. Please consult your health practitioner regarding any specific health concerns and personal care.

Designed by **CAT GRISHAVER**



9 8 7 6 5 4 3 2 1

First Edition
Printed in China

♾ This edition is printed on acid-free paper that meets the American National Standards Institute Z39.48 Standard.

♻ Shambhala makes every effort to print on recycled paper. For more information please visit www.shambhala.com.

Roost Books is distributed worldwide by Penguin Random House, Inc., and its subsidiaries.

Library of Congress Cataloging-in-Publication Data

Names: Hammer, Amy, author.

Title: How to grow a baby: a science-based guide to nurturing new life, from pregnancy to childbirth and beyond / Amy Hammer; illustrated by Michelle Lassaline.

Description: First edition. | Boulder, Colorado: Roost Books, [2021] | Includes bibliographical references and index.

Identifiers: LCCN 2020035307 | ISBN 9781611808704 (trade paperback; alk. paper)

Subjects: LCSH: Pregnancy—Popular works. | Childbirth—Popular works. | Infants—Care—Popular works.

Classification: LCC RG525 .H355 2021 | DDC 618.2dc23

LC record available at https://lccn.loc.gov/2020035307

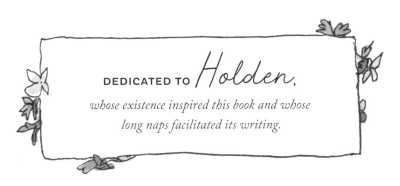

DEDICATED TO *Holden,*

*whose existence inspired this book and whose long naps facilitated its writing.*

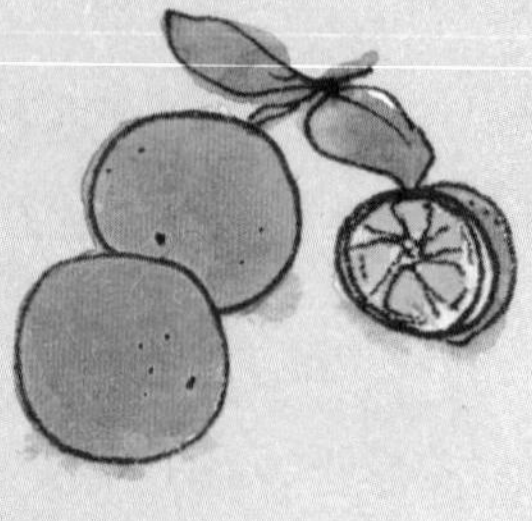

# Contents

# Prologue

I THOUGHT A LOT about E. O. Wilson, the famous entomologist who is known as the father of biodiversity, while I was pregnant with my son. Specifically, I thought about this quote of his: "The love of complexity without reductionism makes art; the love of complexity with reductionism makes science." Wilson understood that the study of the natural world and its creatures, including humans, requires science to reduce phenomena into disparate elements that can be measured and quantified. He also understood that the creative process we may call art is required to reassemble these elements into an integrated metaphor or story that is relatable. Like Wilson, I find that the blend of art and science is essential and helps us navigate and negotiate the uncertainty we face as humans.

When I was pregnant, I wanted to understand what science could and could not tell me about pregnancy, birth, and growing my baby. Science helped me understand the details of my son's development and my changing endocrine system, and it told me when my blood volume would increase and by how much. It guided me as I learned about the functional anatomy of the pelvic floor and the wondrous, diverse ecosystems of the various microbiota on my skin, mouth, gut, and vagina and how they are affected by food and pregnancy.

I noticed the undeniable blend of science and art when I researched and read stories about birth. As much as I could learn and understand this upcoming event, I could not science my way through it, and the stories my mom and other people told me about birth acted as a more relatable guide. Birth is mysterious. It transports us out of the thinking mind and into the feeling body, from study to experience. As an elaborate physiological process and an immensely personal and transformative life event, birth is both science and art.

"Ecology" comes from the word *oikos*, or home, and *logos*, the study and understanding of this home. I wrote this book to explore the home we create in our bodies for our babies. I explore how the external environment and choices we make shape our internal environment and how our internal environment then shapes the babies we grow. Part 1, "Getting Ready to Grow Your Baby," explores the magical moment in time when we start thinking about renting out that downstairs apartment known as the uterus. For as long as you can remember, perhaps for most of your life, the door to the apartment has been locked, and while the door's been knocked on, it's never been opened. When the lock is removed and all types of birth control are thrown out the window (into a responsible waste receptacle, of course), there are steps we can take to support ovulation, replenish potential nutrient deficiencies, and take care of the systems in the body that allow it to function well as a whole.

In the chapter on movement and the pelvis, we dive into the pelvic basin and swim around in its functional mysteries, including the impact of emotions, trauma, high heels, culture, and different types of movement on pelvic health and function. I talk about my favorite movement, one that takes us across landscapes, through forests, up and over mountains, and along sidewalks: walking. I believe that walking through pregnancy and walking with baby allows us to adapt to the changes in our bodies and minds and recalibrate our connection to the world.

Throughout the book we will examine our deepest and most long-term codependent relationships—and I'm not talking about the one between me and my cats. We live in codependent symbiosis with the microbial populations present on, in, and around our bodies. The trillions of bacteria that coevolved with us challenge what it means to be an individual, as we are truly a galaxy of ecosystems. Growing, birthing, and raising babies involve sharing and passing along the bacterial communities that form our microbiome. We have an opportunity to make choices about how we live that impact which bugs we nourish and share with our progeny.

In part 2, "Conception, Growing Your Baby, and Birth," we explore the journey from the union of the sperm and egg, to zygote, all the way to fully developed fetus. This section is rich in information about the science of fertilization and fetal development. Throughout the book I challenge you to consider how you impact the environment and how the environment impacts you and your baby, and I discuss ways to minimize exposure to toxins and support hormone and endocrine changes. We'll discuss movement and fetal positioning, birth and birthing, and the power of the stories we listen to and tell ourselves in the context of this big event.

After the birth we transition into our new role as a parent and learn through hands-on experience the person that is our child. We learn their grunts, the faces they make when they poop, and their urgent need for nurturing and nourishment. The placenta's job is done and the breasts take over growing the baby. Breastfeeding or chestfeeding is a complex physiological and chemical act that provides nourishment, immune and digestive system development, and connection between parent and baby. As scientist and writer Sandra Steingraber said of her baby and breastfeeding, "No one has ever enjoyed my breasts more. Faith [Steingraber's daughter] is the consumer. I am the consommé."

While your baby enjoys your breasts for many hours during the day and night, their brains grow and your brain changes. If your partner is intimately involved in caretaking, they also experience hormonal and brain changes that improve their ability to care for the baby. Part 3, "Growing Your Baby on the Outside," examines the composition of breast milk and how your environment, your experience of parenting, and the food you eat impact your healing body and baby's growing brain. We'll examine how we can nurture our senses during the postpartum period in ways that support the relationship between parent and baby at the physiological and neural level. Finally, we'll examine birth spacing, the integration of the parental and erotic self, and how the stories we choose shape our experience of parenting.

People have probably told you (usually over and over) that having a baby can be hard. Pregnancy can be uncomfortable, birth almost unbearably painful, breastfeeding challenging, and nights long and sleepless. And while some of these were true for me and there were many dirty diapers and hours spent breastfeeding, I found that knowing some of the why behind the sensations in my body and my baby's behavior helped me foster tolerance, respect, and patience. Coming back to the foundations of this book—movement, nourishing food, supportive communities, and taking care of our shared environment—helped guide and ground my choices as a new parent.

Understanding my invaluable, incredible, monumental role in the development of my son's inner ecology built within me a sense of wonder and confidence in my new job as his mother. My desire to learn what science and research had to teach me about growing my baby acted as a bridge to accepting the multitudes of unknown complexities the art of growing a person requires.

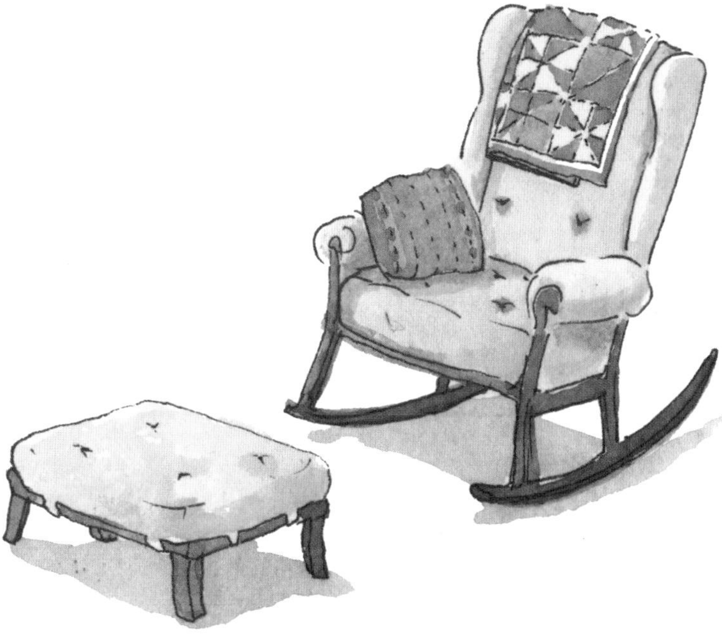

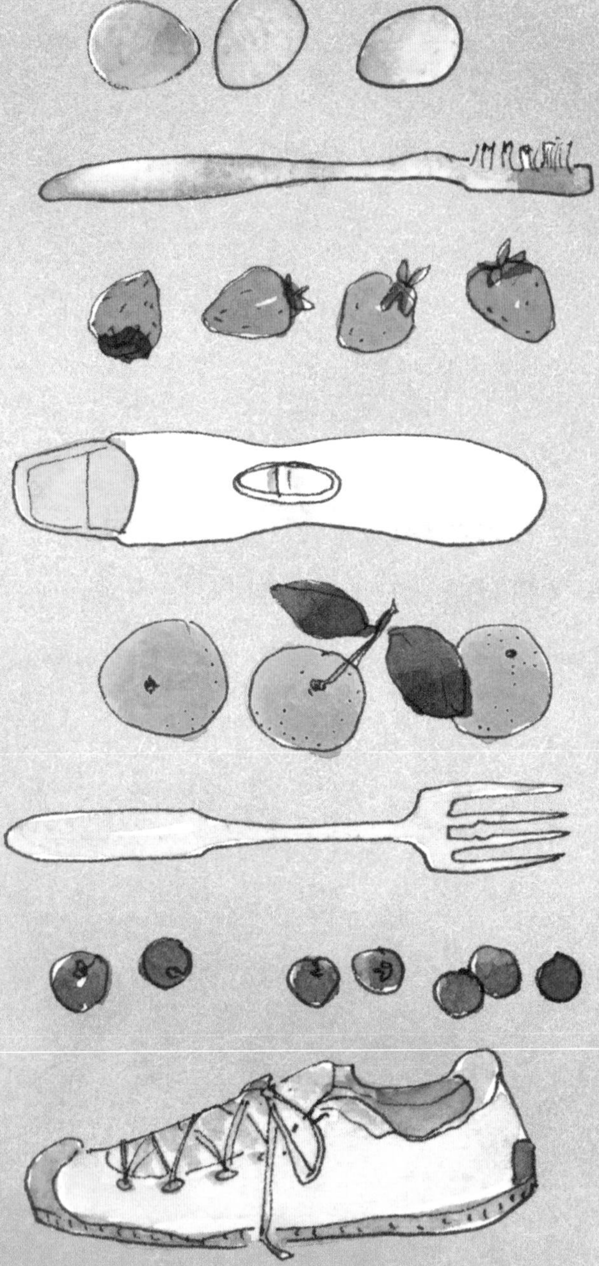

*Part One*

# GETTING READY *to* GROW YOUR BABY

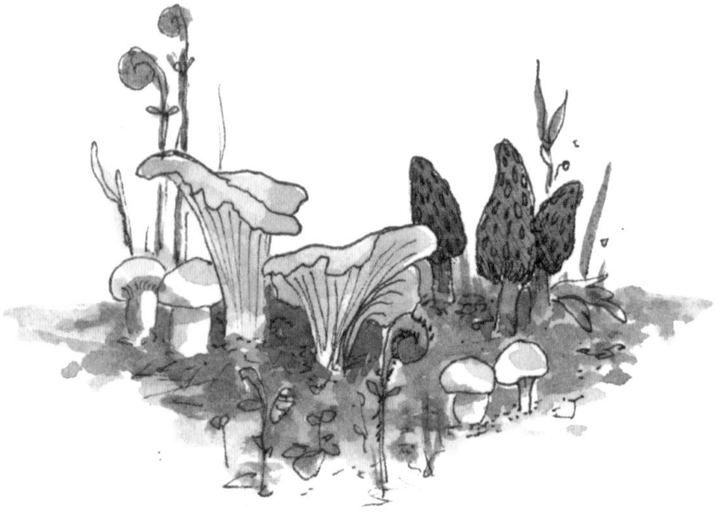

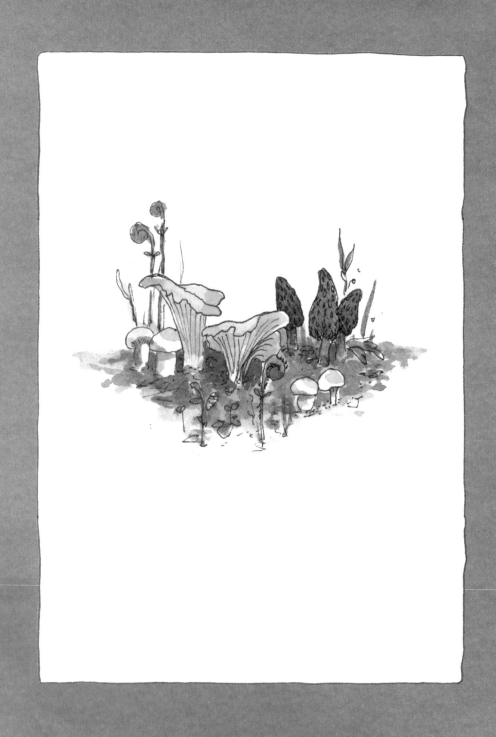

CHAPTER ONE

# New Beginnings

**MY SON WASN'T AN ACCIDENT,** but he wasn't necessarily planned. My partner Max and I were trying out doing *it* right and experimenting with a unique method of conception: not *not* trying. It turns out, if you do *it* right during the right time of the month, you might get pregnant.

I took one pregnancy test and it showed I was pregnant. I took another pregnancy test, which, instead of showing a plus sign, told me in plain English, "Pregnant." I read the test result over and over and over again. I stared at it, trying to let the word my eyes were reading sink into my brain and body.

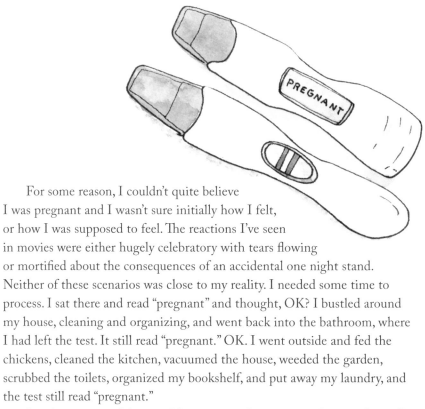

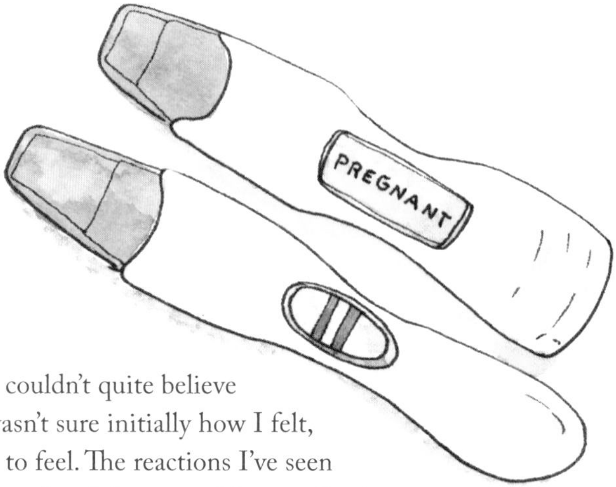


For some reason, I couldn't quite believe I was pregnant and I wasn't sure initially how I felt, or how I was supposed to feel. The reactions I've seen in movies were either hugely celebratory with tears flowing or mortified about the consequences of an accidental one night stand. Neither of these scenarios was close to my reality. I needed some time to process. I sat there and read "pregnant" and thought, OK? I bustled around my house, cleaning and organizing, and went back into the bathroom, where I had left the test. It still read "pregnant." OK. I went outside and fed the chickens, cleaned the kitchen, vacuumed the house, weeded the garden, scrubbed the toilets, organized my bookshelf, and put away my laundry, and the test still read "pregnant."

I took a picture of the test. If it was in a photo on my phone and it still read pregnant, it must be real. I questioned my sanity, but still I looked at the picture of the test on my phone, and it still showed the same result. I was excited in a way that felt distant, almost removed, since I couldn't feel anything yet, or if I could, I wondered if I created the feeling with my new knowledge.

I thought about the last few weeks and realized all the signs were there. On a recent visit to San Francisco, when my partner was giving a talk at an event, I felt something in my energy and body that I couldn't define. I felt impulsive and introspective. While he was at the event, I walked up the steepest streets, trudging through the city until I found some peace and greenery in a park on top of a hill. I sat in the grass and looked out at the city, and I could feel the whisper of a thought in my mind, but I wasn't ready to listen to what it was saying.

For my whole adult life, I made an effort to avoid pregnancy, and when I experienced pregnancy scares, it felt like a threat to life itself. My period would eventually arrive, bringing sensational relief, like a beacon of my ongoing freedom. From a young age, I knew I wanted to experience pregnancy and have children. It felt like a story that was already written in the narrative of my future life. But, I still had to adjust to the reality that this story was now officially starting.

I devised my own process that acted as a pathway toward accepting the reality of change in my body. I started by writing in my journal. My first entry read, "On June 26 I took two pregnancy tests that were positive. This means, unless something happens, that I am pregnant. Between June 10–26, this occurred." I followed this purely factual and unromantic entry with poetry. First, I wrote down "The Whistler" by Mary Oliver, a poem she wrote when she realized that her partner, whom she had lived with for thirty years, could whistle and she understood that we never fully know or possess the people we love. I wasn't sure if my body was the whistler, someone or something I thought I knew for thirty years, capable of such a simple and lovely thing as whistling, or in my case pregnancy, or if I was thinking of Max and our future child, both people I live with and love and will never fully know or possess. The next poem I wrote down was "The Mushroom Hunters" by Neil Gaiman. The last stanza of the poem reads,

The scientists walk more slowly, over to the brow of the hill
and down the water's edge and past the place
where the red clay runs.
They are carrying their babies in the slings they made,
Freeing their hands to pick the mushrooms.

These words gave my journey a destination, my body a job, and my hands a purpose.

When I first wrote to my growing baby, I referred to him as an embryo, as in "Dear Embryo," and told him about the science of his development. I told him that I took two pregnancy tests because I am the kind of person who wants to Know with a capital K, but also that I knew before I knew because I felt my breasts grow tender and something like sureness and intangibility deeper in my body.

I told Max I was pregnant on a sunny afternoon on our upstairs deck. A quiet, surprised grin spread across his face. "OK," he said, still smiling. "OK, wow," and I could see the wheels turning in his head, processing a new future, and I could feel his deep calm mixed with excitement.

## THE PILL

Six years earlier, when I was twenty-two years old, I stopped taking hormonal birth control. I started taking it when I was sixteen because I struggled with acne. At that time in my life I wasn't concerned about the importance of ovulation or my menstrual cycle; I was miserable because of my skin. It seemed like nothing worked. I went to a few dermatologists and they prescribed topical treatments like benzoyl peroxide, which burned my skin and made it feel raw and painful.

I'd never stick with their treatment plans because the products made my skin feel so bad. Then I started taking the pill and my skin cleared up. It felt like a miracle, and I was grateful. For six years I took the pill and didn't think twice. One day I decided I didn't want to take hormones that came from outside my body anymore. It wasn't for any distinct reason other than I felt a vague sense of separateness from myself that was hard to explain.

I figured I should use some kind of birth control, so I got a nonhormonal copper IUD. This T-shaped copper-coated frame is inserted into the uterus and prevents pregnancy by eliciting an inflammatory state that is toxic to

# The Endocrine System

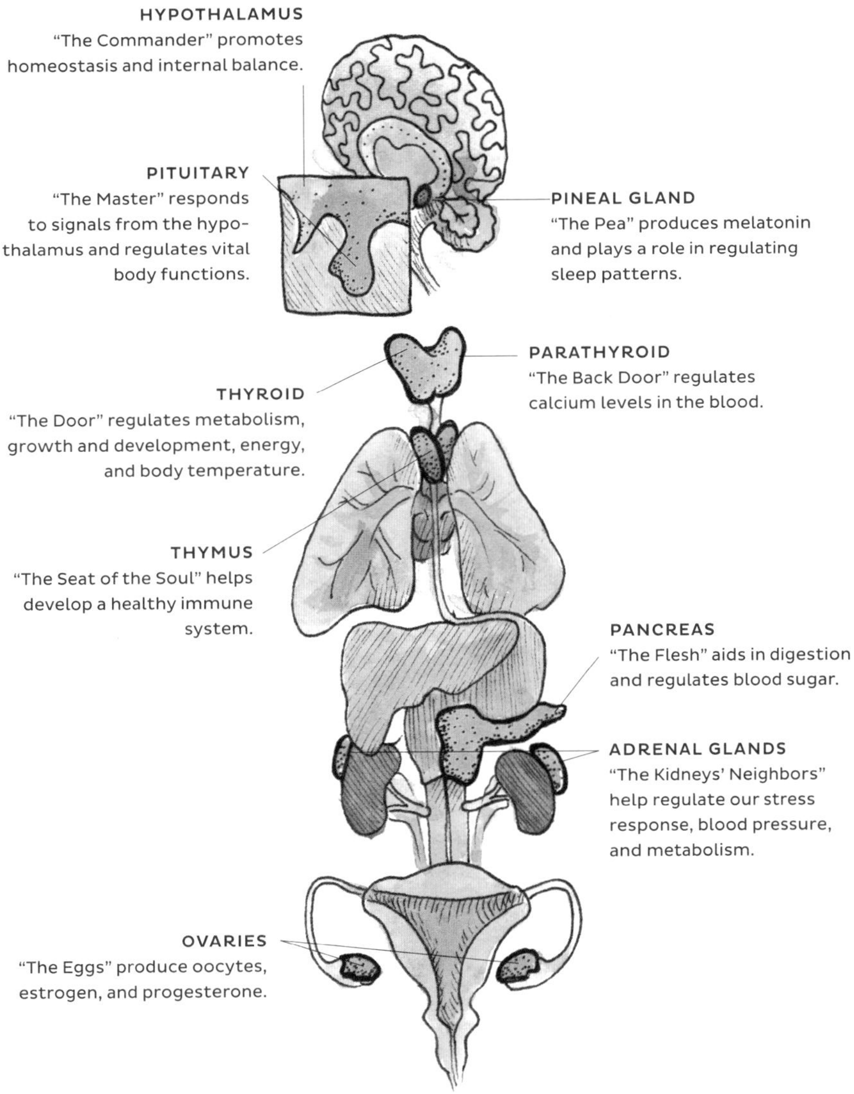

**HYPOTHALAMUS**
"The Commander" promotes homeostasis and internal balance.
**PITUITARY**
"The Master" responds to signals from the hypothalamus and regulates vital body functions.
**PINEAL GLAND**
"The Pea" produces melatonin and plays a role in regulating sleep patterns.
**PARATHYROID**
"The Back Door" regulates calcium levels in the blood.
**THYROID**
"The Door" regulates metabolism, growth and development, energy, and body temperature.
**THYMUS**
"The Seat of the Soul" helps develop a healthy immune system.
**PANCREAS**
"The Flesh" aids in digestion and regulates blood sugar.
**ADRENAL GLANDS**
"The Kidneys' Neighbors" help regulate our stress response, blood pressure, and metabolism.
**OVARIES**
"The Eggs" produce oocytes, estrogen, and progesterone.

# The Hypothalamic Pituitary Gonadal Axis

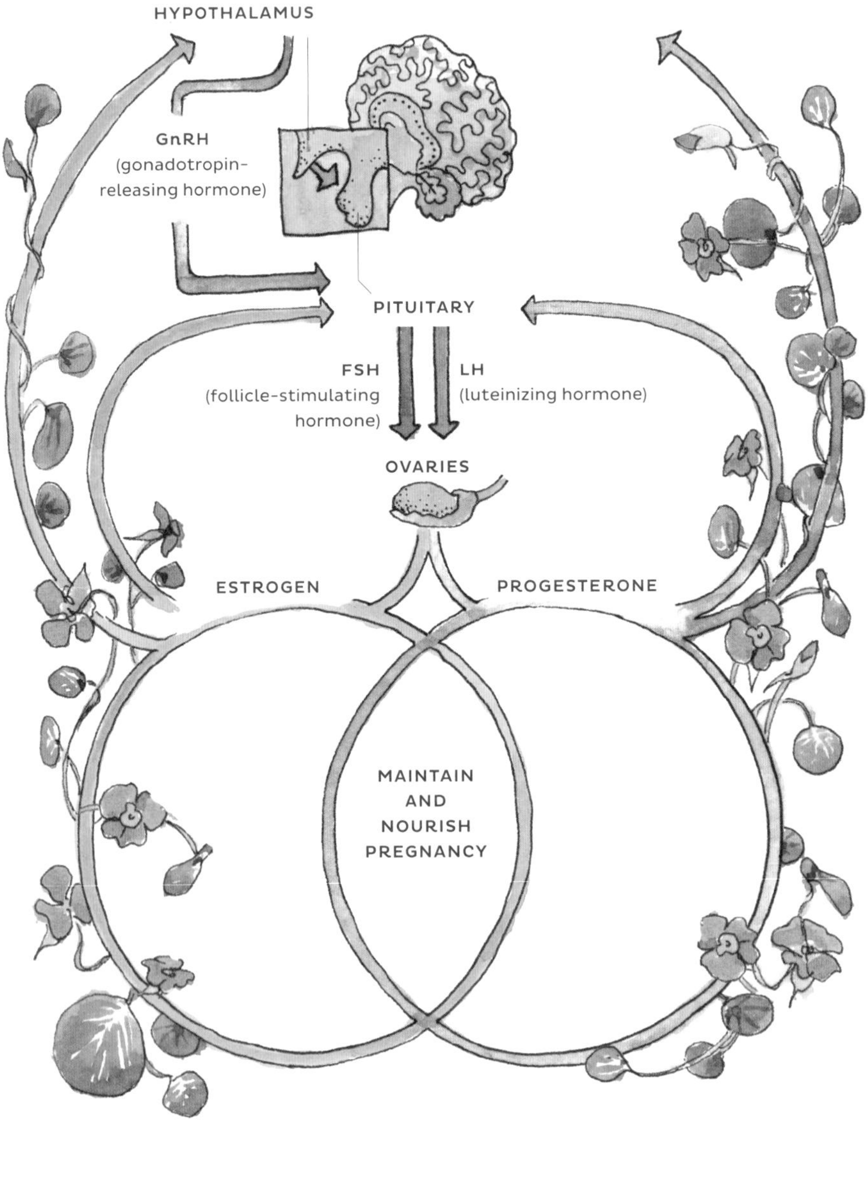

both sperm and eggs. I heard "long-term, nonhormonal birth control" and jumped at the opportunity, missing the fine print about side effects, like severe menstrual pain and heavy bleeding. It had seemed like the perfect option: it was hormone-free, and many of my friends loved their IUDs. Alas, it wasn't for me. Maybe I didn't give it enough time, but after a few months of the forewarned severe pain and heavy and unbearable periods, I figured I might as well try nothing for a while.

This timing was both painful and perfect. My long-term boyfriend and I split up after six years of dating, so I was suddenly single and had some time to get to know my body again during a period of reflective abstinence.

The first thing that changed was my skin. I felt like a teenager again as acne, especially around my jawline, emerged and seemed impervious to my various efforts to cover or eradicate it, instead getting worse, as if it were rebelling against those years of suppression. It turns out, when you stop taking the pill, your body experiences dynamic hormonal shifts, and the production of androgen hormones, like testosterone, may suddenly go into overdrive. Androgens are part of the hormonal waterfall that initiates puberty, and they play an important role in skin health. However, excess androgens cause excess sebum production. Sebum is a waxy, skin-lubricating substance produced by sebaceous glands. Skin cells, from normal cell turnover, can combine with sebum and plug hair follicles. The plugged-up follicles get infected and inflamed, and we call those obnoxious blemishes pimples.

Hormonal contraceptives help clear up acne because they decrease sebum production. I took a combination pill, or a low-dose estrogen and progesterone pill, which is the most common oral contraceptive. These hormones are synthetic versions of the real thing, and they drastically decrease the body's production of endogenous hormones, or hormones of internal origin, specifically estrogen and progesterone.

How do they do this? Well, they communicate with the commander and the master of our hormonal production, respectively known as the hypothalamus and the pituitary gland. The hypothalamus receives information about the body and its hormonal state and sends instructions to the pituitary to perform its crucial role of maintaining the tight hormonal range of the body. The pituitary responds by sending a signal down to the ovaries in the form of

FSH (follicle-stimulating hormone). FSH does exactly what its name says it does. It tells the ovaries to start stimulating some follicles, or eggs, for the big event: ovulation.

When we take synthetic estrogen and progesterone, the communication pathways between the hypothalamus, pituitary, and ovaries are interrupted. The ovaries stop waiting by the phone for FSH to call, and they shut down. Without enough estrogen and progesterone, the cushy, thick endometrial lining—the place where a fertilized egg implants—thins and becomes inhospitable. Finally, the cervical mucus, a viscous and elastic sign of fertility that creates channels for sperm to swim up through the cervix, becomes thick and impassable.

The ingestion of synthetic hormones suppresses our body's production of essential reproductive hormones and thus suppresses ovulation. Because our hormones are complex and have many roles, the pill has systemic effects on parts of our body we don't generally connect to reproductive health, like mood and skin oil production. Estradiol, one of three naturally occurring estrogens in the body, is a hormone made from cholesterol that plays an essential role in ovulation and other endocrine functions, like insulin sensitivity. Progesterone, another hormone we associate mainly with reproductive health, also impacts our immune, enzymatic, and muscular function and helps us sleep and feel less anxious.

Ingesting the synthetic version of these hormones, thus decreasing the amount produced naturally in the body, can lead to a variety of side effects, like depression; blood clots; hair loss; vaginal dryness; painful intercourse; hypertension; thyroid issues; vitamin, mineral, and antioxidant depletion; altered microbiota; metabolic changes that can cause weight gain; and on and on.

When I stopped taking the pill it wasn't because I wanted to get pregnant. But years later, when I learned more about my cycle, the importance of ovulation, and the role of the hormones I had suppressed for years, I was worried about my reproductive health. I was also confused about what the pill meant for me in the narrative I had constructed about my right as a woman to make decisions about my body. The pill had come to represent my power as a woman to choose when I wanted to have babies, and it felt like a safeguard against worry.

It doesn't feel like that anymore. I took the pill without knowing anything about the power and phases of my menstrual cycle. I took it without acknowledging or fully knowing about all the side effects, and I tuned out and suppressed a story—the story of my body and how it works—that I've now spent years relearning. I am fiercely protective of my right to make decisions about my body, and I don't want to make them blindly. It is our right to choose what kind of birth control we want to use, to receive information and education about how our bodies work, and to deeply understand the pros and cons of our choices. When you become pregnant, or if you're thinking about it, you have the opportunity to learn a different story about your body and make choices that will make you feel more aligned with yourself and more powerful.

## OVULATION CELEBRATION

I like the word "ovulation"; it reminds me of other happy words like "salutation," "congratulation," and "sensation." Ovulation is central to menstrual health, overall health, and fertility, and it is the most exciting and loaded event we get to relearn when we stop taking the pill and wake up the connection between our brain and our ovaries.

Ovulation is the release of a mature egg from an ovary into the fallopian tube. Right before we ovulate, estrogen levels peak, which causes a dynamic upsurge of luteinizing hormone (LH), which tells one of the ovaries to release an egg. After we stop taking the pill, we experience a transitory state of recalibration that affects our hormone levels and fertility.

In her book *The Fifth Vital Sign*, Lisa Hendrickson-Jack recommends waiting at least eighteen months before trying to get pregnant after you stop taking the pill. This suggestion is based on optimizing fertility, and this time frame demonstrates the toll of time hormonal contraceptives can take on the body. When we give our bodies enough time to repair the communication pathways that mediate our reproductive hormones and replenish the nutrients

# *The Menstrual Cycle*

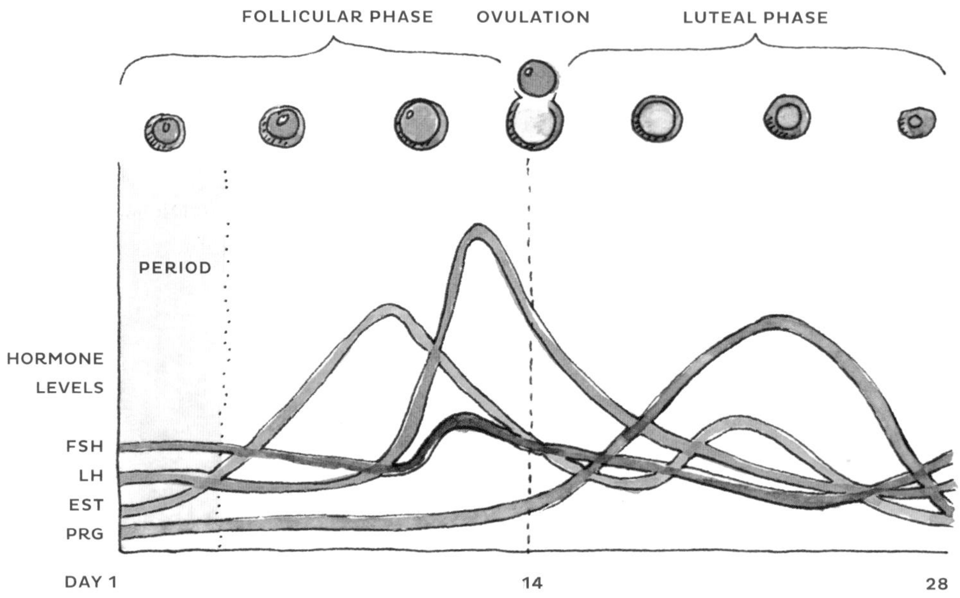


This graph shows a 28-day menstrual cycle with ovulation occurring on day 14. However, it is essential to note that the timing of ovulation is highly variable between individuals and from cycle to cycle in the same individual. A normal cycle length is around 24–35 days with the follicular phase lasting, on average, 16.9 days. Ovulation happens on only one day in the cycle, and the most likely days of conception occur within a six day fertile window, with the highest rates of conception occurring the day before ovulation and the day of ovulation.

the pill depletes, it is like putting in a foundation for the house we want to build. It takes a long time, but it allows us to build a healthy, strong base.

The pill shuts down the communication between the brain and the ovaries. This pathway plays a role in reproductive function as it regulates ovulation, but synthetic hormones also affect the functioning and structure of the brain. Receptor sites for estrogenic, androgenic, and progestogenic sex hormones exist throughout the brain and limbic system and affect emotional processing and development. This means that coming off hormonal birth control is a dynamic process that affects every system in the body, including the way we think.

Is this why, when I stopped taking the pill, I felt compelled to go on walks every night and observe the owls that seemed to speak to a part of me I had lost? Surely it wasn't wise to go out on my own past dark to hike around in the high desert with the potential threat of animals, both human and non-human. But I couldn't resist. I was recovering from a broken heart and experiencing shifts in my body I didn't understand at the time and I wanted to be alone, moving through the night, with the owls' *hoot! hoot!* to surprise me out of my ruminations and into my body that felt delighted by the wildness of the night.

It was around this time that I started working on an organic farm. Maybe my body knew that birth control had depleted key nutrients and led me back into the soil and deeper into my connection with food. I'd wake up with the sun, bike to the farm, and work until early afternoon when it was so hot the air itself felt suffocated by heat. Sweaty, dirty, and dehydrated, I'd bike home, always in a headwind, with barely enough time to shower and get ready for the catering job I worked at nights.

My body ached and I barely made enough money, but when I worked in the garden in the mornings, when it was still cool and quiet, I had space to feel changes in my awareness. I thought about how the history of hormonal contraceptives is told as a great feminist achievement, but it seemed to me that the cost of taking the pill was the suppression and regulation of my hormones, which told a story of fertility and cyclicity in my body.

Hormonal contraceptives impact our ecosystem by altering reproductive health, but they are also linked to nutrient deficiencies and can cause issues with mood, skin, thyroid, and liver health. Fortunately, we are not a stagnant system. We are the primary influencers of our inimitable biomes, capable of making choices that support our inner ecology, bolstering its resilience and nourishing our health, so that we create a sustaining environment when we decide to grow a baby. The choices we make about how we move our body, what we feed it, and how we interact with the world have implications for our health and the health of our babies, and these choices trickle down into our communities and the greater world in which we live.

My favorite choices I get to make that affect my hormones come in the form of dark leafy greens, avocados, mushrooms, yogurt, dark chocolate, oysters, pastured meat and eggs, and organ meats, like liver, from grass-fed cows. I enjoy sitting down and choosing to drink a mug of green tea or bone broth, or to devour roasted kale and brussels sprouts right off the baking sheet, or to tuck into a sweet potato slathered in butter and sprinkled with salt and cinnamon for dessert.

I like to think about food and nourishment as meals that I'll share with my friends and family that incidentally also support my reproductive health and important systems like my thyroid and liver. No one eats just nutrients; we all eat food. Nutrients are singular, and industry can manipulate and isolate them. Food is complex, interesting, cultural, delicious, and magical. It contains stories, traditions, and rituals, and unlike isolated nutrients, it can be grown, harvested, and shared with those we love.

## FEEDING THE THYROID AND LIVER

If I were writing a cookbook for your thyroid to enjoy, I'd include certain key ingredients to bring it both delight and optimal health. The ingredients would include iodine-containing foods, which are essential for creating thyroid hormones, like seaweed, seafood, oily fish, dairy products, and eggs. Some foods, like soy products, can block the thyroid's uptake of iodine, so for these foods to make it onto the ingredient list, they need to be fermented,

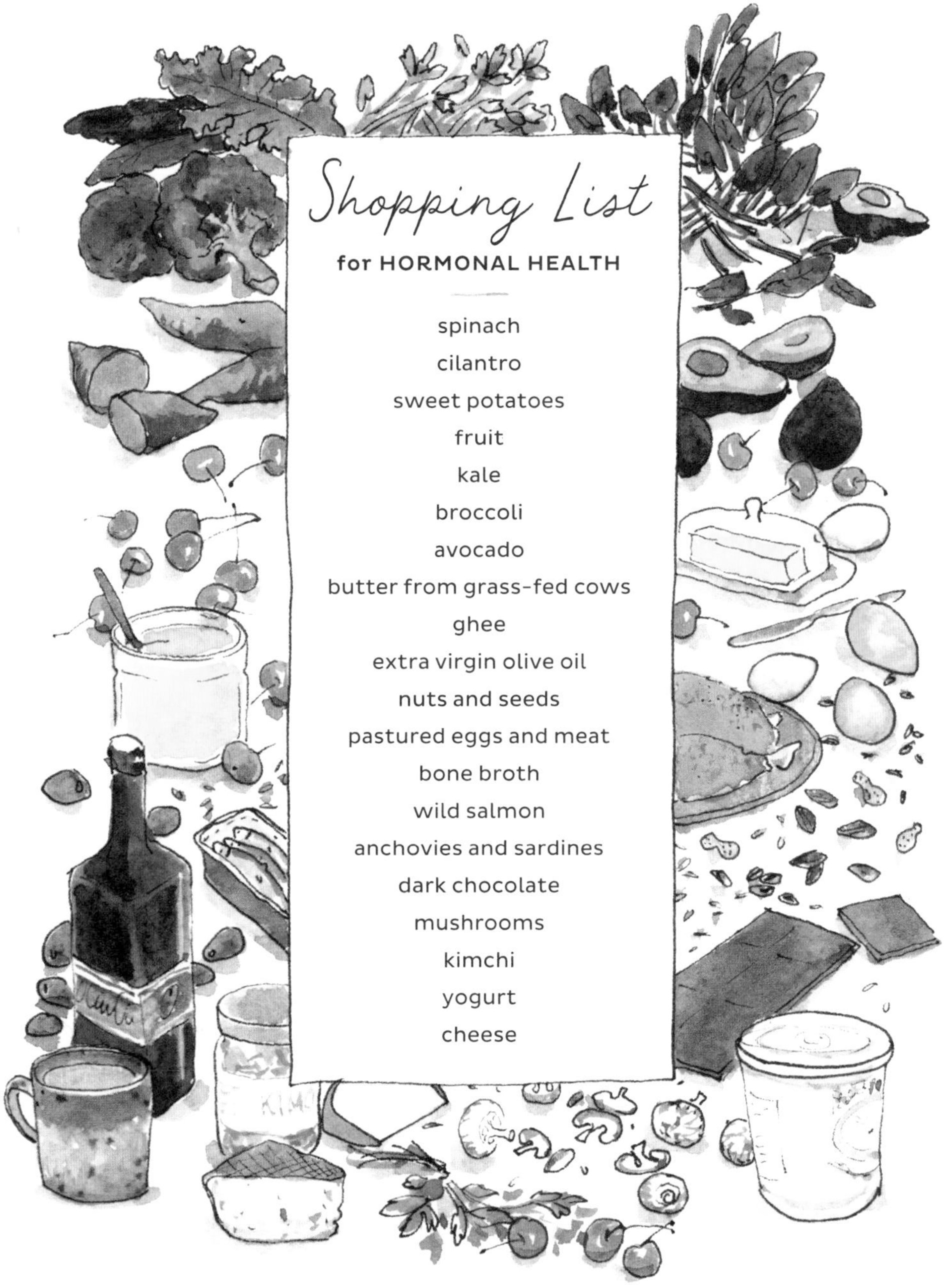

# Shopping List

## for HORMONAL HEALTH

spinach
cilantro
sweet potatoes
fruit
kale
broccoli
avocado
butter from grass-fed cows
ghee
extra virgin olive oil
nuts and seeds
pastured eggs and meat
bone broth
wild salmon
anchovies and sardines
dark chocolate
mushrooms
kimchi
yogurt
cheese

# Replenish Key Nutrients

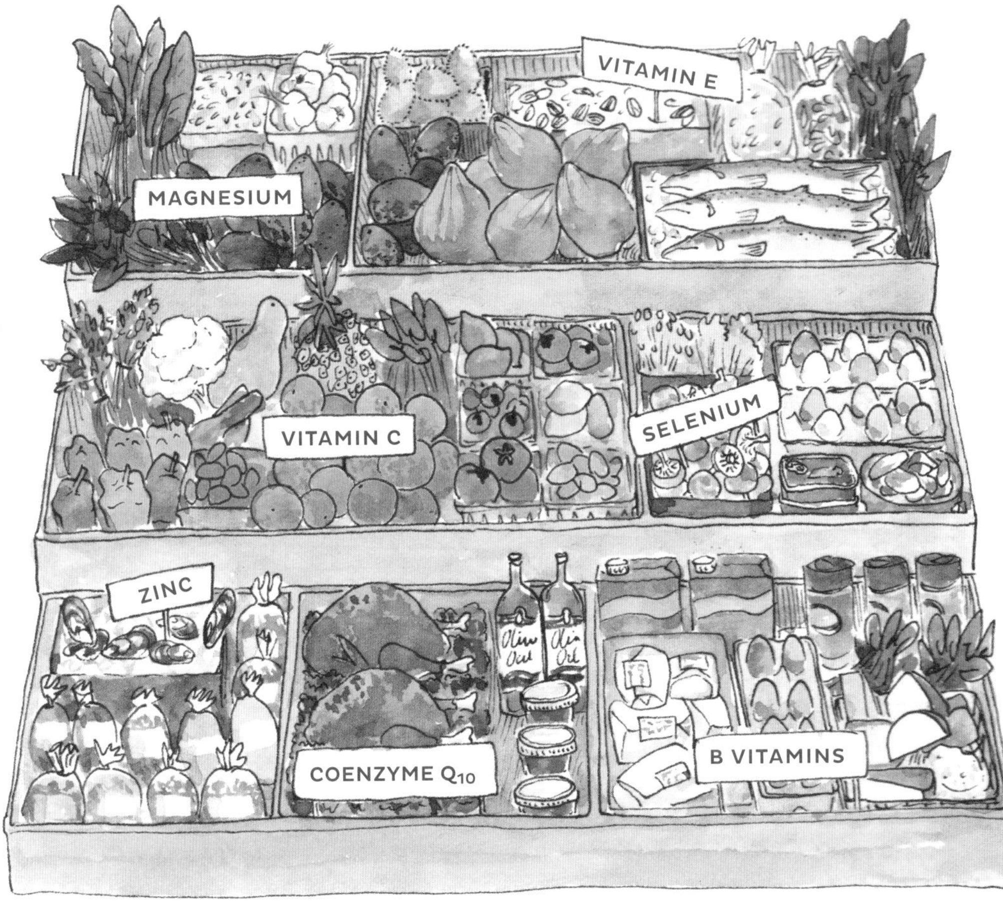

**MAGNESIUM** is an essential mineral that improves energy and cellular functioning, is a cofactor in 300+ enzymatic reactions, and supports a balanced mood. Its sources include spinach, chard, collards, avocado, garlic, yogurt, pumpkin seeds, almonds, and cashews.

**VITAMIN E** is an antioxidant that promotes cardiovascular health, supports and interacts with vitamin C, and protects cells from oxidative damage. Its sources include wild salmon, trout, mango, kiwi, avocado, spinach, sunflower seeds, almonds, peanuts, and pine nuts.

**VITAMIN C** is an antioxidant that supports collagen synthesis and UV protection and is essential for skin health, wound healing, and tissue repair. Its sources include citrus fruits, bananas, strawberries, pineapple, tomatoes, bell peppers, parsley, kale, cauliflower, brussels sprouts, sweet potatoes, and squash.

**SELENIUM** is an antioxidant that supports the health of the thyroid, immune system, and nervous system and protects against cancer. Its sources include Brazil nuts, seafood, organ meats, mushrooms, and eggs.

**ZINC** is an essential trace element that acts as an anti-inflammatory and supports thyroid health, immune health, healing, and the production of GABA (a calming neurotransmitter that promotes restful sleep). Its sources include oysters, seafood, grass-fed beef, pastured poultry, pumpkin seeds, hemp seeds, and pine nuts.

**COENZYME $Q_{10}$** is an antioxidant that supports cellular production of energy and supports immune function. Its sources include oily fish, organ meats, grass-fed beef, pastured pork and chicken, and extra virgin olive oil.

**B VITAMINS** promote energy production and enzymatic reactions; support cardiovascular and nervous system health, cognitive function, and metabolism; feed beneficial microbial communities in the gut; and support fertility and fetal development. Their sources include leafy greens, organ meats, eggs, brewer's yeast, bone broth, sprouts, wild game, pastured meats, and cheese.

which lessens their goitrogenic, or iodine-blocking, effect. Tyrosine, an amino acid with a strong showing in poultry, yogurt, and cheese, and selenium, which is present in Brazil nuts, salmon, mushrooms, and other foods, also support thyroid health.

Thyroid hormones primarily affect our metabolism and are involved in protein synthesis, neurological function, and fetal development. The hormones from the thyroid influence libido, fertility, and reproduction. I keep tabs on my thyroid functioning through lab work because I have a family history of hypothyroidism, and some people may develop thyroid issues following pregnancy.

Vitamin D, movement, and stress management nurture thyroid health. Your thyroid doesn't want you eating junk food from a drive-through as you hurry throughout your day. Thyroid wants you to slow down, feel the sunshine, taste your food, and enjoy the moment. If I were cooking a romantic meal for my thyroid tonight, I'd make it buttermilk roast chicken with cranberry sauce, roasted asparagus, and a big green salad with a few chopped Brazil nuts and cheese on top and a simple dressing of lemon juice, sea salt, and extra-virgin olive oil. If things went well, the morning after we'd drink bone broth with seaweed and eggs stirred in to make a nourishing soup, and then we'd go on a meandering outdoor walk.

The thyroid is the little gland with big impacts mainly on the body's metabolic functions, but the liver is a giant organ that has more than five hundred separate functions in conjunction with other organs and systems. It is central to fetal development, as it is the main site of red blood cell production until thirty-two weeks of gestation, and it plays a role in growth during childhood development. Insulin and other hormones are broken down by the liver, and toxins are conjugated and primarily excreted in urine or bile. Bile is also central to digestive health, as it emulsifies fats and improves absorption of the fat-soluble vitamins A, D, E, and K.

The liver and thyroid are functionally interrelated. Liver enzymes play a role in processing thyroid hormones and in metabolism. Thyroid hormones give back by supporting liver function and bilirubin metabolism. When the thyroid is dysfunctional and our hormone levels are suboptimal, liver function is affected and issues with the thyroid arise. These two either work together like industrious old colleagues, or they encourage the other's demise.

The liver likes strong flavors like garlic, onions, cabbage, and egg yolks. It isn't scared of a little flatulence and enjoys cruciferous vegetables, fruits and vegetables high in fiber, herbs like cilantro, fermented foods, turmeric, berries, bitter greens, and beets. It will enjoy the same meal as the thyroid, but add in some roasted broccoli with garlic and throw some sauerkraut, cilantro, and bitter greens on top.

There are many liver detox diets, but the liver likes the gentle and slow approach and doesn't trust those young guns selling you powders and pills and quick fixes. Curmudgeonly though it may seem, the liver is principled. Consistently choosing healthy food, avoiding inflammatory foods like sugar, alcohol, and refined carbohydrates, moving more, and keeping toxins off our skin and out of our homes are the kind of responsible behaviors the liver respects.

Supporting liver function helps clear endocrine-disrupting chemicals and toxins from our system. Hormonal contraceptives, exposure to environmental toxins, excessive alcohol, and certain medications can have a deleterious effect on the liver, but if we do well by our livers, they tend to take care of us, capable even of regeneration.

## CHOICE IS PARAMOUNT

There's a good chance that if you're reading a book about growing a baby, you're already pregnant. Pregnancy introduces us to what we experience frequently as parents: relentless choices and concern about the consequences of our actions combined with some guesswork. We learn information and make choices that make sense in the moment, then we learn new information that impacts our future choices and sometimes makes us lament our past choices. We live in an ongoing cycle of consideration and growth.

For example, I wish I had had my vitamin D level tested before I became pregnant. Instead, I had it tested after I worked night shifts for a month and the number was dismal. I was stressed and worried about the impact of my low vitamin D on my baby, and I wanted to quit my job and spend the rest of my days walking in the mountains and eating fresh, wild fish, making sure I got all the vitamin D I needed. Instead I negotiated with my boss to stop working nights for the rest of my pregnancy. I increased my consumption of vitamin D–rich foods, took vitamin $D_3$ supplements, and spent lots of time outdoors on my days off.

My experience with vitamin D taught me that information acts as a gateway to change and self-advocacy. Going through something new or challenging, like pregnancy and birth, is an opportunity for profound learning. I found that the answers to so many of my questions and anxieties were waiting for me in the form of research and stories from those who had walked the path before me.

A middle stanza of Gaiman's poem reads, "Observe childbirth, measure the swell of bellies and the shape of breasts, / and through experience discover how to bring babies safely into the world." Experiences, mistakes, and journeys build the narrative arcs of our lives and connect us. No matter what happened before this moment, we are capable of observing and making choices moving forward that help us build up our own power and bolster the health of the babies we grow.

# TAKE ACTION

Replenish your body with key nutrients, especially if you have a history of hormonal contraceptive use. Focus on high-quality, diverse, real foods. Dark leafy greens, fruits and vegetables, fermented foods, pastured meats and eggs, wild fish, and healthy fats like olive oil or butter from grass-fed cows create the building blocks of hormones and support optimal hormonal health.

Relearn the cycles of your body. Growing a baby gives us an opportunity to learn a new story about our bodies. Learn about the physiological changes that happen during pregnancy so that you can make informed decisions and approach pregnancy with calm empowerment.

Nourish your thyroid, liver, and overall health with habits like enough sleep, movement, and nourishing food. Avoid drugs, harmful chemicals, alcohol, and processed food. Sounds simple enough, but a daily effort to take care of yourself—your body, mind, and baby—is grounding and essential.

Observe your body, nature, and habits and feel empowered to make choices moving forward that support the health of your body and your baby. Approaching new information and events with an open mind and a willingness to learn from those who came before allows us to approach pregnancy and parenting with confidence and humility, empowerment, and the understanding that we can't control or know everything. This is the first lesson of parenthood.

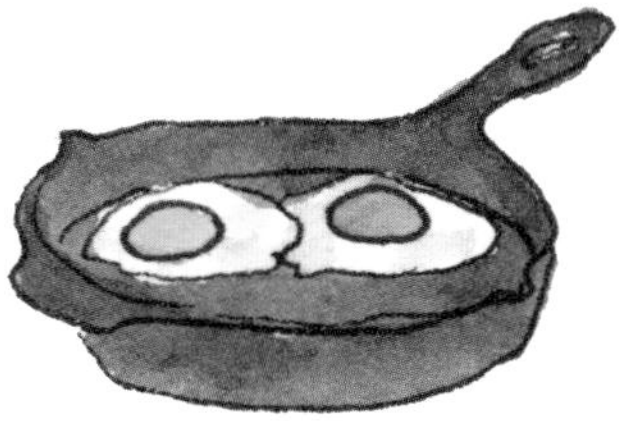

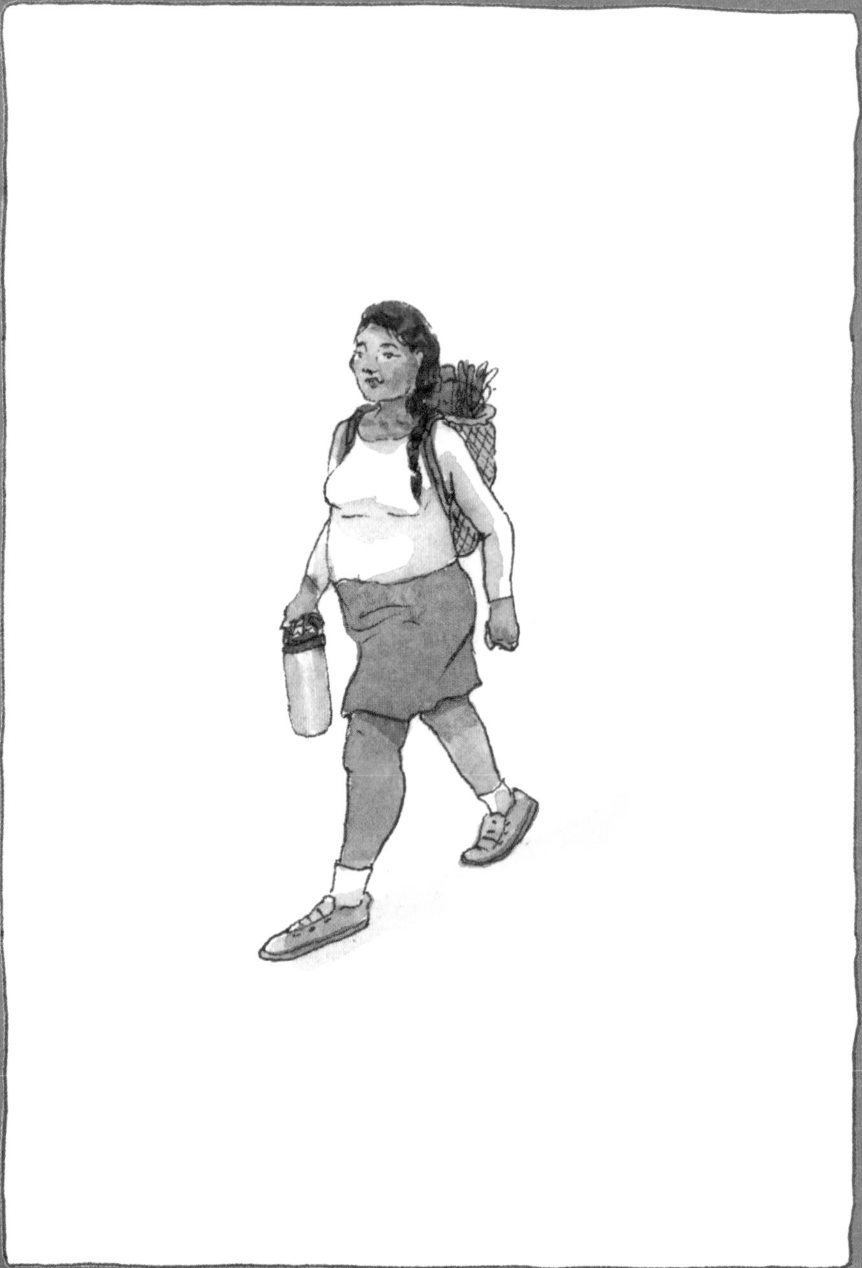

CHAPTER TWO

# Movement & the Mighty Pelvis

**WHEN I WAS PREGNANT** with my son, I worked as a nurse on the seventh floor of the hospital in a busy cardiac intensive care unit. Each morning I climbed up eight flights of stairs. I was diligently committed to avoiding the elevator. I tightened the straps of my backpack, loaded with my second breakfast, first lunch, second lunch, snacks, and water, like I was preparing to climb a mountain. At the beginning of my pregnancy, I kept my pace, and when the rare doctor, nurse, or pharmacist entered the stairwell behind me, I confidently made it to my destination without stopping and without experiencing my nightmare: getting passed.

One morning, sometime in my second trimester, I started my ascent and felt winded right away. As I stopped to gather myself, a doctor entered the stairwell just one flight below. This wasn't just any doctor. He is a rock climber, a sinewy, fit, long-legged mountain man with energy to spare, and he started galloping up the stairs, two at a time. When I saw him, I picked up my pace and attempted an air of casual lightness and grace as my heart pounded and I overheated. It occurred to me after the fifth floor that he must be working on my unit today, and I had to continue my facade of ease for a few more flights. He bounded up behind me as I opened the door to the unit. "Nice clip," he said and disappeared around the corner, a flash of muscle and pure energy. My face was flushed, my heart pounded, and I slowly caught my breath. I decided that from then on, I'd leave my ego at the bottom of the stairs and just make it up, one step at a time.

I took the stairs, but they were my master. With my scrubs it was hard to tell that I was pregnant, until it became obvious the last few months. I fought the urge to explain to people who passed me on the stairs that I was pregnant and that's why I was taking a break to watch the sunrise, that's why I was wearing my T-shirt in winter and sweating, that's why I was huffing and puffing and pausing and using my arms to pull myself up the stairs. I faced my changing body each morning and noticed when my heart started to beat faster because of the increase in my blood volume. I noticed when it felt hard to catch a deep breath, or when my son was kicking or hiccuping or dancing in my belly. I had never sought validation for my stubborn stair habit, but during the last two months of my pregnancy I relished the praise of my coworkers as I continued to put one foot in front of the other.

Some days almost felt easy. Others felt impossible, and I tried different tactics to trick myself up the stairs, like counting to ten in French over and over (*un, deux, trois, quatre, cinq, six, sept, huit, neuf, dix*) and imagining legions of fans cheering me on as I summited the last few steps. I hiked, climbed mountains, and walked frequently during my pregnancy. When I was fourteen weeks pregnant I climbed the Grand Teton in Jackson, Wyoming, a 13,776-foot climb with 7,000 feet of elevation gain, but the stairs were my proving ground, and they proved much more challenging. Each morning the top of the staircase was a small celebration that got bigger as my belly grew.

I took the stairs every day I went to work until I stopped going to work and had my baby.

The stairs taught me about the value and reward of moving and continuing to move throughout my pregnancy. Giving birth is a physical event that requires strength, stamina, and overall alignment. Movement during pregnancy, like walking and climbing stairs, strengthens the body as it gains mass and supports the function and health of the pelvic floor.

The purpose of movement is to keep the whole body healthy and working together, and we continue to need movement while we grow babies. Movement helps create space in the body and supports the development and positioning of the growing fetus. In practice, the movements I performed during my pregnancy were remarkably simple, if not remarkably easy. I walked and hiked outdoors, squatted, sat on the floor, stretched, helped remodel our home, planted and harvested food from the garden and cooked meals, cleaned the house, climbed a few safe trees, played with my niece and nephew, and took the stairs instead of the elevator. I also rested. Some days, when I felt especially tired, I neglected my garden. Sometimes I only went for a walk around the block and felt winded, while other times I hiked miles up a mountain and felt like a champion. My level of movement varied, and that was OK.

We all have different starting points and have moved differently in different bodies over our lifetimes. It makes sense that when we get pregnant, we start at different points of alignment, strength, and endurance, and the way I choose to move isn't the way you have to choose to move. It just matters *that* we choose to move. Exercise can at times feel prescriptive and like it doesn't meet us where we're at. Movement, on the other hand, has the potential to change the way we live and challenge our leanings toward convenience and sedentarism. The message is not "Do not exercise"; it is "Move more, more often, and in more ways."

Max and I attended a two-day intensive childbirth class because I felt that we should and I didn't want my birth to be his first viewing of this event. While the class was informative and the teacher said sweet things about birthing, like "Your body is having a baby, let it," what I remember most were the videos of women quietly giving birth with Enya playing in the background.

I wanted to have a nonmedicated vaginal birth, but I was pretty sure mine wouldn't be a quiet, nonstrenuous affair.

I moved because it felt good, and I moved because I wanted to do anything I could to increase my chances of having the birth I wanted and to decrease the time I spent pushing out my baby. How we move and our alignment affect baby's position, and position may affect how long it takes to push a baby out of your body. There are no promises when it comes to birth, and expectations can lead to disappointment, but movement supports not only birth but also the pelvic floor and the overall health of the mind and body. It helps us recover after the baby is born and improves our long-term health.

## KEGEL? NO THANK YOU.

The pelvis is composed of the ischium, ilium, pubis, sacrum, and coccyx. This bony structure houses our reproductive organs, the lower urinary tract, and part of our small bowel and colon. The pelvis allows us to walk upright and is shaped like a basin and supported by connective tissue and muscles. The group of muscles that span the bottom of the pelvis and support the pelvic organs comprise the pelvic floor, which is like a living, breathing dome that finds synchrony with the up-and-down movement of the thoracic diaphragm. As we inhale and exhale, the pelvic floor moves down and up. The pelvis and pelvic floor support the bladder, uterus, vagina, colon, rectum, and anus. When the bladder, uterus, or rectum are full of pee, baby, or poop, respectively, the pelvic floor adjusts. When the muscles in the pelvic floor relax, we pee and poop; when they contract, we don't.

These muscles also play a role in determining whether we feel pleasure or pain during sex, contribute to stability, and assist in lymphatic and venous pumping. The intricately designed pelvic floor counteracts the forces of gravity acting on the body, and intra-abdominal pressure from actions like lifting and coughing. The functioning of the pelvic floor depends on its flexibility, movement, relaxation, contraction, suppleness, strength, elasticity, length, and

# Pelvic Floor Anatomy

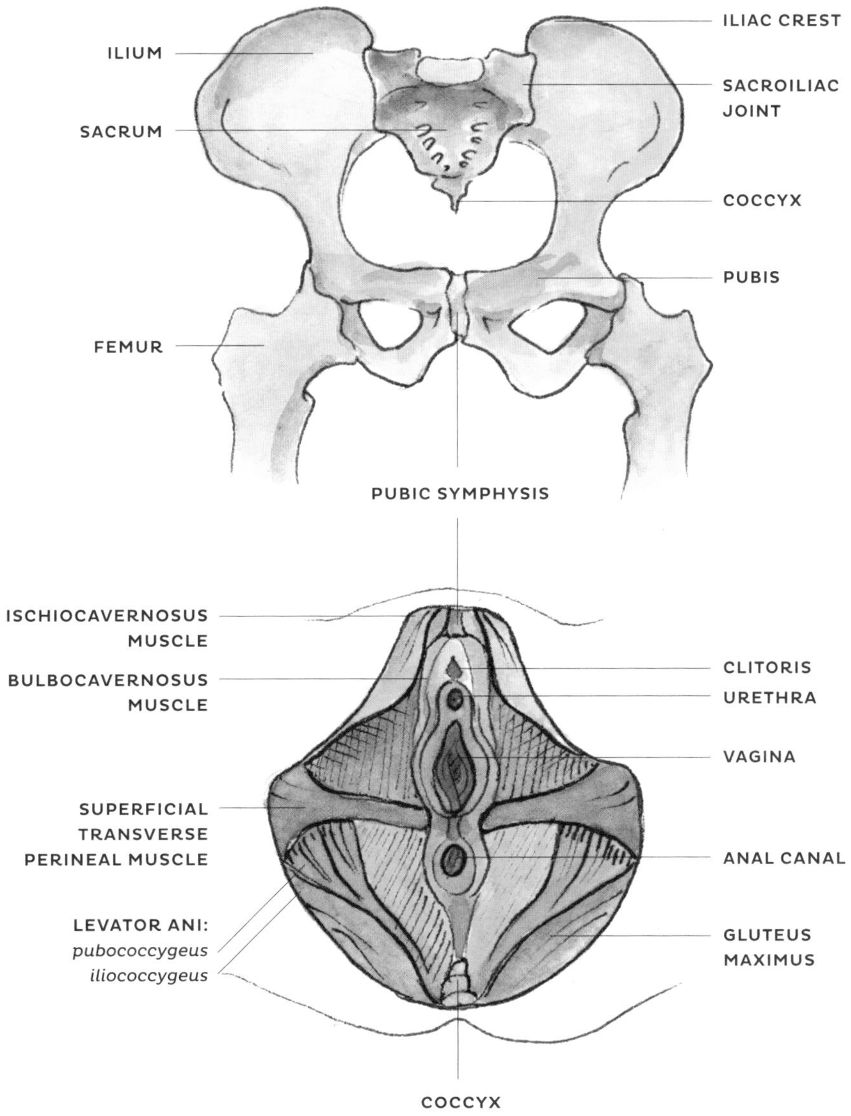

ILIAC CREST
ILIUM
SACROILIAC JOINT
SACRUM
COCCYX
PUBIS
FEMUR
PUBIC SYMPHYSIS
ISCHIOCAVERNOSUS MUSCLE
CLITORIS
BULBOCAVERNOSUS MUSCLE
URETHRA
VAGINA
SUPERFICIAL TRANSVERSE PERINEAL MUSCLE
ANAL CANAL
LEVATOR ANI:
*pubococcygeus*
*iliococcygeus*
GLUTEUS MAXIMUS
COCCYX

# *Pelvic Floor Roles*

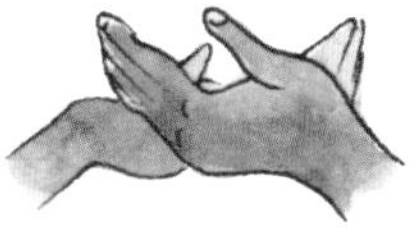

**SUPPORT:** The pelvic floor muscles support the pelvic organs, including the bladder, rectum, and anus, against abdominal pressure and gravity.

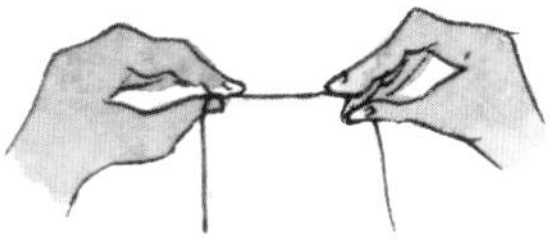

**SUSPENSION:** The muscles, fascia, and ligaments that compose the pelvic floor suspend the vagina, urethra, and other structures in the pelvis, allowing them to function optimally.

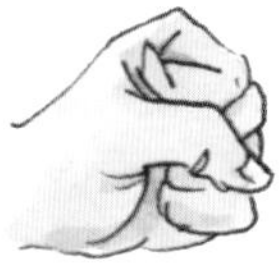

**SPHINCTER:** Wrapping around the opening of the bladder and rectum, the pelvic floor muscles help prevent leakage when we jump, sneeze, cough, or laugh. These muscles also relax and lengthen so that we can pee and poop.

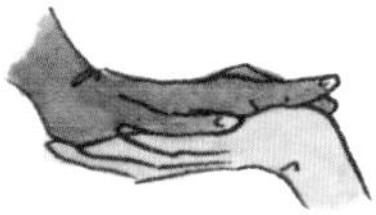

**STABILIZER:** The pelvic floor muscles are our true deep core. They attach to the hip and pelvis and help coordinate muscle movements with the hip, back, and abdomen.

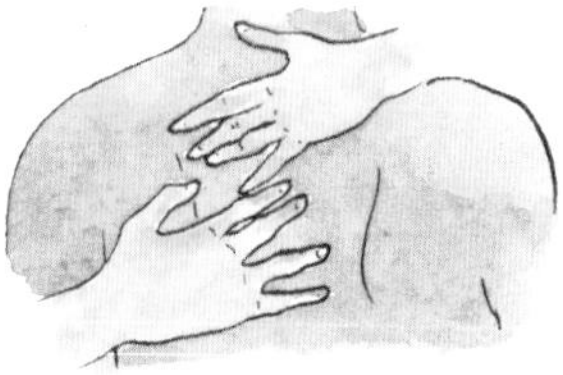

**SEX:** Flexible and strong pelvic floor muscles contribute to sexual functioning, including the sensations experienced during sex. Flexible pelvic floor muscles are important for comfortable sex, and strong pelvic floor muscles contract rhythmically during an orgasm.

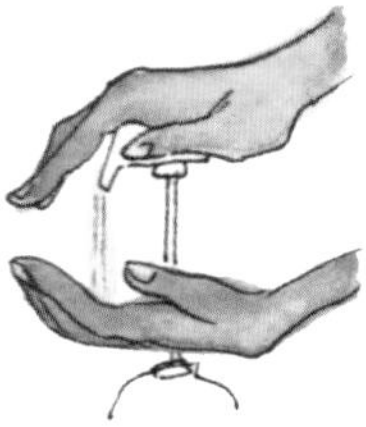

**PUMP:** Pelvic floor muscles act as a venous pump for the pelvis. This essential role minimizes congestion and swelling.

resilience. Unfortunately, many of these traits are not considered, as maintaining pelvic floor health has been reduced to the performance of a single prominent exercise: the infamous Kegel.

Dr. Arnold Henry Kegel was an American gynecologist who published an article in the 1940s about toning the pelvic floor muscles after childbirth to prevent incontinence, a common pelvic floor disorder people may experience after birthing babies. His work was important because it acknowledged the pelvic floor and the experience of those who give birth, but his exercises, which were specifically designed for incontinence, were generalized and recommended to everyone. We don't all have the same pelvic floor. Some of us hold tension and need lengthening, while others need strengthening and contraction. Kegels target the pubococcygeus (PC) muscle and reduce the purpose and function of the pelvic floor to just two of its several complex roles: strength and contraction.

Early on in my pregnancy I saw recommendations for Kegels everywhere I looked. Kegels are an oddly marketed exercise that encourage us to imagine squeezing an object in our vaginas and stopping the flow of urine during convenient moments throughout the day, like when we are sitting in traffic, waiting in a doctor's office, or watching TV. As my guilt over always forgetting to Kegel while I was driving shifted into a wholehearted rejection of the exercise, I wondered, did our ancestors ever do Kegels? Then I discovered the work of writer and biomechanist Katy Bowman, who helped shift my Kegel rejection into informed obstinance.

Bowman shines a light on the reductionist thinking American culture applies to movement and how it promotes segmental, isolated exercises like Kegels for pelvic floor function instead of considering the body as a whole. She explains that when Kegels are performed in a body that spends a lot of time sitting, or even exercising but not moving in diverse ways, this exercise can actually promote pelvic floor weakness, imbalance, and general discomfort. The whole body is involved in pelvic floor health, so choosing one muscle to contract repetitively does little to improve the structural imbalances that perpetuate dysfunction.

When the pelvic floor is overly tight and we then repeatedly Kegel and contract these tight muscles, it can pull the sacrum forward and out of alignment. There are issues with a sacrum that is out of alignment and overly constricted, and the first one that concerns you is pain, especially during pregnancy. This pain may be expressed as sacroiliac joint pain, or the tension in the pelvic floor and sacrum can lead to back and neck pain or headaches. The next issue that concerns you is birth, especially vaginal birth. Tightness and immobility in the sacrum and sacroiliac joints affect the ability of the pelvis to open, and you need this to happen to its full extent because the baby needs to go through this passage on their way to your arms. The sacrum, like the pelvic floor, requires a balance of strength and flexibility. There are movements you already know how to do, that you learned as a baby, that support these functions better than any isolated exercises developed by professionals. These include walking, squatting, climbing, and sitting on the ground instead of in a chair.

What does a lot of movement look like in my real life? Well, currently I'm writing this book balanced and bouncing on my yoga ball. I shift my position frequently from cross-legged, to sitting on my knees, to standing, to a deep, wide leg squat, and sometimes I lie on my belly or sit in a groin stretch. Because I am prone to sitting too much for too long, every day I have to figure out how I'm going to move more in my environment. The effort is ongoing, and some days I don't move enough, but I keep trying.

At work when I was pregnant, I walked a lot as a function of my job. I squatted and stretched and snuck into empty conference rooms to do gentle inversions with my knees up on a chair and my forearms on the ground. More than a few times my coworkers asked if I was going into labor, reminded me that the labor and delivery unit was just a few floors down, and told me their own stories about pregnancy and growing babies. In our home we use Squatty Potties in our bathroom so we can assume the best physiological position for daily evacuations. Sometimes I pee outside in the tree-tangled corners of our backyard or on long hikes in the forest or desert. Working in my garden gives me the opportunity to squat, reach, pull, dig, crawl, shovel and turn compost, and climb trees to pick fruit and prune.

Moving more doesn't mean we can't also exercise; it just means that in addition to exercise, we also try to spend more total time moving throughout the day, instead of feeling like an hour or two of exercise means we're done with movement for the day. This kind of movement is not always low impact and easy. It is challenging and loads the body in diverse ways, but it also includes the sacred art of resting.

The starting point of all this movement is our feet, and the way we move is impacted by what we put on our feet. The shoes we wear change the way our bodies move from the ground up. Any amount of heel changes the geometry of the body, including the position of the ankles, knees, hips, pelvis, back, abdomen, and rib cage. One of the simplest changes we can make to improve the alignment and health of the pelvis is to spend less time in heeled shoes. This might mean walking barefoot more around the house, adopting a zero-drop or negative heel shoe for walking and exercise, or gently transitioning from a high heel to a low heel to no heel during pregnancy.

I love beautiful shoes, especially my heeled leather oxfords, and I resisted giving up wearing my clogs at work because they were the only ones I felt that I could wear for fourteen hours without too much pain. But about halfway through my pregnancy, I started experiencing low back pain, deep pelvic pain, and calf cramps, and I noticed my hamstrings were always tight. I changed my footwear to a minimal, barefoot shoe and put my heeled shoes and clogs up high in my closet. At the same time, I focused on my alignment and posture, specifically my feet. Following Bowman's alignment advice, I worked on creating straight lines with the outside edges of my feet. Imagine the outside edges of both feet pressed up against a wall, with the fifth toe all the way down to the heel making contact with the wall's surface. At first I felt knock-kneed and awkward, but after a few days of wearing minimal shoes and walking with my feet more aligned, my back and pelvic pain disappeared.

My movement patterns changed too. I noticed the muscles in the outside of my hips were more engaged, and this engagement increased the stability of my pelvis and abdomen, which made me feel more grounded and stronger in my body even as my belly grew bigger. Pelvic pain during pregnancy is called lightning crotch because it feels like your pelvis has been struck by lightning. As much as I love heeled shoes, I hate lightning crotch more, and it was worth taking a break from my favorite shoes to feel more comfortable in my body.

Bowman recommends that anyone who wants to regain and retain the health and function of the pelvic floor and digestive system, and the mobility

# High Heels and Geometry

Your feet are the base of your body's posture and movement. High heels impact the alignment of your whole skeleton and change the geometry of your body. Spending more time barefoot or transitioning to a shoe without a heel helps improve alignment and decrease tension in the pelvic floor, low back, and hips.

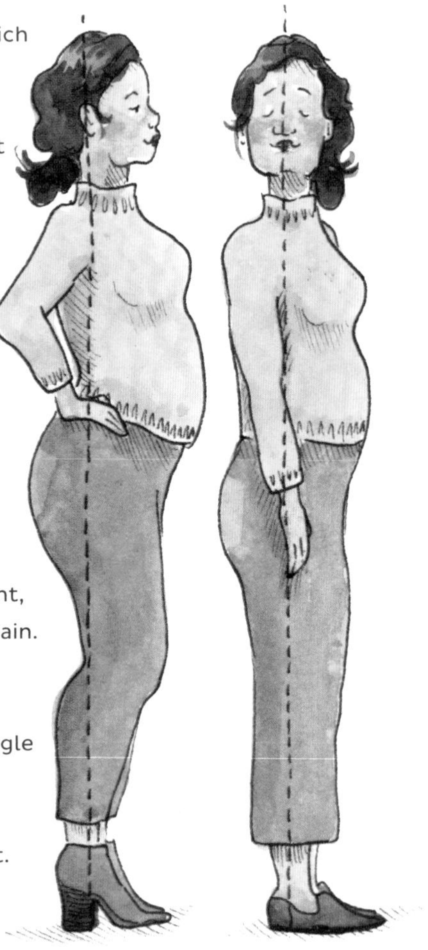

Heels change our posture and alignment, which affects breathing. The abdomen naturally wants to stick out, and sucking it in causes upward pressure on the diaphragm (so it can't fully expand) or downward pressure on the pelvis (increasing tension in the pelvic floor).

The back hyperextends to maintain balance, which can cause chronic back pain, spasms, and compressed and degenerated disks in the spine.

The knees, hips, and pelvis shift forward, increasing stress and pain in the hips, thighs, butt, and groin. An out-of-alignment pelvis and hips shift the whole body out of alignment, weaken the pelvic floor, and can cause neck pain.

High heels shorten the Achilles tendon and stiffen the calves, and the change in ankle angle alters the angle of the pelvic floor.

Weight shifts forward to the balls of the feet. This can lead to joint and nerve damage and foot deformities.

of the hips and lower back, should ditch their heels. All the symptoms and pain I experienced with my heeled shoes made sense, since heels, as Bowman writes, "shorten the muscles down the backs of the legs, which then pull on the pelvis, tucking it under." Tucking the pelvis, or standing with the pelvis shifted forward over the feet, changes the loads placed on the body, creating more loads and pain in the lower back and compromising how we use our glute muscles. By untucking the pelvis and stacking it over the ankles, our bodies are better able to support us, and we might notice less pain in our backs and hips. Pain during pregnancy is common, but it is not necessarily normal. The way we carry our bodies, our alignment and posture, can contribute to either more or less pain. If pain is part of your experience, changing your shoes just might take the lightning out of your crotch.

## MESSAGES FROM DOWN BELOW

When I was seven years old I was horrified that someday I would grow breasts. I didn't want them. I was dismayed when they grew in during high school, and for many years I would hunch my shoulders forward, actively trying to reduce my chest. I didn't know I was hunching until I was recovering from shoulder surgery and a friend who practices Rolfing, a system of structural bodywork, called me out. I then realized that the way I felt about my body changed the way I held my shoulders and was the cause of my neck, shoulder, and back pain. I still have to correct myself when I fall back into the habit, and I'm a little insecure about having a large chest, though breastfeeding has validated these inconvenient monuments of my womanhood.

In the same way that our deeply held beliefs and insecurities shape how we move and hold ourselves, stress, trauma, tension, and suppressed emotions impact our bodies and alignment. Stress may come from relationships, our careers, the messes our partners make, sitting in traffic, or seeing trash on the side of the road and reading about the environmental crisis we're facing and then feeling like maybe we're really irresponsible to bring babies into this crazy world, but we're mammals and our biology is strong and we decide we'll do our best to raise ecological babies who love and protect the world and make it a better place.

Stress crops up and stays in the body when it has no place to escape and therefore cannot run its natural course through movement and release. Trauma also lives in the body, especially in the pelvis, whether from an abusive relationship, serious violations like rape, or accidents and injuries. Feelings of shame, guilt, anger, and embarrassment impact the way we feel, move, and experience pleasure. The connection between the fascia, nerves, and muscles and our emotional energy is not some fringe mind-body ideology. There is a real, physiological connection between our emotions and our bodies.

My loading zone for stress and insecurity is my shoulders, but the jaw, neck, back, and pelvis are also common places for us to carry tension. For the body to be healthy, which means supporting its functions like strength and flexibility, we must move often and in many different ways. When we start to hold tension in our body, we restrict certain types of movement, which impacts the function of the whole. For example, if we restrict or hold our breath, or don't breathe fully and deeply, the thoracic diaphragm doesn't move to its full extent, which leads to a shortening of the pelvic floor. The pelvis also experiences tension when we clench our jaw. I felt this during labor. It was hard not to clench my jaw, because pushing a baby out of your body is hard work, but it was essential to my labor to relax my jaw because it made the process one degree more doable.

The body is shaped by how we move it and how we feel about it. We can move all day, squat to pee outside, eat the healthiest food, and still experience dysfunction and discomfort if we feel anxious, carry a suppressed story of shame or trauma, or feel relentless stress that travels with us in the body, fed by the cycles of our mind.

It is challenging to address subconscious or habitual movement patterns. We can start by paying attention to how we're moving and breathing, the thoughts we have about our bodies, and how we're holding ourselves when we usually don't pay attention, like when we're cooking or working on the computer. It can help to work with someone who specializes in alignment and movement because they can see the story your body tells without being wrapped up in the narrative. Somatic Experiencing practitioners, mind-body mentors and coaches, Rolfers, massage therapists, osteopathic manipulation therapists, and pelvic floor physical therapists are among those who manipulate tissues to target tension, and some even help you discover the origin of the tension.

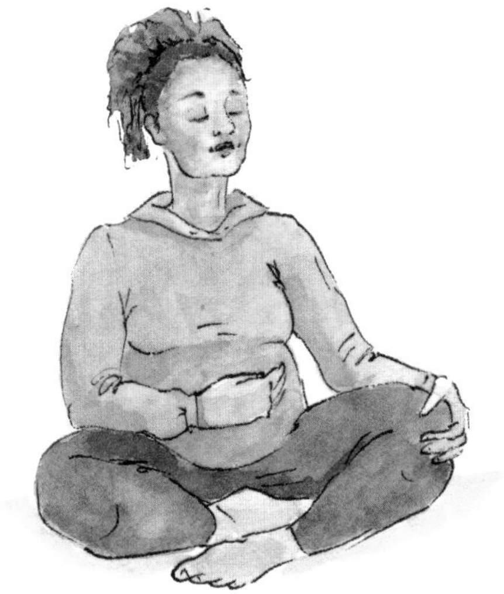

## Meditation for the Pelvic Floor

Sit on your sit bones, relax your jaw and shoulders, lengthen your spine, and soften the muscles in your eyes and face. Close your eyes and feel the gentle inhale and exhale of the breath, letting it come and go without effort. Once you feel settled in your body, start imagining your pelvic floor as a bright light that is deeply connected to the earth. Feel yourself rooting down as you simultaneously expand and lengthen upward. Stay in this space for 5–20 minutes and allow thoughts to enter and exit your mind without judgment. Notice the changes in your body and mind as your baby grows, and give yourself enough time to find quiet stillness.

I appreciate bodywork because touch therapy offers support without words. But the cost can be prohibitive. Healing does not have to happen in the hands of a professional you pay. Writing or journaling, talking to people, doing breathing exercises, and engaging in reflective movement like walking and meditation also create space to understand how the mind is working and affecting the body. Deep breathing is a free and tangible starting place. Unclench the jaw, relax the neck and shoulders, close your eyes, sit on your sit bones, and breathe, allowing thoughts to come and go. Meditation is a reprieve that allows you to come home to yourself. It helps the brain find space and the body find peace.

Reflecting on how our ancestors lived helps me gain an appreciation for humans' capability of movement. Hunter-gatherer tribes moved to survive. Gathering materials to build shelters and community structures, hauling water, chasing, harvesting, carrying and processing animals, foraging food, carrying babies, walking barefoot or in minimal shoes over diverse surfaces, climbing trees, squatting to pee and poop, and building fires were just some of their daily activities.

Modern culture has largely placed these activities into two categories: camping and exercise. We go away from our daily life to camp and spend time outdoors interacting with the landscape in some of the ways our ancestors did. We try to make our bodies strong in the gym with special machines and tools that we pay to use. We pay people to grow, make, and process our food and to build our houses. Appliances toast, bake, broil, microwave, chop, mix, whip, grind, pit, slice, and dice our food. Water comes out of our sinks, preheated, and dishwashers clean our dishes.

These cultural conveniences allow us to drive to work, work all day (usually sitting in a chair looking at a computer) and then drive home, make dinner in thirty minutes or less, and watch TV until bedtime, where we sleep on comfortable mattresses in temperature-controlled rooms.

Maybe you don't entirely relate to that cultural story. When I get grouped into a cultural norm, I rebel and think, "My life doesn't look like that!" I don't own a TV. I grow food in my garden, grind my own coffee beans, and hike up and down mountains. Even with my best efforts, many of my movements are outsourced because I still live in a culture of convenience, and I learned not from my hunter-gatherer ancestors but from my parents, who learned from their parents, who are removed both physically and ideologically from how humans lived for thousands of years. There is no blame in this information, just a reminder that we are physically capable beyond what we imagine, and imagination may be the key to increasing movements in our life.

## THE SLOWEST WAY FROM HERE TO THERE

Walking is my favorite essential movement. It brings us outdoors, can be sustained for hours, and acts as a moving meditation that allows us to process change and find peace in our decisions. It can bring us to the top of mountains, around the next bend, or down oceanside trails and into the water. Walking cured my broken heart after breakups, and it was on the top of a mountain, after a hike, that Max proposed. I walked during my pregnancy—sometimes short, slow strolls around the neighborhood, and sometimes deep into the mountains.

During the last few days of my pregnancy, it started snowing. I trudged through the snow, taking careful slow steps and deep breaths, wondering when my baby was going to start his journey into the world. During my early labor, I walked around outside, pausing during contractions and holding on to trees through the intensity of action in my body. After the birth of my son, I felt joy when I took my first extremely short and slow walk around the block with him in my arms. As the months passed, we walked farther distances, and now he leads the way, walking me toward his adventures and curiosities, teaching me the magic of moving through the world with a changed perspective.

In her book *Wanderlust: A History of Walking*, Rebecca Solnit writes that walking "is a state in which the mind, the body, and the world are aligned, as though they were three characters finally in conversation together, three notes suddenly making a chord." This chord gives us a kind of peace and freedom within ourselves, each rhythmic step orienting us to both the place we're walking and our thoughts.

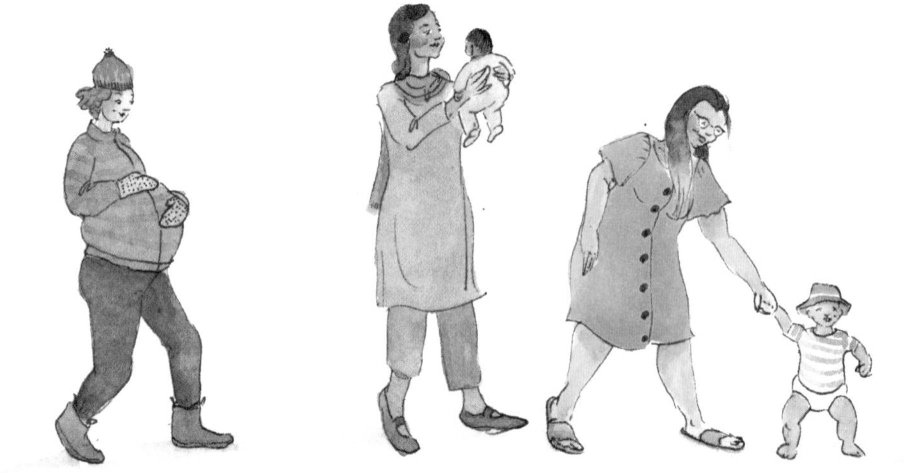

Walking, especially if you are meandering, is, in our modern culture, inefficient, purposeless, and unproductive. It is in these happy, useless moments where pleasure and surprise live and the mind functions best. As Solnit says, "I like walking because it is slow, and I suspect that the mind, like the feet, works at about three miles an hour. If this is so, then modern life is moving faster than the speed of thought, thoughtfulness." The connection point between the ground and the body are the feet, and they are a good place to start when exploring the biomechanical and anatomical action of walking.

Walking bipedally is an evolutionary innovation that builds strength and resilience in the body. We benefit from walking in diverse places, on diverse paths, trails, and surfaces, with diverse loads, and in diverse environments with diverse company, either alone or with a group. In each human foot there are thirty-three joints, twenty-eight bones (including the sesamoids), and more than one hundred muscles, tendons, and ligaments. The foot and ankle are intricately related, and together they provide structural support for repetitive loads. The foot is rigid when flexed and pointed and flexible when walking on soft surfaces like sand, where it acts as a shock absorber and propels us forward. Pathological or structural changes, like rigid footwear or high heels, affect the functions of the foot and ankle. The foot moves on three planes around three axes and involves the muscles of the lower extremities to accelerate and decelerate the foot and to stabilize and support dynamic loads and movements.

Shoes reduce and redistribute heel pressure and increase pressure under the toes. A narrow toe box compresses the foot and can cause foot pain. Heels increase forefoot pressure, and higher heels decrease ankle joint motion, alter our gait, and can lead to Achilles shortening. This discussion of feet, ankles, and walking brings us back to the pelvis. The position and mobility of the ankles is connected to, and affects, the position of the pelvis and the function of the pelvic floor, including muscle activation and contraction. Fortunately, walking far and frequently acts as a natural stabilizer of the sacrum and pelvis and supports pelvic floor function.

Solnit describes the pelvis as "a secret theater where thinking and walking meet," as it is the key to upright walking and the place where babies' brains grow and develop. Intelligent structures and systems exist outside the brains in our heads, and I want to talk about the space between the head and the body and how it relates to walking and birth.

I'm not referring to an anatomical location, such as the neck. I'm talking about the space between the mind, or consciousness, and the experience of the body as distinct from the mind, also known as the somatic experience. Walking acts as a mode of transport across physical distances and from the thinking mind to the experiencing body. It is in this way a moving meditation that connects us to our bodies and our place in the world. This idea of somatic experiencing and trust in the intelligence of the body is essential to birth. Pregnancy and birth happen in the body. The mind prepares, consumes information like this text, plans, visualizes, worries, fears, dreads, excites, wonders, ponders, theorizes, idealizes, expects, and imagines outcomes and situations. The actions of the mind affect the body, and the body affects the mind. Birth requires a certain relaxation of the mind so that we can take direction from the body.

Walking is a way to get from here to there and thus a connection point between places, whether geographical locations or between the functioning of the mind and movement of the body. Reconsidering the distances we consider walkable, such as the grocery store one mile away, challenges our cultural sedentarism. Walking through uncomfortable weather exposes us to heat and cold that were previously considered detrimental to our health and homeostasis. Now we're finding that our bodies can adapt over time to environmental

# *Bare Feet and the Brain*

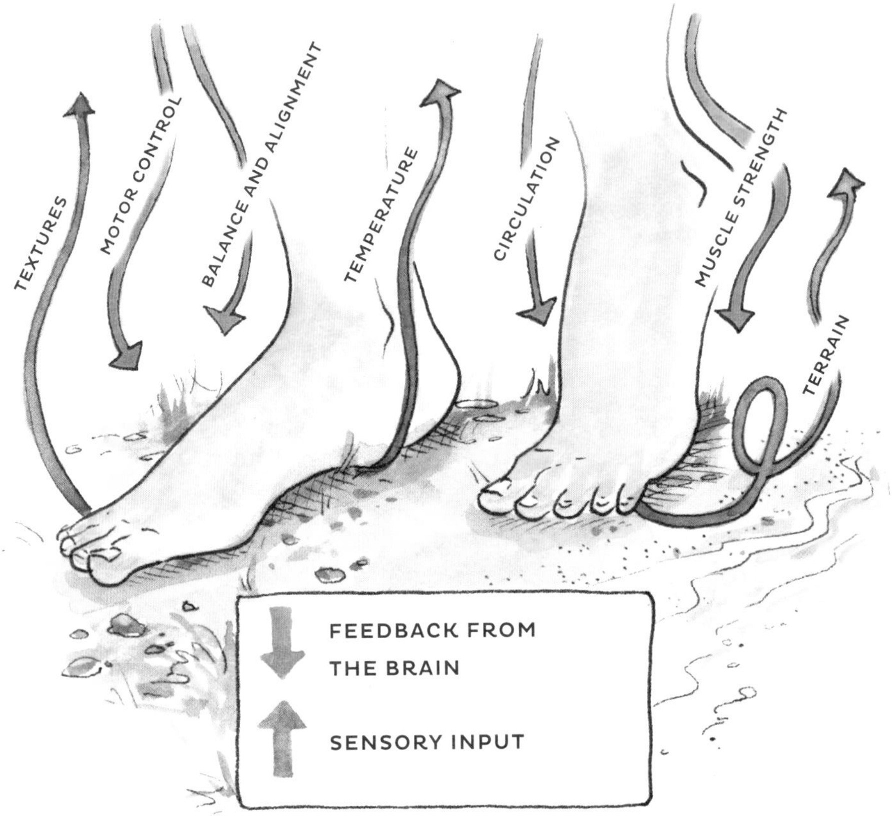


Walking barefoot sends sensory feedback from the feet to the brain. The result is improved balance, motor control, muscle strength, circulatory flow, and alignment. The sensation of feeling the earth with your feet builds stronger neural connections between your brain and your feet and improves awareness of your body in space, or proprioception. Additionally, the more you walk barefoot, the more healthy calluses you form, which we evolved to develop in order to protect our feet from hot or sharp objects without disrupting our gait or sensitivity to the ground.

extremes and that exposure may have significant benefits for cardiovascular and general health. Exposure to cold induces physiological changes, including an increased amount and activation of brown fat, which is more metabolically active than white fat. Cold exposure dramatically increases the release of the neurotransmitter norepinephrine, which is involved in focus and positive mood, and may reduce inflammation and improve immune function.

I want to make it clear that I'm not suggesting rapid and dramatic changes like walking barefoot in no clothes up a mountain through a snowstorm or in extreme heat. Our bodies like slow changes that build our fitness or resilience gently. My point in this discussion of walking and movement is that we are capable, and our bodies are able to adapt and support us. Our culture can make us feel disempowered during pregnancy and treat us like we're not capable of moving or making rational decisions, or it can expect too much and not honor the biological changes in the body and push us to do all the same things we've always done.

When you move far and frequently, the incremental increase in load strengthens muscles and connective tissue, and in this way pregnancy acts as its own training program. Walking supports our mind and body, as previously discussed, but it also gets us to stop sitting. It takes a long time to walk many miles, and it helps us progressively adapt to a growing pregnant body.

## WHAT ARE YOU SITTING ON?

Speaking of sitting, are you sitting in a chair? We live in a world where sitting in chairs for hours is normal, even expected. As kids we jump, swing, hang upside down, climb trees, sprint, and play all day, and then we rest, exhausted at the end of the day. As teenagers we might continue moving and playing if we participate in sports, but school starts to encourage more sitting, compliance, and hours of homework. As we enter college and graduate school, or the workforce, we sit more, and people in an office spend six hours sitting on average. We sit to drive, to eat dinner, to watch TV, to study, and to work or play on the computer. All this sitting is like an adult rite of passage in our culture, but our sedentarism is an outlier from all of human history, and getting older does not negate the need for diverse movement for our health.

This is relevant to pregnancy because if we want to have a "natural" birth, which in this book I define as an unmedicated vaginal birth, we need to acknowledge that our bodies are experiencing pregnancy in an unnatural, sedentary culture. If we expect our bodies to perform unmedicated, vaginal birth because birthing is a natural phenomenon, then we might consider aligning the rest of our lives to a natural—that is, normal, in the context of human history—amount of movement, which turns out to be way more than the prescriptive thirty to sixty minutes of exercise per day.

Unfortunately, we have adapted to sitting and to insufficient movement because it is normalized. As a human animal, we seek comfort, rest, efficiency, and simplification. The problem is that we now have access to conveniences that eliminate movements that our bodies depend on to be healthy. So why is sitting for hours in a chair so bad for the body? Any position, held for too long without change, has adverse effects on the body. Our bodies benefit from frequent natural movement, and pregnancy does not exempt our bodies from needing to move. Sitting, or sedentarism in general, for long periods of time affects the body at the cellular level.

Even while we are still, our intestines digest, our eye muscles move, our tissues repair, and our core temperature adapts to its environment. We are in perpetual motion because we exist with the force of gravity. How we move in relation to gravity promotes well-being or disease. If we don't move, gravity harms us and promotes disease and physical deterioration like muscle wasting and decreased aerobic capacity (think astronauts in space). This is because diverse movement, with diverse loads and positioning, supports diverse functions in the body that are essential for survival and wellness. These functions include, but are not limited to, the movement of blood, the transport of oxygen and fuel for cells, the removal of cellular waste products, digestion, immunity, reproduction, coordination, and balance.

The environment we live in, and the internal environments we create via movement and food, affect our bodies and genetic expression, and they affect the environment, movement, and genetic expression of our babies. This is because movement places loads on the body, or on the cells, that cause cellular adaptations. These adaptations include changes in density, shape, strength, and functionality. The body responds to the input it receives, so if sitting in one position for hours is the input, the body responds by adapting. The body doesn't need to be strong and robust to sit because the gravitational loads are placed on the chair.

When we spend too much time in one position, the body adapts to that specific position at the expense of adapting to other positions. In other words, some parts of the body get stronger with overuse, and other parts of the body get weaker with underuse. The more disparity there is between these overused and underused parts, the more potential there is for tissue damage when we move from sitting to standing to running.

The point of this section on sitting is not to say we should never rest and never sit. The point is to examine how often we sit in the same position without moving. One way to move more while sitting and resting is to move off the couch or chair and onto the floor and do what we might call natural, or self-supported, sitting. One reason sitting on the floor gets us to move more is because we get uncomfortable faster and reposition frequently. This repositioning creates different loads on different parts of the body and requires different types of mobility and flexibility.

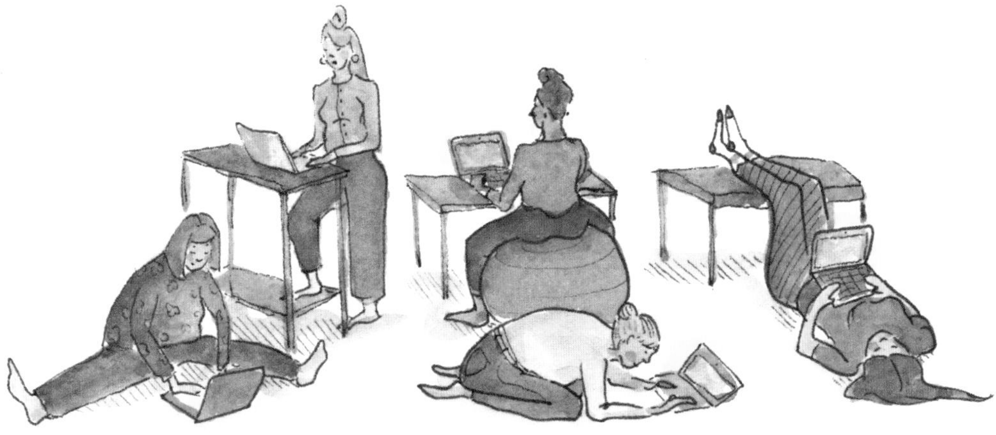

Getting up off the ground into a standing position requires full-body strength, mobility in the joints, and coordination. This ability to get up off the floor is such an important movement that it is used to predict all-cause mortality. Mobility, flexibility, and strength are important for all people, and this includes pregnant people, who are also capable of sitting on the floor and standing up, even with big bellies. In the next section, we'll cover more specific information about birth anatomy and how it relates to mobility, symmetry, muscle functioning, and alignment, but for now, stop sitting all day long.

## SQUAT ON

My son has a beautiful wide-leg sumo squat. He spends a lot of time in a deep squat with his spine perfectly aligned and strong legs supporting his body as he examines different objects in his hands, like shells, special rocks, flowers, acorns, and other treasures. I think of it as his scientist position. His deep squat is also his pooping position.

Squatting is important for some people during childbirth. I gave birth to my son during the longest squat of my life, and I've never been more grateful for my ability to maintain this position. Squatting is a range of movements that requires knee and hip flexion, strength, balance, range of motion, coordination, and adaptability to changing loads. Because most of us don't spend much time squatting, it's important to pay attention to how we squat. Try squatting down to the floor. Notice if your heels are in contact with the floor, if your feet are straight or turned out, and if your knees are stacked over your ankles. Did you hold your breath or bear down? Could you hold this squat for a few minutes, or is it uncomfortable?

Come back up. If you can't press your heels into the floor, spend some time stretching your calves. If your feet are turned out, your lower body is holding tension, in which case slowly start to bring the outside edges of your feet straight and engage your glutes. A stronger butt and less lower-body tension will also allow you to stack your knees over your ankles, and soon you'll be able to hang out in a low squat for longer. Take it slow. Squatting more doesn't mean you start with one hundred reps today; it means checking in with your body and taking gradual steps. Squatting this way supports the functioning and tone of the pelvic floor, improves core strength, aids in stability, and improves hip flexibility. These functional movements help support the body and prepare it to birth a baby.

Instead of doing a set number of squats each day, I try to incorporate them the same way my son does, often and without thinking about them as an exercise. I squat a lot to play with him, but also when I'm working on my computer, or outside in the garden. As the body gains mass during pregnancy, consistent squatting allows the ligaments that stabilize the joints in the pelvis, knees, and hips and that hold the pelvic organs in place to be supported by strong muscles.

Squatting builds strength in many muscle groups, and I want to focus on the glutes specifically. The glutes act to stabilize the sacrum, which plays a role in the functioning of the pelvic floor. The glutes also support the body during walking by working with the hips, legs, and the rest of the body to move one leg forward while holding up the body on the other leg. During pregnancy, the body gains mass in the front and center as the baby grows. As you go about your day walking in shoes with no heels, squatting frequently, and naturally sitting and moving with pleasurable diversity, the whole body adapts to the changing loads by gaining strength and resilience. Part of this adaptation includes increasing the mass and strength of the glutes so they can balance the growing mass on the front of the body.

Your strong butt will help you counteract cultural and media messages about how pregnant people move and behave. The image of a woman sticking out her pregnant belly, waddling, and needing to lie back with her feet up, pelvis tucked under, and complaining of her discomfort is thrown at us in movies, other books about pregnancy, and advertisements. All these positions undermine the structural and functional integrity of human bodies and lead to back pain, misalignment, and other discomforts that we associate with pregnancy.

While our center of gravity does change, our hips widen, and our stride length decreases so that we move with more stability on a wider base and keep our feet on the ground slightly longer during each step to support our extra mass, we are not hopeless victims of our changing bodies. We are, in fact, the opposite. Through incredible adaptations, including stronger butts, our bodies adjust to the increased load and support it by building strength and moving in a way that promotes balance and stability.

We live in a culture of extremes and reduction, but the movements that support graceful and gradual adaptation in the pregnant body are complex, integrated, and biologically normal. The anatomical and biomechanical information we can learn about the body is fascinating because it tells us about how the body works in concert with all its parts connected. But we don't need a background in science to squat more, stop sitting so much, walk far and often, or imagine ways we can incorporate more movement into our lives and leave behind some of the stereotypes of pregnancy. We are immensely capable, even while, or especially while, we are pregnant.

## MOVING PAST EXERCISE

I was impacted by Katy Bowman's work in part because it validated my long-term trouble with sitting still. As a kid, I was in constant motion and despised the idea of exercise. I remember when my soccer coach made our team run five miles when we were twelve years old. We all moaned and groaned and wondered why we would go for a run when we could just play soccer.

As a college skier, I spent a lot of time in the gym lifting weights, which caused my thigh muscles to grow exponentially. I was serious about exercise at this point in my life and felt guilty if I didn't work out for three or four hours every day. I am not against exercise; I have spent a lot of my life training and thinking about the ways I need to get stronger. But when I stopped ski racing at the end of college, there was suddenly space for new movement that brought back a feeling of lightness, pleasure, and fun.

This pleasure in moving my body drives me to incorporate more movement into my life, and I move more now and feel stronger and more balanced than I did when I was seriously training for my sport. Anatomy and biomechanics help reinforce the need for more diverse movement, but enjoying that diverse movement helps us continue to choose to move.

Exercise fits into the category of movement, but it does not satisfy all the movement needs of the body. Exercise is usually specific. It includes things like lifting weights and jogging but does not necessarily include things like climbing trees, shoveling the compost pile, or getting on hands and knees to scrub the floor.

There are exercise guidelines for pregnant people to try to ensure that we move the minimal amount to stay healthy, which is around thirty minutes of walking a day, but there aren't guidelines about how much to move to be *optimally* healthy. This differs based on your starting point of fitness, but the message is still to move more, more parts, in more diverse ways, more often. While pregnant, our inner ecology changes, and it is worth thinking about the goal of moving more. The goal of exercise may be to stay healthy, not gain too much baby weight, and lose the weight quickly after birth. Certain types of movement may include these goals and also focus on facilitating the birth experience you desire by supporting the functioning of the pelvic floor, the positioning of the baby, and the overall strength of the body.

At this point I'm used to seeing headlines like "Sitting will kill you, even if you exercise," "Your chair is killing you," "7 ways sitting will kill you," "Sitting is the new smoking," and "Is sitting a lethal activity?" These sensationally dire headlines point to research that shows people who sit more tend to die earlier than people who sit less.

I get that our culture responds more to these types of headlines than, say, "Walk, squat, climb trees, and garden more because it's fun!" or "Be bold: squat and pee outside" or "Shovel manure, live a long time," but it seems a little unfair to demonize chairs for our habits, or tell us that sitting is killing us, then offer "solutions" like taking a walk around the office every hour or replacing our chair with a standing desk. This isn't enough. Replacing one all-day position with another all-day position doesn't improve our overall health, only frequent, diverse movement does.

It's hard for these articles to offer solutions because our infrastructure is designed to sit us down and keep us there. We do not, as a society, enjoy equal access to places in which we can move freely. That's why urban farms, groups that advocate for mobility justice, sidewalks, clean streets, city parks, open space, and protected wilderness are so important. It's why advocating for our right to move, and move often, is important where we work, and it's important to teach our kids about their right to move. Movement is something we can build into our life, replacing TV watching with walks to the park, or engaging in what Bowman calls "stacking our life," where we move as much as we need to while accomplishing something we want to or have to do. For example, walking to the grocery store as a family meets the need for movement, family time, and buying groceries.

Moving more requires us to change our habits and reprioritize our time. It forces us to reframe our ideas of efficiency and reevaluate the point of hurrying. Pursuing more motion is worth the effort both physically and socially for the health of our bodies, and it's worth fighting for as our inherent right as humans who grow babies.

# TAKE ACTION

Move your body more often and in more ways. Movement—like water, oxygen, and food—is essential for your body. Through incredible adaptations, our bodies adjust to the increased load of carrying a baby. Diverse movement helps us adapt by keeping us strong and balanced, aligned, and resilient. Taking great pleasure in movement helps us choose this action again and again.

Notice where you carry tension in your body. Our insecurities, trauma, stress, and shame impact how we move and the health of our bodies. Meditation is a tangible place to start repairing and reconnecting to our bodies so that we can move with our whole being without restriction.

Question what you wear. Heeled shoes change our geometry and compromise our physiology. Spending more time barefoot or in shoes without heels allows us to move without increasing tension and pressure in the pelvic floor and other parts of the body. Changing our shoes and aligning our feet may also reduce or eliminate common aches and pains during pregnancy.

Walk long distances, squat often, and sit on the floor. These movements help us fight against our sedentary leanings and also help prepare our bodies for labor and birth. A strong and aligned body supports the health of the pelvic floor and optimizes the baby's position in the womb. As humans who grow babies, we are immensely capable and have the right to move.

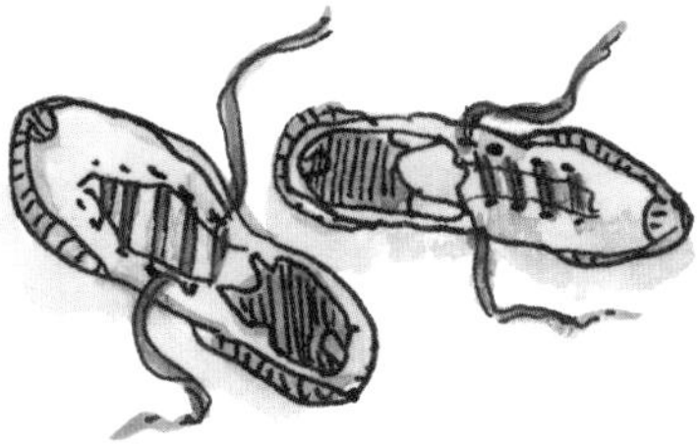

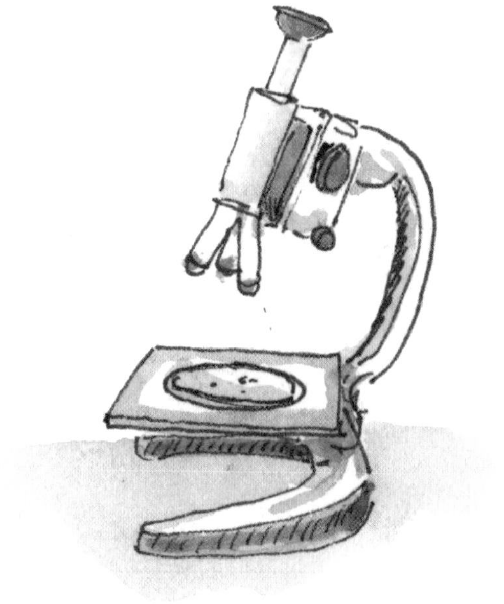

CHAPTER THREE

# Cultivating Your Baby's Microbiome

**ALTHOUGH IT DOESN'T QUITE WORK** this way and is far more complex, I like the idea of mothering, and being mothered by, our microbiota. If we think of all these ecosystems of microbes as our own legions of children, it allows us to ask some questions about how we want to raise these tiny organisms. If our body is their nursery, college dorm room, and retirement home, how do we create an environment that promotes their health throughout their lifetime? What can we feed them that allows them to be contributing members of society who strengthen immune function and help prevent invaders, allergies, and autoimmune disease?

Just as we would never intentionally poison our own children, we may also feel fiercely protective of our internal residents and avoid antibiotics unless absolutely necessary and other medicines that confer more harm than benefit. Just as it is with our human babies, all our actions and choices matter and affect the health of our microbial children. Water quality; exposure to pollution and secondhand smoke; toxic chemicals in paint, makeup, and household cleaners; nonstick cookware; and the pesticides, herbicides, insecticides, and antibiotics on and in industrial food all impact our microbes and their ecosystem. Even as we learn more about our microbiota, there are still so many mysteries. But if we approach them as we approach our babies—with an open mind, curiosity, and a willingness to take care of them—we can foster communities through our choices that contribute to our own health and the health of our human babies.

Rising estrogen and progesterone levels during pregnancy change how our guts function and the composition of our gut microbiome. Each trimester comes with progressive adaptations in the gut microbiota that allow our bodies to undergo the necessary metabolic changes that support pregnancy. These metabolic changes include weight gain, changes in insulin sensitivity, and altered metabolic hormone levels. During early pregnancy, our bodies focus on increasing nutrient and fat storage to meet the needs of late pregnancy and lactation after birth. Late pregnancy, on the other hand, is marked by increased insulin resistance so that more glucose is available to the growing baby. Microbes that excel at extracting energy from food populate the gut during pregnancy.

The compositional changes in the microbiome impact our baby's weight gain and future body composition, immunity, and health. Your microbiota may be one of the most important influences on you and your child's health after birth. This is why obesity, which creates different microbiota changes and impacts metabolic hormones differently, may increase the risk of obesity for our children. When we go through pregnancy undernourished, or don't gain enough weight, we may experience increased infections and preterm deliveries. The indispensable fat stores our microbes help us build nourish our babies while they are in the womb and shape their long-term health.

# Maternal Microbiome

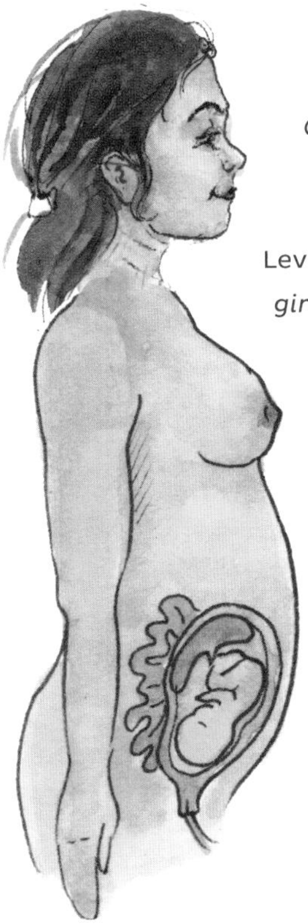

### MOUTH

*Oral health is connected to fetal health.*
Microbial counts in all stages of pregnancy increase.
Levels of pathogenic bacteria (*Porphyromonas gingivalis*, *Aggregatibacter actinomycetemcomitans*, and *Candida*) increase.

### GUT

*Changes in the gut microbiome maximize energy transfer to the fetus.*
Overall bacterial load increases.
Overall bacterial richness decreases.
*Proteobacteria* and *Actinobacteria* increase. These bacteria are associated with inflammation, weight gain, and reduced insulin sensitivity.

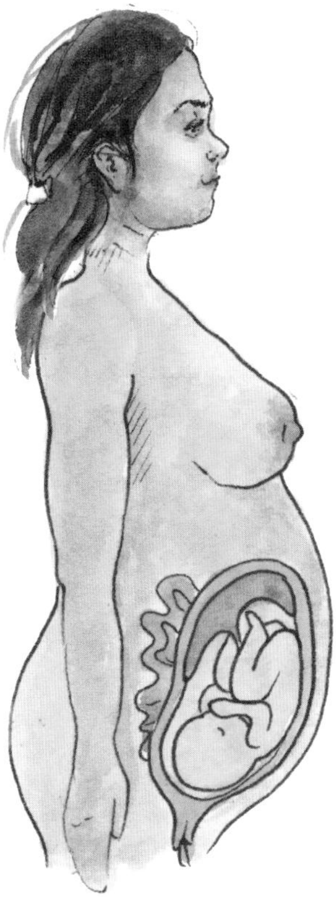

### VAGINA

*The vaginal microbiome defends against viral and microbial infections and disease. Microbial populations vary with gestational age and ethnic group.*
*Lactobacillus* species increase.
Microbial stability increases.
Overall microbial diversity decreases.
Vaginal pH decreases.
Vaginal secretions increase.

# *Fetal Microbiome*

**FETAL MICROBIOME** (inherited from birthing parent) → **INFANT'S MICROBIOME**

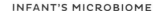

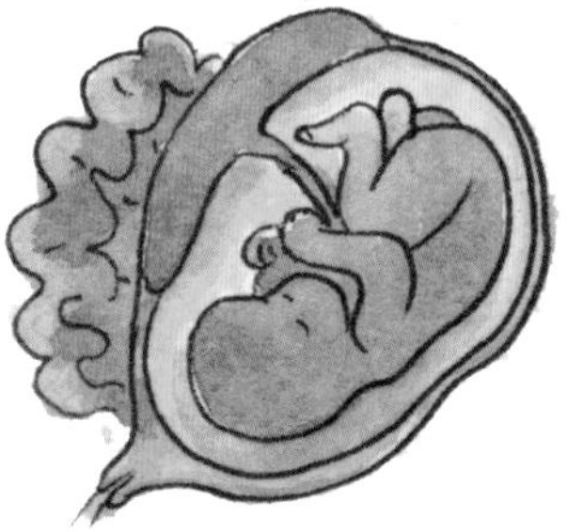

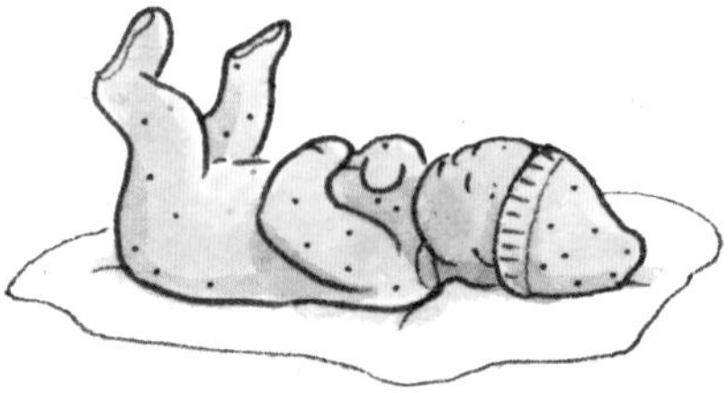

Maternal antibodies, microbiota, food intake, and environment → Development of the infant's gut, immune system, metabolic function, and microbiome

↓

Long-term health: weight gain and body composition, immune function and response, and neurodevelopment

## THE GUT HABITAT

We tend to hear the most about the gut microbiome. This incomparable habitat starts where food enters and ends where it exits. Within this habitat live trillions of bacteria that are impacted by everything we eat, our genes, and the environment. The intestines are the most diverse portion of the gut microbiome. The bugs in the intestines help turn food into parts we either use or discard and assimilate essential vitamins and minerals. Along with the liver, our microbes help detoxify the body and they maintain the function and integrity of the intestinal wall. The small intestine is where nutrients are absorbed from the food we eat, while the large intestine is where fiber is fermented, water is absorbed, and undigested food moves through on its way out.

Our bacterial populations respond to what we eat and what we put on our bodies. They impact our metabolism and influence our appetite, mood, and how we respond to toxins and drugs. The choices we make consciously and the habits we perform subconsciously are all influenced by our relationship with our invisible residents. The majority of serotonin, the neurotransmitter implicated in almost every human behavior from eating to sleeping, is synthesized and regulated by bacteria in our gut.

My son spends a lot of time in the chicken coop, getting licked by dogs and cuddling cats. He went through a phase where he'd stuff big handfuls of sand and dirt in his mouth. I'd watch him curiously, attempting the ever-present balance of allowing him to learn on his own while protecting him from danger. He ate greens in the garden that had bugs on them, and he still regularly eats the food he drops on the ground. We adults wash and scrub and sanitize and try to teach kids to be less messy. But we have much to learn from their unhygienic habits. As children interact with the world, they necessarily get their clothes dirty, but they may also bolster the abundance and diversity of their microbiota, which determines their risk of developing certain diseases, their susceptibility to common infections, and their ability to bounce back after illnesses.

The information researchers are learning about microbiota and the microbiome every day has profound implications for how we look at the most common ailments of industrialized societies and how to treat them. Obesity, inflammatory intestinal diseases, diabetes, allergies and asthma, depression, arthritis, and other chronic diseases are challenging to treat and painful to experience, which makes the science surrounding our microbial communities so exciting. It offers hope where hope may seem scarce and wonder at the potential of our relationship with our microorganisms.

When it comes to the science on the gut microbiome, the impact of healthy food is one of the more evidence-backed findings. Our microbes adapt to what we eat, and they impact the place where the food enters: our mouths.

## THE BUGS IN OUR MOUTH

Your mouth is complex. Its overall health is impacted by genetics, ethnicity, stress, age, toothpaste and toothbrushing, how you were born, what you were fed as an infant, and what you've been putting in your mouth since then. During pregnancy, and especially during early pregnancy, you have higher oral microbial counts compared to nonpregnant people.

There is also an increase in overall bacteria, especially pathogenic bacteria that can contribute to issues with oral health. Oral bacterial imbalance (dysbiosis), periodontal disease, and infections are correlated with an increased risk of preterm birth, so it is essential to take care of your mouth during pregnancy.

I like my dentist, but we don't talk about diet, saliva, the oral microbiome, or hormones and how these things affect my teeth. I want to know what dentists learn during their many years of school and training and to chat with them about the intricacies of oral health, but the dentist's office is a place we typically go with apprehension, and if we leave without a cavity or something more sinister, like a root canal, it feels like a narrow escape of doom.

Away from the dentist it's easier to ponder the oral microbiome with wonder. The nooks and crannies of the mouth house more than seven hundred species of microbes that create interactive biofilms. Every surface sheds and changes, except for the teeth, which are covered in a thin outer layer of enamel. Enamel is the hardest tissue in the body. It gives our teeth shape and protects the inner layers of the teeth from decay. The balance between demineralization (the wearing away of enamel) and remineralization (the restoration of enamel) contributes to our ability to avoid cavities and gum diseases. Talking about enamel and oral health requires a consideration of saliva and its unique functions.

For more than two thousand years, saliva—its thickness, smell, taste, and sensation in an individual's mouth—have been used as diagnostic markers by Traditional Chinese Medicine doctors. It is called the brother to blood, and changes in saliva indicate wellness or disease in the body. Saliva contains enzymes, hormones, and other compounds that allow us the sensation of taste, keep our mouth clean by controlling microbial populations and growth, regulate pH, and protect the teeth.

The stuff of our saliva tells a story about what we've eaten, how hydrated we are, the drugs we've taken, our stress level, and our ability to taste. It solubilizes, or breaks down, our food so we can taste it, and binds it into a slippery mass that glides down the esophagus. It carries away food debris through flushing and starts the process of starch digestion. We swap it with our lovers, and spit it out, and when its flow rate slows down at night, we wake up with bad breath. It offers a feast of nutrients to the microbial communities in our mouth, nourishing their environment and contributing to a healthy, balanced living situation.

When the bacterial communities in the mouth are optimal, they promote health and protect us from disease. The mouth is deeply vascularized, meaning your lips, gums, tongue, and oral mucosa receive a rich blood supply that supports their functions and healing. This network of blood vessels also allows bacteria and other harmful substances to enter the bloodstream. Cavities form when acid-producing microbes beneath plaque get a hit of sugar and drastically lower the pH in the mouth. This starts the dissolution process of the minerals in enamel. While saliva clears away sugar and acid, maintaining an ideal pH, salivary flow varies, so some zones are more vulnerable to decay than others.

Certain foods protect the teeth and the overall health of the mouth. Foods that provide abundant bioavailable, essential minerals and vitamins include protein-rich foods like fish, pork, beef, and other meats. Cultured dairy, like yogurt, cheese, and butter, helps neutralize highly acidic foods and happens to create some of my favorite food combinations, like wine and cheese, coffee and cream, and fruit and yogurt. Raw and cooked vegetables feed our beneficial microbes. Healthy fats like bone marrow, bone broth, fish, eggs, and other organic, pastured animal products support absorption of fat-soluble vitamins. Seaweeds are rich in minerals, and fermented foods (like kimchi and sauerkraut) and lacto-fermented foods support microbial diversity and abundance.

The food we eat is important, but so is the physical act of chewing. Our teeth adapt to the mechanical stresses placed on them. Softer diets full of processed foods fail to stimulate the normal development of the jaw and face, resulting in crowded, crooked teeth that are prone to decay and dental-arch abnormalities. Chewing tough, fibrous food for more time throughout the day encourages the development of strong, healthy teeth and jaw muscles. It helps that the foods that require a lot of chewing—raw vegetables, tougher cuts of wild game, grass-fed meat, or dried fish—also benefit our overall health.

The way we breathe also impacts our health. Breathing in and out of the nose benefits oral health, while mouth breathing slows down saliva production and can contribute to both structural and bacterial oral imbalances.

Our brushing habits matter too. Brushing your teeth right after eating acidic foods like citrus fruits or coffee can damage enamel that's been softened as a result of the pH changes these foods induce; instead, wait thirty to sixty minutes before brushing. Swooshing water around in your mouth after eating helps reduce the acidity and isn't damaging to the enamel. And of course, the basic oral care instructions you learned as a child apply: brush your teeth every day, twice a day, applying a gentle massaging pressure with a soft-bristled brush for two whole minutes, without missing your gum line. Brushing this way breaks up the plaque on the teeth and maintains an oxygen-rich environment for your health-promoting microbes.

Finally, toothpaste matters. Some toothpastes and mouthwashes contain antibacterial chemicals like triclosan, which has endocrine-disrupting properties and kills off the bacteria in your mouth instead of nurturing the good guys, or sodium lauryl sulfate and other surfactants that provide the satisfying foaming-at-the-mouth effect but also negatively impact the phospholipids on the tongue that support the function of our taste buds and may promote cancer and canker sores. Other toothpastes look to sweeten up the toothbrushing experience by adding artificial sweeteners, which are bad for microbial health in the mouth and gut.

When I went to the dentist during my pregnancy, I avoided X-rays and kept the seat up a little higher or moved to my side and took breaks to sit up and move around when I was uncomfortable. Foods high in sugar, or very cold water, made my teeth hurt, so I cut down on sugary treats and drank room-temperature or warm water, as increased blood flow to the gums and hormonal and microbial changes can make your teeth more sensitive.

# Protecting the Mouth Biome

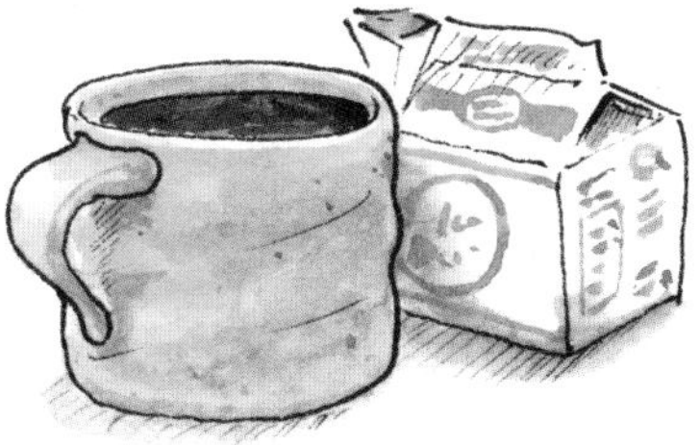

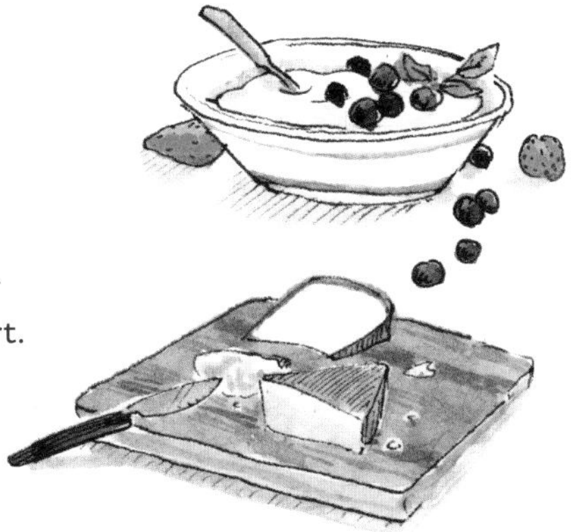

Neutralize acidic foods with calcium-rich foods like cheese and plain yogurt.

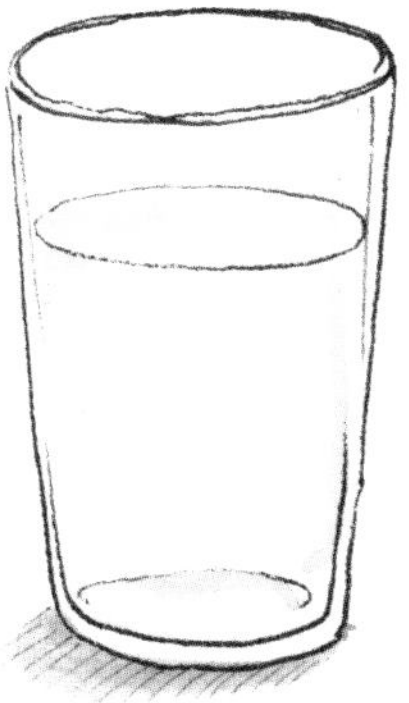

Rinse your mouth with water after eating and wait 30–60 minutes before brushing to protect enamel.

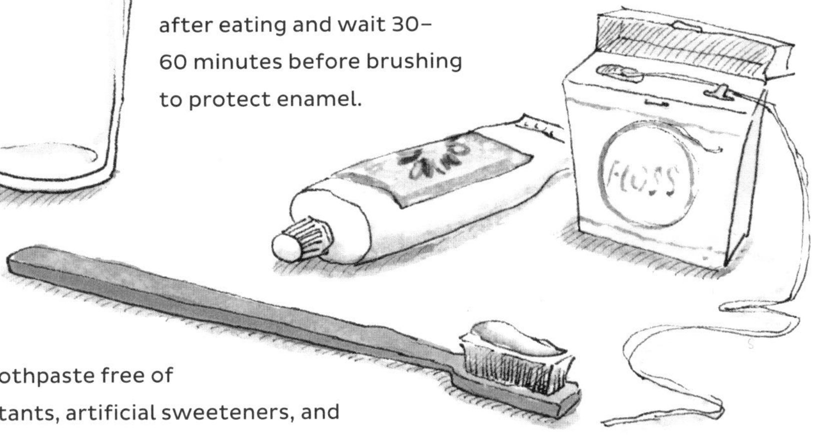


Use toothpaste free of surfactants, artificial sweeteners, and antibacterials like triclosan.

Avoid sticky and hard candy (especially sour candy), starchy foods like chips, alcohol, and carbonated drinks.

Brush for 2 whole minutes twice a day, and floss once a day.

## FLORA'S FAUNA

During pregnancy, the changes in our physiology and bacteria extend beyond the gut and mouth. The vagina, the place of initial entrance of the sperm and eventual exit of the baby, is a dynamic environment. The outer layer of the vagina is composed of loosely connected glycogen-filled cells that are permeable to microbes and particularly adept at thwarting off infections. This layer is created by the sloughing of cells on the vaginal surface, by immune mediators, and through the action of *Lactobacillus*, bacteria that maintain an acidic pH through the production of lactic acid.

Increased estrogen and progesterone during pregnancy drive more glycogen into the outer layer of the vagina, which increases the population and stability of *Lactobacillus*. This stability may play a key role in preventing infections that could harm the environment of the developing baby. Vaginal dysbiosis, or bacterial imbalance, is associated with pregnancy complications like pregnancy loss and preterm birth. The bacteria in the vagina are stable, but they aren't static. Our stress, diet, antibiotic exposure, body composition, and genetics impact *Lactobacillus* abundance. The vagina may act as a key source of bacteria during prenatal development that shape your baby's gut microbiome, so supporting the health of the vaginal microbiome supports baby's health. Promoting a balanced, *Lactobacillus*-rich home in the vagina means eating a diet that promotes bacterial diversity. It also means avoiding deodorants, harsh cleansers, and the antifeminist practice of douching and manipulating vaginal odor. The perpetuation of douching and ridding the vagina of its natural odor promotes insecurity about and mistrust in the body and can lead to dysbiosis that actually causes malodor and health issues, including a heightened risk for infections and damage to developing babies.

The vagina is its own intelligent design with self-cleaning properties, including cell turnover, mucus production, and the aforementioned health-promoting microbes. Wearing loose clothes and cotton underwear, gently washing with water, and the occasional breeze help maintain the natural balance of the vulva and vagina by encouraging optimal bacterial communities and healthy functioning of the lower genital tract.

## YOU ARE NOT ALONE

We exist in codependent relationships with invisible organisms. If learning about microbial ecosystems in your body doesn't challenge how you see yourself and your body in relationship to the world, having a baby who depends on you for growth, safety, guidance, and microbial inheritance almost certainly will. Our unseen comrades, commensals, and hitchhikers give us the opportunity to shift our perspective and acknowledge that we know very little. There is wonder and humility in this reckoning.

Our microbial ecosystems are unique to our bodies, and the differences between my bugs and your bugs, and your bugs and anyone else's bugs, are vast. Our behavioral, immunological, and digestive differences may be explained by our particular microbial communities. Our uniqueness has less to do with how we view ourselves and more to do with the populations of creatures that call us home.

Reconsidering the uniquely human idea of separateness and individuality has far-reaching consequences for how we think about our relationship to the world. The term "holobiont" was introduced to describe an organism plus its symbiont community it depends on to live. In the book *Arts of Living on a Damaged Planet*, Scott Gilbert explains how "human bodies are and contain a plurality of ecosystems." The volume of our microbial organisms is similar to the volume of our brain and is as metabolically active as the liver. The vast microbiome is its own organ system, living on and within us, shaping who we are.

We humans have about twenty-two thousand different genes. This seems like a big number until we consider that bacteria from various environments—our birthing parent's body and skin, the birth canal, breast milk, the world we live in—bring around eight million more genes into the picture. *Eight million!* Our development into who we are and who we could be is shaped by, and depends on, our symbionts.

During pregnancy, our metabolism and microbiome change to support the growing baby. The bacteria in our digestive and reproductive systems are different at the end of pregnancy because it is important for certain bacteria to be present for the baby in the birth canal. This cometabolic state extends to breast milk, which helps form gut capillaries and lymphoid tissue in the baby. Birth is not so much the creation of a new individual as it is the cultivation of a new community of relationships that symbiotically exist with your baby. Your role as the keeper and cultivator of these bacteria is immensely important and largely left out of the story our culture tells us about growing babies. Gilbert writes that when babies leave the womb and enter the world during birth, they are not gaining independence. "There is no such thing as 'independence,'" he says. "It's mutual dependency all the way down, and birth is the exchanging of one symbiotic system for another."

## LOOKING BACK TO LOOK FORWARD

Many of the studies on the microbiome and its changes during pregnancy have been performed on animals, and so much of this science is brand new. The interaction between you and your microbiome is complex. Add a baby to the picture and the ensuing physiological, endocrine, metabolic, bacterial, and behavioral changes, and relationships become more intertwined, more interesting, and more mysterious.

When we have babies, we have the opportunity to look back and look forward. Whenever I see the phrases "lack of studies," "need for more research," or "lack of evidence" at the end of scientific studies that are careful not to make causal claims, it helps me to remember that our human ancestors have been having babies for millions of years. We join a lineage of billions who have carried and birthed babies, and the cumulative experience and stories of these birth-givers is invaluable.

During the last few million years, we learned from other parents and coevolved with our microbiota, and we continue to live on a planet that is full of parents and microbes. What has changed dramatically is the way we live, what we eat, how much we move, and our environmental conditions. Naturally, this has implications for how we experience pregnancy and how we give birth and raise babies.

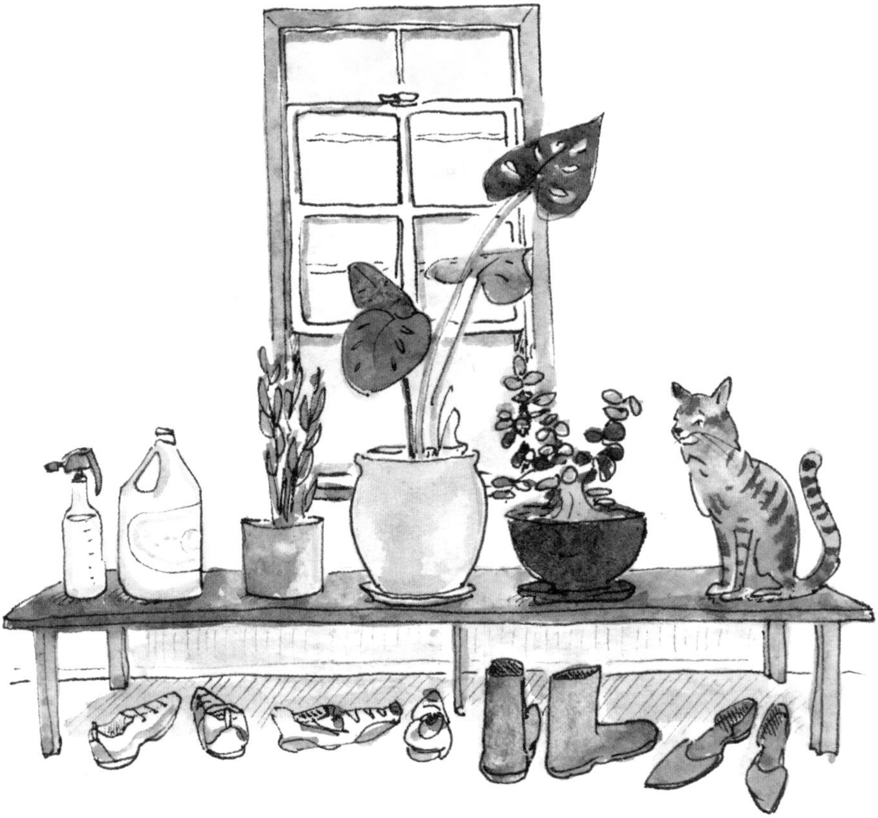

# Microbiome Restoration

Move often, especially outside and in nature.

Manage stress and improve your sleep.

Spend time with plants and animals.

Eat diverse, nutrient-dense, fiber-rich, and fermented foods.

Eat less sugar and fewer processed foods.

Drink clean, filtered water.

Avoid toxic body care products.

Avoid taking antibiotics unnecessarily.

Care for your home's microbiome:

- Use nontoxic cleaning products.
- Take your shoes off inside.
- Avoid pesticides and antibacterial products.
- Add houseplants.
- Open your windows.

Traditional diets and lifestyles supported great microbial abundance and diversity, which helped build fitness and resilience. The urbanization of our world, including our housing, population density, clothing, personal care products, chlorinated water, soaps, toothpastes, separation of our homes from the environment, and relationship to food and how it's grown, has impacted our microbiota by reducing diversity and creating a mismatch with the requirements of our coevolved biology.

This mismatch and its impact on our microbial diversity reduce our ability to come back to full health after illness and our resistance to pathogens. Over the millions of years of mammalian evolution, babies have been exposed to fresh air, the vaginal and skin microbiome, and breast milk, which bolster their microbial communities with diverse and abundant bacteria they evolved to inherit. Today interventions of sterility are commonplace after birth, which creates an unnatural environment, especially for new parents and their new babies. Modern medicine is a modern miracle, but it has much to learn from the past. You can't control the way your baby is born, but you can advocate for their rightful inheritance of the microbiome you tended to throughout pregnancy through actions like skin-to-skin contact and skipping the soapy baby bath.

Fortunately, we can make choices that help improve our microbial communities, and so many of these choices are wonderful and bring great joy, meaning, and connection to our lives. Spending time outdoors, moving often, and eating healthy food support our bacteria and overall health. These actions nurture our relationship to the world, which in turn nurtures our growing babies.

# TAKE ACTION

Consider your microbial comrades and cultivate a diverse microbiome. Our microbiome impacts our babies' body composition, immune function, and overall health. Our microbes respond to what we eat and put on our bodies. They affect our metabolism, inflammatory response, cravings, and behavior. Go outside and eat sustainably grown food. When we interact with the world and don't scrub it off with harsh, antimicrobial soaps, we cultivate microbial residents that build our health and resilience.

Care for your teeth. Our teeth and gums may become more vulnerable to dysbiosis during pregnancy, and our oral health impacts our babies. Eating foods that provide abundant bioavailable and essential vitamins and minerals helps keep our mouths healthy. Brush twice a day and avoid sugary and starchy foods and toothpaste with ingredients like triclosan, sodium lauryl sulfate, and artificial sweeteners, which disrupt microbial health in the mouth and gut.

Trust your vagina. The unique structure of the vagina and the microbes that live there are particularly adept at thwarting off infection, which is good for you and your baby. Avoid harsh cleansers, soaps, and douching. Reduce stress, eat nourishing food, and minimize the use of antibiotics whenever possible.

Restore your connection to the world. Forming a relationship to our local place and the food we eat, either by growing our own or buying from local farmers, brings great joy to our lives and nurtures our microbes. When we care for our microbes, we take better care of our bodies and protect our environment.

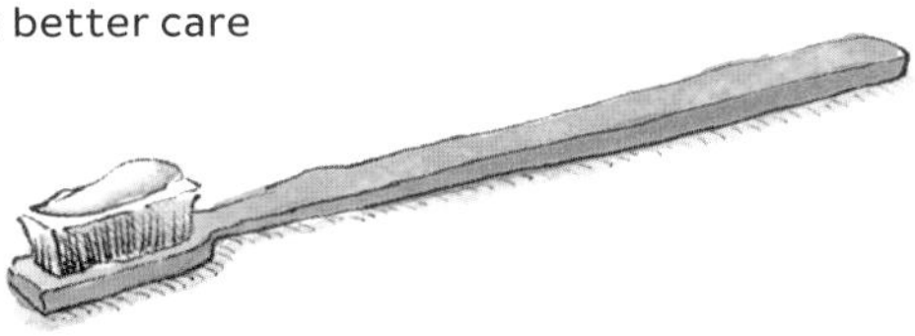

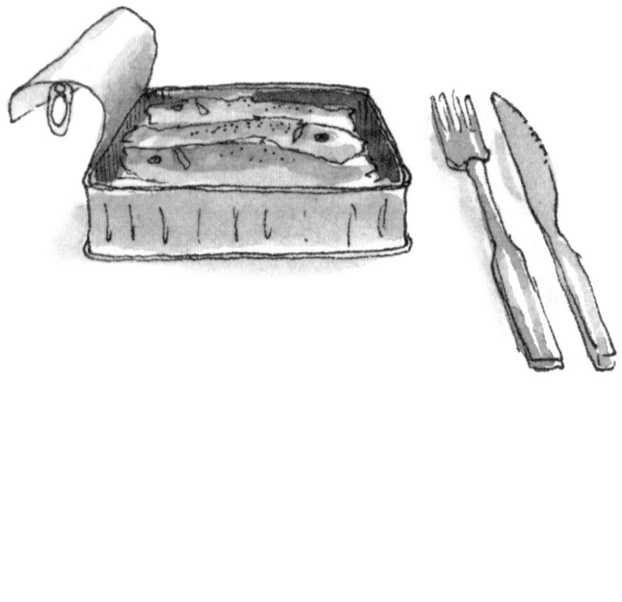

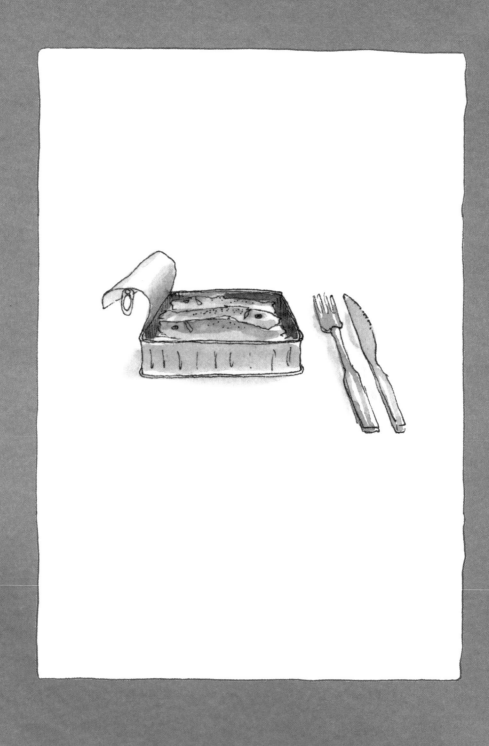

CHAPTER FOUR

# A Sperm's Tale

I LIKE TO JOKE WITH MAX that we waited many years before procreating because I needed that time to get his sperm into tip-top shape. I'm sure they were decent, but after years of my cooking, I like to think my efforts put a little extra skip in his sperm cells' proverbial step. He grew up eating fifty shades of beige and ramen noodles. In college he finally started eating basic vegetables, but not ones that were too threatening. He was an obstinate and picky eater as a child, but he's grown into an open-minded man who, thankfully, trusts me and loves my cooking.

For all humans, reproductive health matters and is shaped by the food we eat and the way we live. While individuals planning for pregnancy are encouraged to take a prenatal vitamin before, during, and after pregnancy—because we know nutrient deficiencies impact the health and development of the baby and we are encouraged to live as if our children's future matters—nonbirthing partners are simply warned about the impending onslaught of diaper changes and encouraged to enjoy their last moments of freedom.

Sperm don't get a lot of recognition or attention in the story of reproduction and growing babies. Before people contribute their sperm in the process of making a person, they are generally not counseled on nutrition and lifestyle and how their choices impact sperm quality and fertility. This is important because some studies have shown that cisgender men's fertility rates in developed nations have declined over the last five decades. Impotence is not related to traditional masculinity, but it is related to environmental and lifestyle factors. These factors include exposure to environmental toxins like herbicides, flame retardants, air pollution, and cigarette smoke and to endocrine disruptors like plastics, fragrances, cleaning products, radiation, and heavy metals.

Endocrine disruptors interfere with how our body makes, transports, uses, and eliminates hormones. This interference can mimic or block hormonal effects, which impacts our reproductive, neurological, metabolic, immune, cardiovascular, and developmental health. Endocrine-disrupting chemicals are ubiquitous in our synthetic landscape, and sometimes we like to slather them on our body. For example, when the word "fragrance" is listed on an ingredient list in products like perfumes or colognes, deodorants, lotions, shampoos, household cleaners, or makeup, it might be made from phthalates, a developmental and reproductive toxin.

The way these products cause harm in our bodies is complicated and has to do with factors like how much and how often we're exposed and what age we are when we're exposed. For example, babies, because they are small and their body systems are immature, may experience devastating health consequences when exposed to endocrine disruptors, whereas adults may not be harmed to the same degree. When we are exposed, we don't always have an immediate health consequence. There is a lag time between exposure and outcome, and exposure to many types of these chemicals has a synergistic or additive effect.

# The Making of Sperm

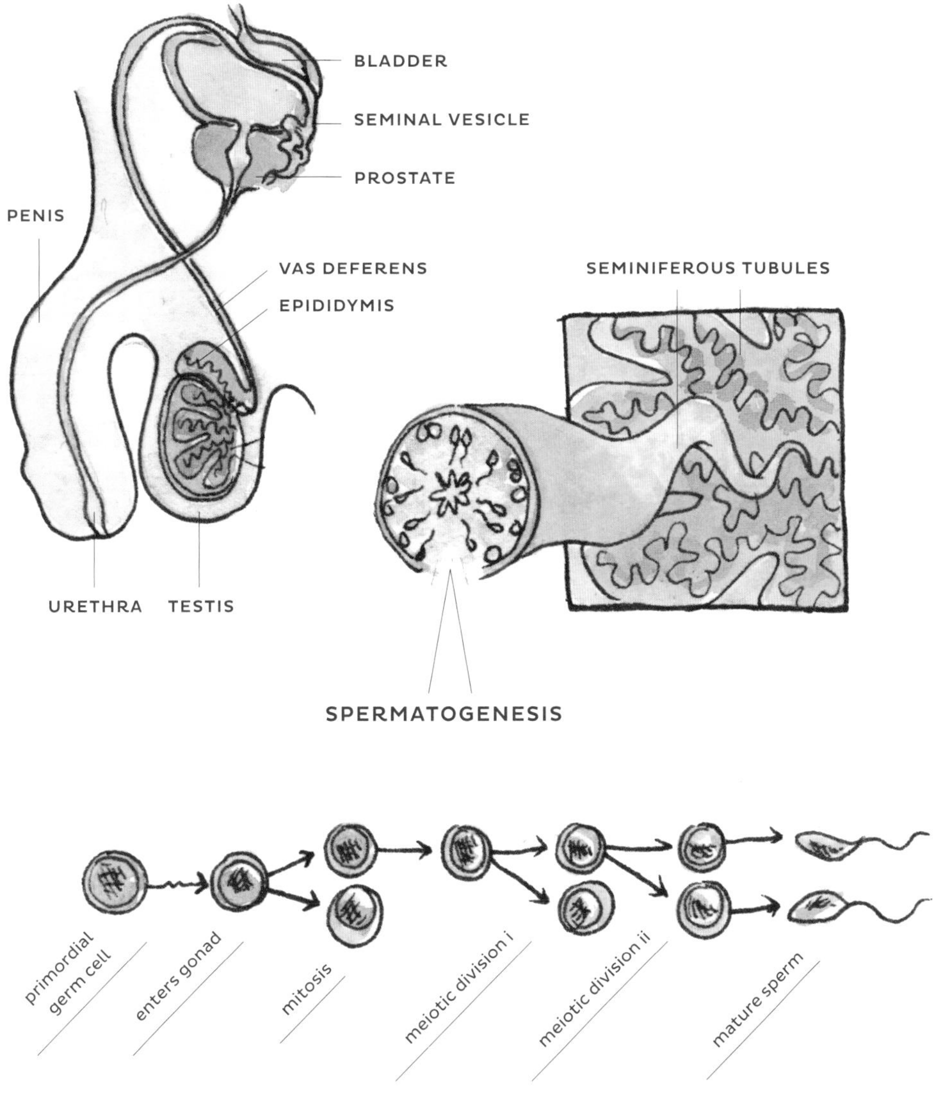
BLADDER
SEMINAL VESICLE
PROSTATE
PENIS
VAS DEFERENS
EPIDIDYMIS
URETHRA
TESTIS
SEMINIFEROUS TUBULES
SPERMATOGENESIS
primordial germ cell
enters gonad
mitosis
meiotic division i
meiotic division ii
mature sperm

# Sperm Morphology, Motility & Count

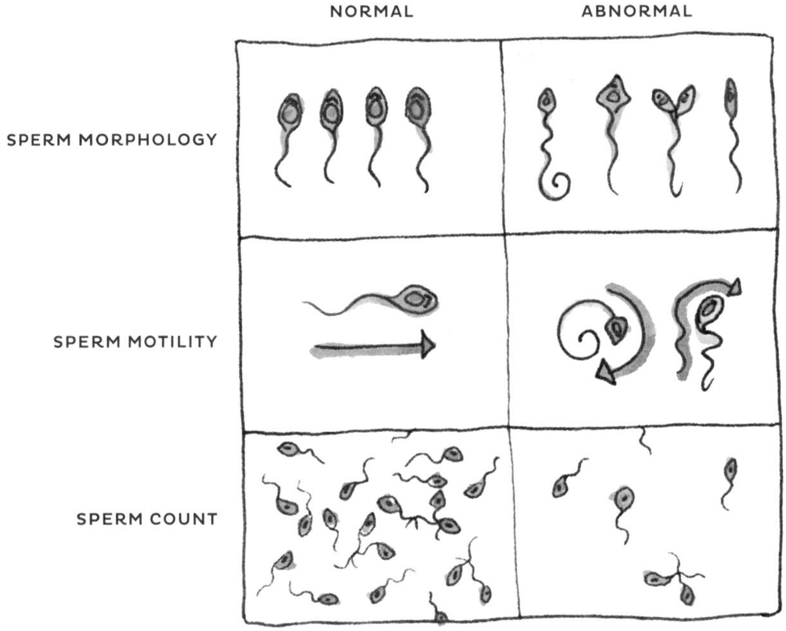


For a long time, we were told that exposure to low levels of endocrine disruptors wouldn't harm us, but now we've found that even minuscule levels of exposure to some of these chemicals can have monumentally potent effects, and they can cause mutations in our DNA that get passed on to our kids.

Environmental and lifestyle factors change the way genes are expressed, both in our own body and those of our future children. The study of these changes is called epigenetics. The DNA inside the sperm cell isn't malleable, but the way DNA is transcribed and expressed *is*, and this is influenced by the way we live, and by how our parents lived, and their parents, and so on.

When the sperm cell and egg join together during the process of fertilization, the zygote, also known as your future baby, has a differentiated epigenome, and the old patterns are wiped clean, in a sense. But some imprinted genes bypass this reprogramming and impact your baby's development with these inherited gene changes in place. It is thought that these imprinted genes are more sensitive to environmental signals like diet, hormones, and toxin exposure.

We are accustomed to hearing that we should eat a healthy diet, manage stress, and exercise, but we're not as used to hearing about the importance of the preconception paternal diet and how it impacts the health of the sperm and the ability of the sperm to join with an egg to create a viable embryo, or how the health of the nonbirthing partner at the time of conception affects the long-term health of the baby created. The big three characteristics that define sperm health are shape, mobility, and count. When too many sperm cells are misshapen or are inadequate swimmers, or when sperm count is reduced, fertility is compromised. Sperm are vulnerable to their environment. Some ill effects of exposure to products containing endocrine disruptors, toxic chemicals, and synthetic plastic solvents include low sperm count, issues with morphology and function, DNA fragmentation, and the stimulation of reactive oxygen species, which stress the body and can also damage DNA and cause issues with sperm production.

## PROTECT THE GONADS

A few weeks before Max and I made our son, he and a few friends biked over three hundred miles from our house in Reno, Nevada, to Inyo County, California. They stopped and climbed up mountains and skied down along the way, ending the trip with the long ascent and decent of Mount Whitney, the tallest peak in the contiguous United States. Along the way he inhaled diesel fumes as trucks and cars whizzed by. He rode on what he called his Sierra saddle, a leather bike seat that took some breaking in before it stopped feeling like it was damaging his goods. I thought he was crazy, but I didn't worry about his sperm or know that sitting for long periods of time on a bike can stress the gonads as they are squeezed, overheated, and compressed. I didn't know that, in response to high heat, germinal cells produce heat-shock proteins, which can create more oxidative damage.

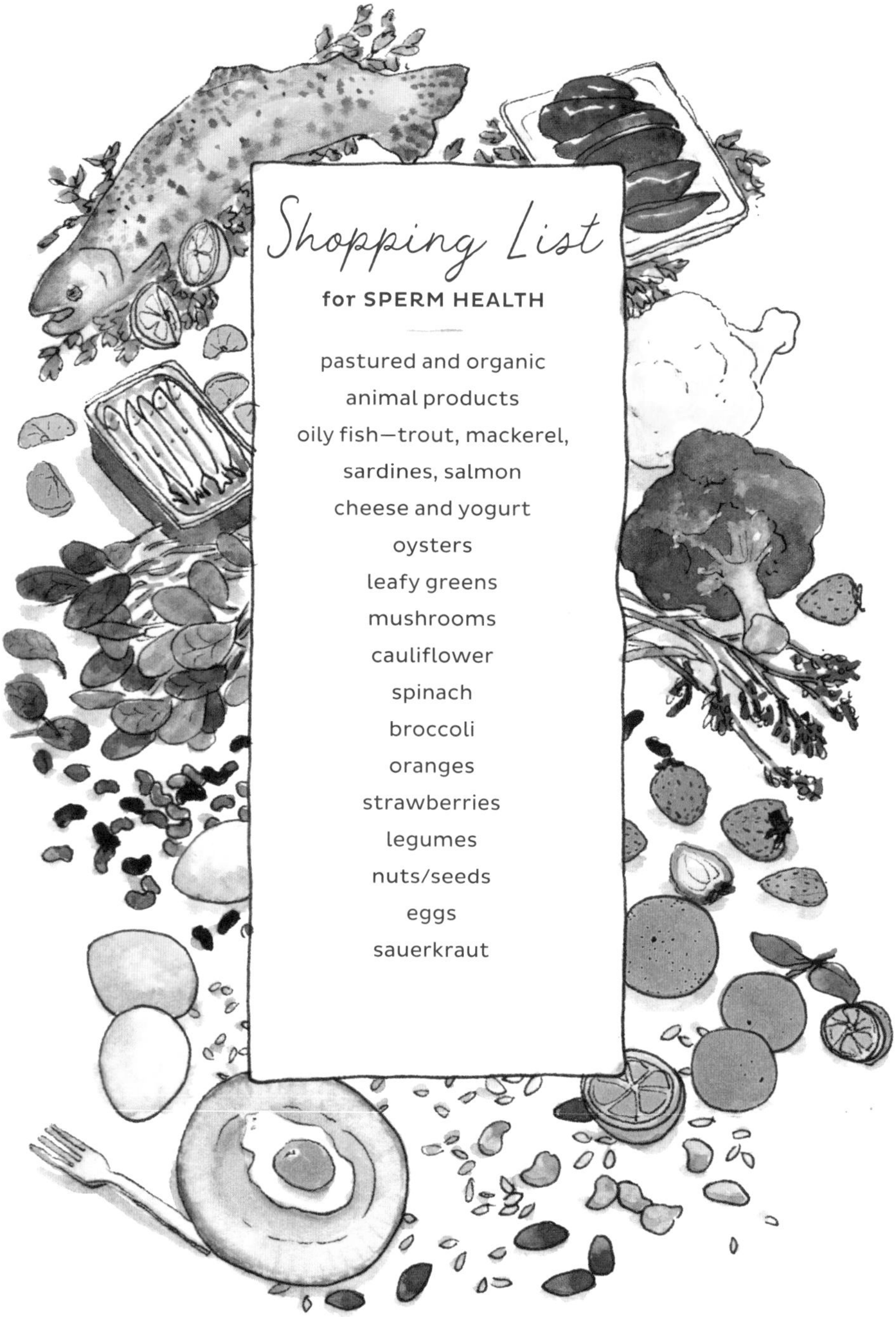

# Shopping List

**for SPERM HEALTH**

pastured and organic
animal products
oily fish—trout, mackerel,
sardines, salmon
cheese and yogurt
oysters
leafy greens
mushrooms
cauliflower
spinach
broccoli
oranges
strawberries
legumes
nuts/seeds
eggs
sauerkraut

If I had known a little more about sperm health, I might have yelled, "Take care of your gonads!" as I watched him bike away. In the same way Max was exposed to diesel exhaust emissions and gonadal stress, we are each exposed to the bad stuff in the air, food, and water every day. It can be overwhelming to consider the bad, but it can be delightful to consider the good. During his bike ride he ate wild salmon and sardines, avocados, seeds, nuts, fruits, and vegetables, and these foods, rich in antioxidants, vitamins, and minerals, are known to improve semen quality and balance out oxidative damage. He spent abundant time moving his body with his friends, supporting his reproductive and mental health. And he didn't smoke cigarettes, do drugs, or drink excessive alcohol, which can introduce cell mutagens and, when combined, damage sperm.

Max despises tight pants, which can overheat the gonads, and he rarely has his cell phone on his body, a habit that's frustrating to me but forgivable when I remember that overexposure to cell phones and other devices can impact sperm health and quality. He doesn't work night shifts, and he wears blue light–blocking glasses with dark red lenses when he works on his computer at night. He looks like a combination of a Tour de France bike racer and Robert Downey Jr. (who often sports red-tinted frames on the red carpet), but it helps prevent the disruption of his circadian rhythm, which impacts reproductive health and fertility.

## FERTILE GROUND

If your sperm-contributing partner is like mine, they might learn about how diet, sleep, drugs, electronics, lifestyle habits, medications, and environmental factors affect sperm quality and overall health and reason that the only logical thing to do is to throw away their cell phone, swear off pants, reject all components of the Western diet (except coffee, of course), and decide we should live in the woods, hunt and forage for our own food, and, even though it doesn't quite fit in the story, figure out how to ski and climb every day too.

# Protecting the Gonads

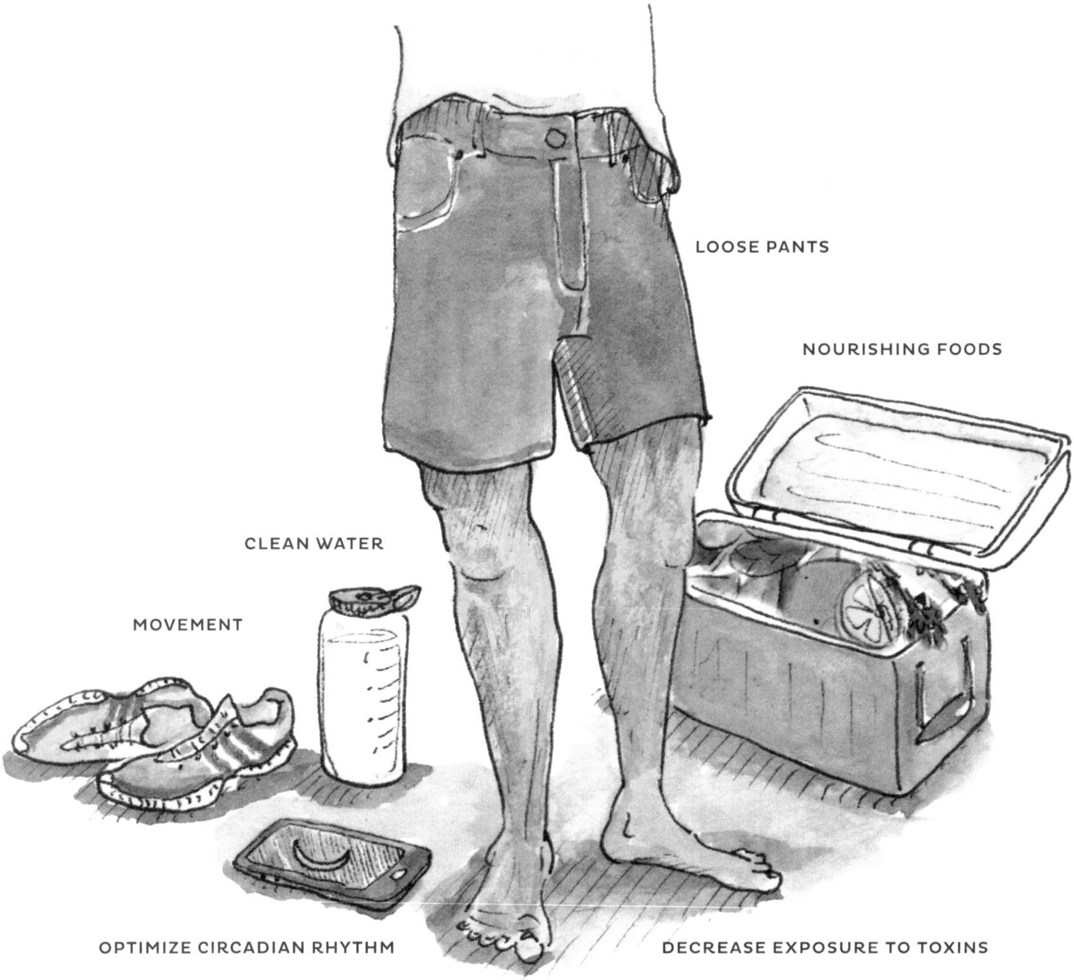

While I appreciate this sperm-protecting immoderation and concern about the health of our future children, I think part of this dream has to do with my partner's love of snow and dislike for pants.

Maybe your partner is on the other end of the sperm spectrum and believes that fertility is the realm and responsibility of the birthing parent. For cisgender men, trouble with sperm quality and fertility often emerges as a threat to masculinity, one that sparks commentary and induces sperm panic as studies continue to show declining sperm counts and issues with male fertility. This is an issue where lifestyle factors meet culture. Low sperm counts are associated with a higher risk for cardiovascular and other diseases. Both the birthing parent and the sperm-contributing parent may experience issues with fertility with advanced age. The biological clock might not tick as loudly in cisgender men's ears, or maybe our culture taught them not to hear it and instead believe in their ageless virility, but sperm producers over the age of forty-five increase baby's risk of prematurity, low birth weight, seizures, and other long-term health issues like cancer.

Even as it becomes more common for people to have babies in their thirties and forties, the terms our medical system has historically used to describe pregnant people over thirty-five make me imagine an old woman, walking with her cane and squinting to read the print on the boxes of diapers she buys as she prepares for the arrival of her baby. When we are pregnant over the age of thirty-five, we are considered AMA, or of "advanced maternal age," deemed "elderly primigravida" if pregnant with our first child, or told we're having a "geriatric pregnancy." Pregnant people over thirty-five undergo intense screening for health risks. Meanwhile, Hugh Hefner (RIP) became a father to his third and fourth children at ages sixty-five and sixty-six, becoming a symbol of inimitable vitality and celebrated for an ageless ability to impregnate.

In the story of growing babies, we often forget the people who provide sperm, but they are one-half of the equation. All people experience threats to reproductive health, as our chemical industry remains largely unregulated and lobbies Congress to avoid regulation of its toxic products. We may all do better by our health by avoiding food treated with pesticides and wrapped and heated in plastic, and avoiding BPA-laden paper receipts, but we'll do best if, as a culture, we stop supporting companies that promote the use of endocrine-disrupting chemicals and demand protection of our future children by caring more about all of our reproductive health and rights.

Sperm health and epigenetics appear to be highly responsive to positive lifestyle changes. Eating well and moving often improve our future children's metabolic and mental health. Taking greater responsibility for reproductive health is an act of caring—or for some, of parenting—before a baby is in the picture. Taking care of our children starts before we have them, with our own bodies, and extends to our partners, families, friends, and communities. Parents who have more support and healthier partners and who nurture their health through diet, movement, and lifestyle tend to have children with greater cognitive and overall health.

Support looks different depending on who you talk to and the dynamic of your relationship with your partner. For me, support is the gift of time so that I can write, work outside, or gather food from the garden or the market and cook. When I was pregnant and working full-time, I felt supported when my partner made an effort to cook food that I would love when I was home late. His support is a glass of water or a cup of coffee in the morning, and it's him listening to me talk about sperm health and living as if the future of our children—their health, relationship to the world, and sense of place in it—truly matters.

# TAKE ACTION

Eat nourishing whole foods. Choosing organic, nutrient-dense food like wild salmon, avocados, seeds, nuts, fruits, vegetables, and pastured and grass-fed meats supports optimal hormone levels and healthy sperm. Avoiding nonfermented soy products, drugs, alcohol, white flour, and sugar supports healthy reproductive functioning.

Optimize your circadian rhythm. The circadian system is the master regulator of almost all physiological processes. Getting plenty of sleep at night, spending time outside during the day, and limiting exposure to blue light at night promote overall health and well-being. Disruption of our circadian clock, through abnormal light-dark exposure, alters the secretion of reproductive hormones and reduces fertility.

Protect your gonads. Tight pants and too much time sitting lead to gonads that are squeezed, overheated, and stressed. Germ cells respond to tight, hot quarters by producing heat shock proteins, which causes even more damage to reproductive health. Looser pants and more time spent moving than sitting give the gonads the freedom they need.

Balance the unavoidable bad with intentional good. We are all exposed to some degree of environmental toxins we can't control. Choosing to move often in diverse ways, spending plenty of time outside in green places, eating high-quality, nourishing food, and avoiding smoking (of any kind) help our bodies build resilience and help sperm contributors produce abundantly healthy sperm.

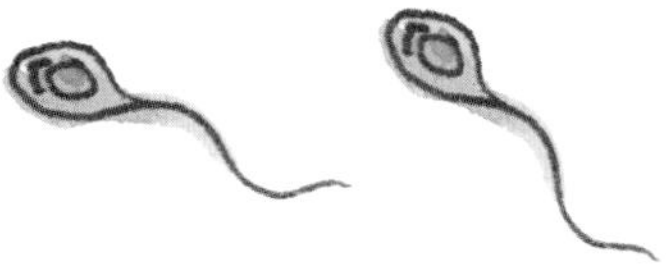

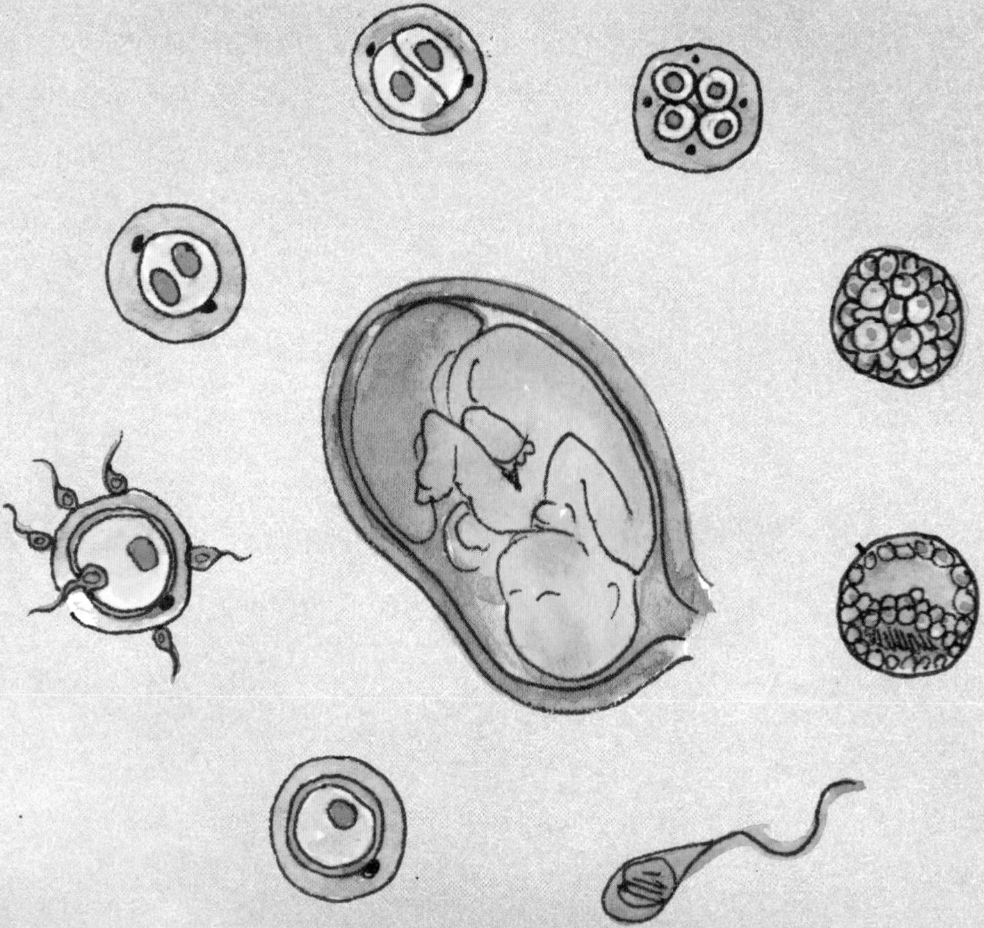

# Part Two

# CONCEPTION, GROWING YOUR BABY & BIRTH

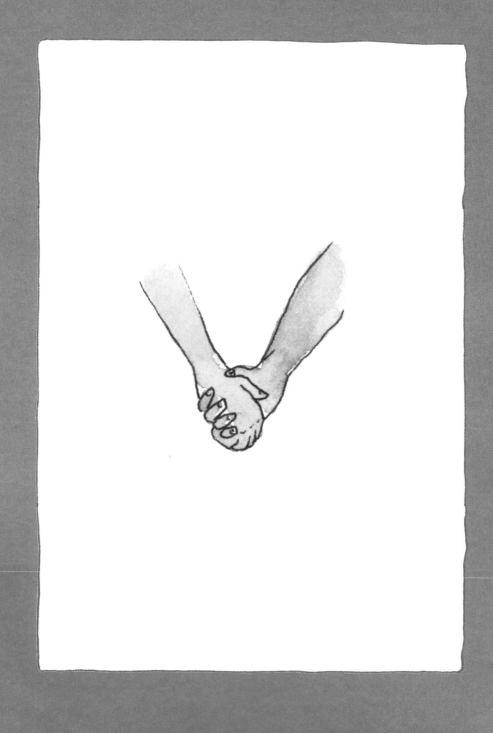

CHAPTER FIVE

# The First Trimester

**SCIENTISTS, TEACHERS, AND PARENTS** have taught us about fertilization, or how you got here, using many stories and metaphors. Parents might say babies are brought in by storks, or they might use the "birds and the bees" metaphor. (Of this problematic interspecies metaphor, a ten-year-old Bart Simpson said, "The sun is out, birds are singing, bees are trying to have sex with them—as is my understanding . . .") While these metaphors attempt to explain reproduction to children and miss the crucial ingredient (sex between humans), other metaphors that leave much to be desired are used by grown-ups to teach other grown-ups about reproduction.

While the last chapter examined the health of people who produce sperm because they are often left out of the story about reproduction and growing babies, there is one key event in which they play the starring role. The story of fertilization, or when sperm and egg meet and join, is a sperm-centric tale shaped by cultural stereotypes of "masculine" and "feminine." The stories we tell and the metaphors we use are important because they reinforce the truths and beliefs we hold as a culture. I propose shifting away from a male-dominated story of fertilization and rethinking the way we visualize the forming of a new person. Perhaps if our origin story is one of interaction and gender equity, our culture and imagination will naturally shift toward an appreciation of balance over domination and nuance over strictly defined gender roles.

For successful fertilization to occur, both egg and sperm actively participate. Despite this requirement of mutual involvement, both mainstream media and scientific literature fall into gendered descriptions and fairy-tale stories to describe this event. The sperm, in this telling, is a superhero or a knight in shining armor. Meanwhile, the egg is a damsel in distress who is waiting for her sperm to rescue her from demise. In almost all medical textbooks, the story of sperm and egg reads much like the Disney version of "Cinderella" or "Sleeping Beauty": handsome, brave sperm journeys to rescue helpless princess. While the sperm is celebrated and applauded for its harrowing egg-penetrating journey, the egg is shrouded in mundane language. When a sperm cell dies, it perishes, but when an egg cell dies, it disintegrates or degenerates—a quiet disappearance versus the tragic loss of the heroic sperm.

Sperm are talked about like the men they supposedly represent (that is, with great reverence and importance), whereas eggs tend to have shorter explanations about their role in fertilization. Eggs are to be fertilized; sperm do the fertilizing. The egg is passive, or worse, a nonparticipatory fortress, while the sperm is all action and bravado. We can't help but attribute masculinist symbolism to sperm and dependent receptiveness to the egg. This metaphor of the soldiering sperm and the helpless egg might seem like a relatable way to tell the story of fertilization. The problem with this telling is that it creates the sense that our innate selves are defined by cisgender and patriarchal stereotypes, with men acting as inherent or deserving conquerors and women as victims who need rescuing. The other problem with this story is that it's not quite biologically accurate.

There's another story with slightly different metaphors you may have heard. When scientists discovered that sperm aren't the speediest swimmers—their forward thrust is weak, while their side-to-side force is quite strong—sperm were described as hapless armies of tiny man-organisms who don't know where they are going and are too proud to ask for directions. Scientists discovered that the egg has distinct physical and chemical properties that influence fertilization. No longer defined by passivity, the egg was now an aggressive, sperm-trapping spider-woman who selects a worthy sperm and imprisons it as it attempts to escape. Now the sperm was the victim and the egg was a woman who trapped a man against his will.

Slightly different gender stereotypes inform this story. The egg's active role is associated with women's power and manipulation, bringing to mind witchery and sorcery to procreate. This idea, even more than the other, frightens our culture that values masculinity and control. Emily Martin, a cultural anthropologist from Stanford, was one of the first people to illuminate how cultural conditioning and gender stereotypes influence biologists' male-centric descriptions of sperm and reproductive health. She argued that this point of view impacts how information and research is interpreted and the kind of questions researchers ask. If scientists assume the egg is passive, they won't look for chemicals it releases or possesses that drive the action of fertilization. If the sperm are in charge and do the penetrating, we won't wonder how the egg is involved in this process. In other words, our stories and stereotypes are shaped by history and culture, and we can't readily ask questions, or see what we're missing, if we fail to imagine that other stories are possible.

In her paper on the subject, written in 1991, Martin looked at the standard textbooks used by premedical and medical students and noticed that the story of reproduction was told using celebratory language for sperm, whose production is admired for its abundance and called remarkable. Meanwhile, words like "debris" and "shedding" described menstruation. Ovulation, a process that is more analogous to sperm production, is likewise discussed with lackluster morbidity. The books celebrated how cisgender men are endless sperm-producing machines and lamented the limited nature of women's eggs, which decline in number over time.

Metaphors and stories aren't the problem. These creative tools help us comprehend biological processes and build an imaginative understanding of events we can't see. But there's a problem when our origin story celebrates traditional ideas of masculinity and minimizes roles associated with femininity. The stories we tell can perpetuate inequality or shift us toward mutual respect and understanding.

In my own undergraduate textbook on anatomy and physiology, the authors said the sperm must "breach" the egg's defenses before the egg can be "penetrated." Even though the book does a good job of explaining that true fertilization occurs only when both chromosomes combine, it can't help but craft a conquering story of adventuring and penetrating sperm and leave out the qualities of the egg.

Biologist Scott Gilbert doesn't describe fertilization as a battle involving the force of the sperm or the wiles of the egg. In the widely used textbook he wrote, *Developmental Biology*, he says fertilization is like a dialogue between sperm and egg. In his chapter "Fertilization," he quotes Walt Whitman and Charles Darwin, indicating that this event is characterized by a mix of poetry and science. I like the idea of biological poetry taking place in my uterus.

Elaborating on the nature of the dialogue between sperm and egg, Gilbert states, "The egg activates the sperm metabolism that is essential for fertilization, and the sperm reciprocates by activating the egg metabolism needed for the onset of development." His description illustrates that the egg and the sperm are both drivers of this process of fertilization and both have essential jobs to perform that depend on reciprocation, not force or domination.

## AN EXCLUSIVE CLUB

Somewhere around 250 million to 280 million sperm enter the vagina during ejaculation, and of those millions, about 200 sperm make it within the egg's vicinity. They are propelled by the action of uterine muscle contractions and are channeled through cervical mucus, and they are allowed to go on, or are held up, based on biochemical interactions. Persistence, competence, and a little luck turn out to be much more important than swimming speed for sperm. Pregnancy that is attained through vaginal intercourse can occur during a six-day window. This window gives the sperm more time to reach the oviduct where the egg resides and become fertilization competent. When sperm first leave home in the testis, they are incapable of taking part in fertilization. Within the reproductive tract, they transform and mature into competent young sperm.

Far from being passive, the egg and reproductive system are intricately involved in guiding and shaping the sperms' journey. While the uterine muscles contract, urging the sperm onward, some regions of the oviduct may slow down sperm and slowly release them back into the reproductive tract. Sperm motility is important once the sperm reach the oviduct, where they become hyperactive. This hyperactivity is influenced by the composition of the sperms' tails, and the way the sperm move is adapted to the viscous fluid present in the oviduct.

The inner depths of the oviduct are highly exclusive. The sperm must interact with the zona pellucida, a transparent membrane surrounding the egg, before it can begin its conversation about the future with the egg. The egg has been busy focusing on its own dance, or meiosis, as it prepares to meet the sperm and present its DNA. The sperm that ends up uniting with the egg may not be left to random chance. Some research is starting to look at the interaction between the egg and the sperm and is finding that the egg may have a bias about which sperm it grants access. The egg may actively select a specific sperm based on its sex chromosomes, genetics, and other biochemical information we haven't discovered yet. When the chosen sperm and egg do join together, through a series of fusions and activations, they unite and start their journey toward the inner womb.

# *The Union*

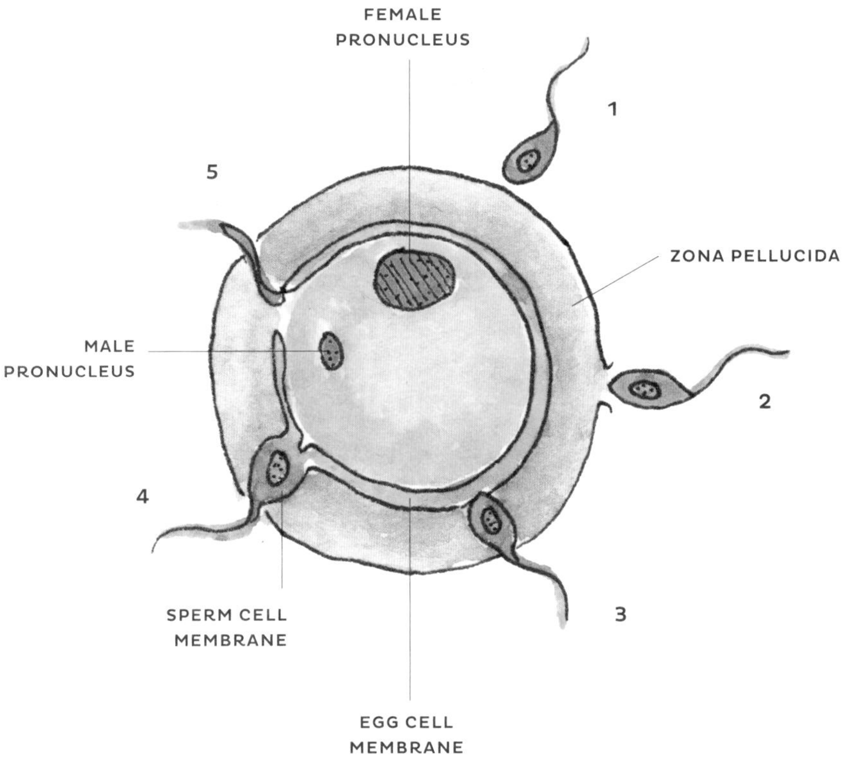


1. Uterine muscles contract and encourage sperm into the oviduct.
2. Sperm binds to the zona pellucida.
3. Contact with the zona pellucida triggers the acrosome reaction.
4. The sperm cell membrane and egg cell membrane fuse. This fusion combines the genes from both parents and creates a new organism.
5. The egg is metabolically activated by the entrance of the sperm nucleus to begin development.

# The Journey and Implantation

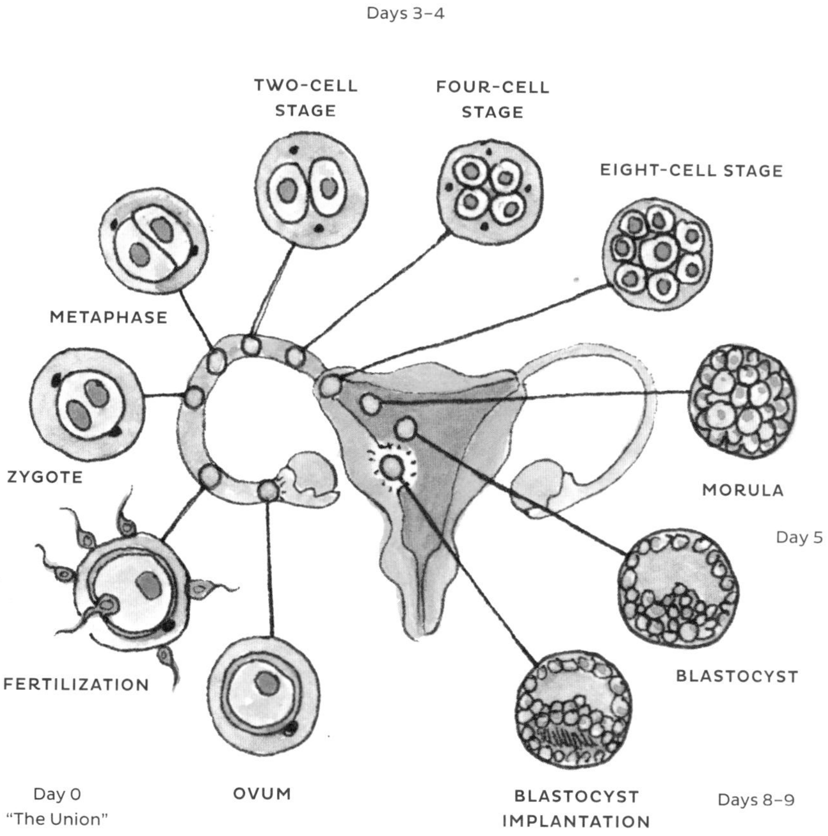

# The Hormones of Fertilization and Implantation

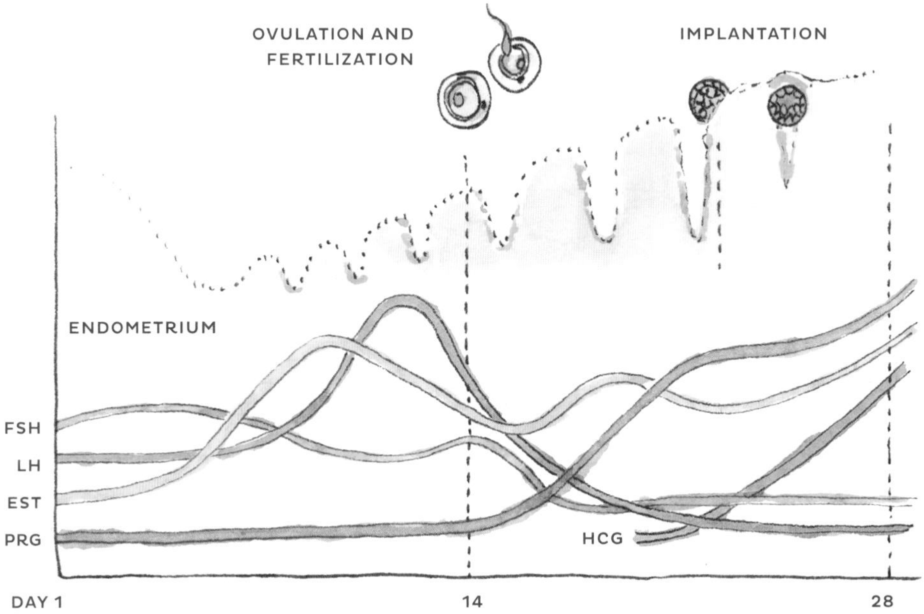


Synchrony between the early embryo and the endometrium is required for successful implantation. The endometrium becomes "receptive" during a specific period known as the "implantation window," which opens around 6–8 days after ovulation and remains receptive for about 4 days. FSH and LH are essential for ovulation, while estrogen and progesterone prepare the body for, and sustain, a pregnancy. HCG, which is known as the first hormonal sign of conception, is one of the key molecules that contributes to endometrial receptivity, and the amount produced increases considerably after implantation.

## JOURNEY TO THE INNER WOMB

The united form of egg and sperm is called a zygote ("yoked together"). The zygote travels toward the uterus and arrives there five or six days after the union. During this honeymoon, the zygote divides and becomes a blastocyst. This tiny cellular mass contains embryonic stem cells, which carry all the information needed to form and develop the cells in an embryo. Small yet full of promise, the mass of cells arrives at its new home ready to lay down roots in the uterine lining and start growing.

A thick, luscious endometrium (*endo* meaning "inner," and *metrium*, "womb") is essential for successful implantation. This part of our body abides by the cyclic rhythm of our internal clock whose hands are set by hormones sent from the hypothalamus, pituitary, and ovaries. A surge of estrogen and progesterone open the inner womb's window of implantation. Right before ovulation, estrogen and progesterone cause one of the layers of the endometrium to grow and prepare for possible implantation. It becomes swollen with fluid and nutrients, creating the perfect environment to support the growth of a baby.

During implantation, the uterus is bustling with invading, dying, and repairing cells. Inflammation helps prepare the uterus, and we feel its effects in the form of fatigue. Implantation takes around five days of flurrying activity. Twelve days after ovulation, just before one of the layers of the endometrium would normally shed, menstruation is prevented by specific hormones. The pregnancy hormone our tests read, hCG, keeps the corpus luteum around and starts stimulating the growth of the placenta. The corpus luteum, or "yellow body," journeyed with the egg and matured into a progesterone-secreting supporter of early pregnancy. HCG levels are generally high enough to tell us whether we're pregnant one week after fertilization, and they reach their peak at ten weeks of pregnancy. Then hCG levels drop drastically as levels of estrogen and progesterone steadily climb.

## TRANSFORMATION

My first trimester was marked by a bone-deep fatigue, or perhaps "uterine-deep" fatigue is more anatomically accurate. I lived through the exhausting, inflammatory stage of my pregnancy during the heat of the summer. As the temperature consistently crept over one hundred degrees in the high desert outside, I laid on the cool tile downstairs in my house and watched as my garden grew miserably because of my neglect. While I usually had the energy to go to work and come home and put in a few hours of physical labor in my yard, I instead returned home and went to bed around 8:30. But as I struggled through crushing fatigue and occasional nausea, I also felt profoundly curious and intuitive, like something inside me was awakening.

Early pregnancy is a moment of great transformation, and it might be marked by emotional swings, fatigue, and morning sickness. Hormones and physiological changes shape these shifts, while our embodiment acknowledges and accepts them. My first trimester changed my relationship with my body and the world. I was determined to connect to this transition, the good parts and the bad, and to embrace the physiological shifts and power of growing a person in my body.

I felt a surge of change and creativity too. I wrote my wedding vows in a flurry of inspired energy, and I wrote in my journal more throughout the first trimester than at any other time while I was pregnant. When I was around five weeks pregnant, I wrote, "I'm tired and introspective. My belly already feels different, like it's considering taking on a new shape, but won't commit to change for a while." When I was six weeks pregnant, I told my little embryo about how his heart was beating rapidly, around 100 to 160 beats per minute, and how his intestines, lungs, pituitary glands, brain, muscles, and bones were all starting to develop. How his neural tube was forming, how his head was enormous compared to his c-shaped body, and his kidneys, liver, bronchi, larynx, and tooth buds were developing too.

I wrote to my embryo that many pregnancy resources insisted on telling me he was the size of a lentil and I decided that if he was a lentil, he must be my favorite variety, the petite French green lentil. At eight weeks, the resources told me my baby was the size of a blueberry, but it was unclear if they meant he was the size of a wild Maine blueberry (very small and sweet) or a big juicy California berry, and thus started my weekly argument with fetal–food size comparisons.

As my newly pregnant body worked to adapt to the presence of a new occupant, my mind went through its own process of adaptation. One benefit to my fatigue-induced downtime and garden neglect was my increased time to find out what was going on in my body. I watched videos and revisited my textbooks on reproduction and developmental biology. I saw art in the images and words, instead of facts I had previously needed to memorize for exams.

As I consumed information about fertilization and implantation, I noticed that the shape-shifting metamorphosis that occurs as the blastocyst becomes an embryo, then a fetus, and as fingerlike shapes and layers become the elaborate placenta, is like watching disparate colors on a painter's watercolor tray become an image of something recognizable. A splash of peach becomes the umbilical cord; a dot of blue, the amniotic cavity filled with fluid; and spots of red and tan, the intricately intertwined placenta. From its snail-like origins, the embryo curves into a recognizable human form. In a complex origami of flesh, nerve, and tissue, layers fold and stack to form the major organs.

The processes that shape this growth are known as induction and migration. Induction is the process of stem-cell differentiation and evolution that results in specific structures and tissues. Migration is the march of cells that builds the growing human organism. In the nervous system, for example, cell migration creates special patterns. Once these cells, specific to the nervous system, settle into their stationary position, only neurites can travel along the cells' path and reach their destinations in the various tissues that compose and connect the system. Brain development is an ocean of complexity and migration is the ship that navigates it, allowing billions of neurons to each form thousands of connections to other neurons.

By three and a half weeks the embryo's tiny heart is pumping blood. The end of the embryonic period is week eight, and the major organs and skeletal muscles are formed and contracting spontaneously. The umbilical cord is delivering blood to and from the placenta. From one cell to a one-inch fetus, the first eight weeks is the fastest your baby will grow throughout all of pregnancy.

## GROWING A NEW ORGAN

The first time I saw a placenta was in the operating room during a C-section birth I observed as a nursing student. I stared at it, amazed. It was richly, exuberantly red, larger than I imagined, and deeply vascularized. Noticing my curiosity, one of the nurses asked if I wanted to see it closer and allowed me to gently touch the incredible organ. I pressed my gloved finger into the disk-shaped placenta, and it felt robust and slippery. The nurse turned it in her hands with great care, showing me the side that looked like a brain with swirling, pooling blood, and then showing me the fetal side, smooth and encased with the attachment for the umbilical cord extending out and recently detached from the baby it helped grow.

When I delivered my placenta after the birth of my son, I didn't have the presence of mind or energy to examine the new organ that supported my son on the inside. My midwife told me later that my placenta was on the large side, and I felt oddly proud of this little fact. The placenta, which means "flat cake," develops when placental cells come into contact with our blood and reshape blood vessels in the uterine wall so that they become a source of oxygen, nutrient transport, and waste removal for the fetus. The placenta is aptly named *decidua*, as it sheds like a leaf after birth, marking a significant change in the season and landscape of our lives.

By the third week of pregnancy, the placenta starts its job as the circulatory provider to the fetus and continues to adapt to the fetus's changing needs and increasing size, becoming a fully functioning organ by the end of the third month. The placental barrier regulates the metabolic process of exchange between you and your baby. From the growing stalk of the fetus sprouts the umbilical cord, swimming in amniotic fluid and attaching to the fetal side of the placenta.

The placental barrier is more like the drip irrigation system in my garden than an impenetrable concrete wall. In my yard, if something too large—say, a large rock—enters the pipes that carry the water to my plants, the object won't get transported through the small holes of the drip system and therefore won't end up in my garden. Similarly, inside a pregnant person's body,

# *Placenta Decidua*

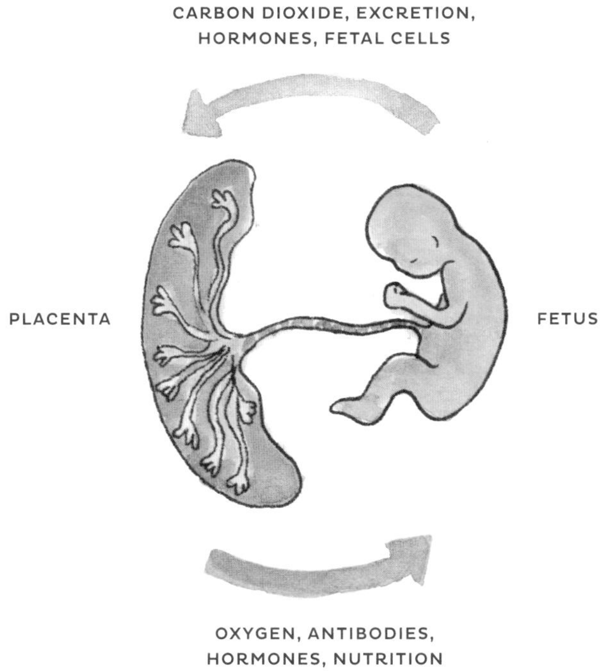


The placenta is the uniting point between the fetus and your body. Its roles include respiration, nutrition, excretion, protection, and endocrine and immune function. The placenta protects the baby, passes along maternal antibodies, and releases hormones into the fetal and maternal circulation that impact metabolism, fetal growth, labor, and birth. It adapts and changes over time to meet the metabolic needs of the baby, and, incredibly, fetal cells are able to migrate across the placental barrier to the birthing parent and become part of their organs and tissues. They may even help repair damage and disease.

large bacteria carried by the blood don't make it to the fetus because they are blocked by the protective transport properties of the placenta. However, the sorting system is based more on molecular size and weight than substance. This means that small, lightweight chemicals that are fat soluble have no problem passing through the pipes. Most drugs also make it through to some degree.

The substances the baby needs, like oxygen, calcium ions, iron, vitamins, fatty acids, and glucose, move across the barrier and influence growth and development. The stuff the baby doesn't need, like low-molecular-weight pesticides, also easily cross the barrier and can hinder growth and development. Not only do some drugs and dangerous environmental toxins cross the placental threshold, but their negative effects are compounded and magnified by the distinct process of placental blood flow and transport. The physical and pharmacological properties of various compounds determine how they are transported through the placenta and the effect they have on the baby.

The placenta might look like a cake, but its branching vasculature, full of blood, acts like a tree of life, bringing in nutrients, taking care of respiration, making hormones, and filtering out waste. The bad comes with the good, and when scientists look at the placenta under a microscope, the history of its various stressors is written in its unique composition.

The size and shape of the placenta affect its ability to transfer nutrients to the baby. This is because weight translates to surface area. Too small of a placenta, and the baby's development isn't well supported. Too big, and there may also be problems. Basically, you want the Goldilocks of placentas: not too small and not too big, but just right.

Both placenta and baby depend on glucose as their primary energy source. The other primary building blocks the placenta transports to the fetus include amino acids, fatty acids, cholesterol, and lipoproteins. The placenta is remarkably adaptable, altering its morphology and functioning in order to optimize nutrient transfer and thus fetal development.

Our body composition and diet directly impact the composition, function, and efficiency of the placenta. This organ is the only one we grow and shed. We don't have total control over our body composition. Each of us struggles with parts of our bodies we wish we could change. I'd like to choose smaller quadricep muscles in my thighs so jeans would fit more comfortably, and a smaller cup size so I could live a bra-free lifestyle. Alas, I depend on a certain amount of stretch in my denim and support for my bust. But we can choose how we move and what we eat. What we eat grows the placenta, which is the only part of us that has direct contact with the baby growing in our belly. The same foods that nourish and grow our babies also grow the placenta.

## SPROUTING THE SEEDLING

The first trimester encompasses both the embryonic period, which lasts for eight weeks, and the transition from embryo to fetus. These divisions are useful for diagnostic tests and prenatal appointments, but the experience of pregnancy is indivisible and organic. Whenever I think about gestation weeks or trimesters, I'm reminded of Nina Planck's view of these divisions of time in her book *Real Food for Mother and Baby*. "Weeks don't matter," she writes. "Even the trimesters—twelve to fourteen weeks each—don't correspond to embryological milestones."

The baby grows and unfolds like a flower blooming. Separating this growth into stages is like trying to break down the moments of blossoming into disparate events. Every time you look away, writing in your notebook or sketching the flower, you look back up to see the shape has shifted again.

Despite her dislike of splitting a time of continuous growth into distinct trimesters, Planck navigates the overwhelming amount of prenatal nutrition recommendations by creating three simplified, manageable categories that correlate with the trimesters. The first trimester is all about growing the fine details, like the liver and toes; micronutrients, from leafy greens, eggs, vegetables, fish, fermented foods, meat, bone broth, and fermented dairy, help grow these parts. The second trimester requires abundant protein and calcium for structures like organs, lungs, and the brain to grow larger. The third trimester is all about fish, healthy fats, glycine, and omega-3s to continue to grow baby's brain.

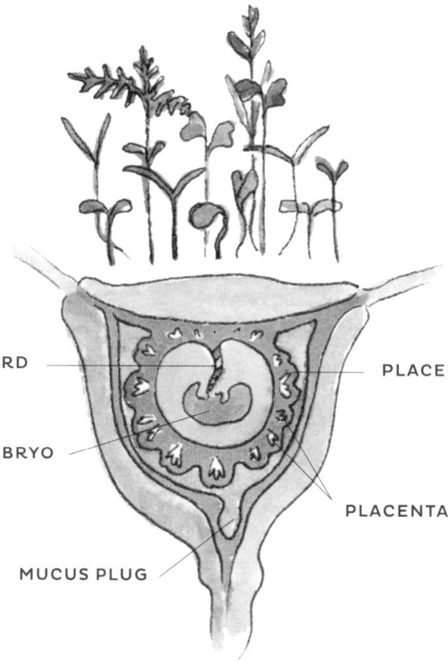


I like to think about fetal development, and the nourishment and care it requires, as a single seed in the soil. The seed starts out tiny, surrounded by a sea of dark, loamy soil teeming with life. The seed is already alive and contains embryonic tissue and a store of nutrients for initial germination. When the soil is adequately moist, there is enough daylight, and the temperature is comfortable, the seed wakes up. The primary root, the radicle, emerges from the seed like an umbilical cord and starts absorbing water, and then the shoot emerges above the soil surface, elongating and finding its structure and sprouting leaves like a backbone sprouting limbs. The conditions surrounding the seed create the eventual plant. To grow to its full potential, the small seed needs food, water, and oxygen.

The seedling's roots are responsible for assimilating micronutrients from the soil. As the radicle dives down into the earth, it anchors the plant in the ground. The more we care for the soil, the more micronutrients there are available for growing the seed. Like the placenta, the root depends on various transport mechanisms, and it can bring the good with the bad.

The preconception diet of the soil is composed of minerals, organic matter, water, and air. Soil health and structure are affected by what the soil comes into contact with and its interaction with the environment. In conventional farming, chemical fertilizers are added to the soil to increase the fertility of the soil, and thus yield from plants. Conventional farming cares about the short-term yield, while organic farming considers long-term soil health and the interconnectedness of our shared ecosystem. In our bodies, conventional agriculture is like eating candy for years, then conceiving and eating some candy enriched with a few vitamins. This type of bandage approach provides an initial burst of energy but just as surely leaves us tired and depleted—an unsustainable sugar crash at the cellular level. By contrast, organic and regenerative farming practices focus on the health of the whole and on replenishment.

Our bodies are garden beds, and they want a continuous influx of nutrient-dense food grown and pastured without dangerous sprays, medicines, and practices. Consistently adding nutrient-dense matter impacts the micronutrient abundance, enzyme activity, and physical and chemical properties of the soil. The result is a robust and resilient seedling that grows into a healthy plant.

The same principles apply to the babies we grow. Fetal growth puts a greater demand on our bodies to regulate DNA synthesis, transcription, and methylation. Our need for vitamins and minerals is higher because of these processes, and micronutrient deficiencies have negative impacts on our babies, such as an increased risk of neural tube defects and preeclampsia. Within the placenta, antioxidant enzymes require micronutrients like vitamin E, iron, vitamin D, selenium, choline, copper, zinc, and manganese to protect the growing fetus and placenta from oxidative stress and damage. Without enough micronutrients, blood flow to the fetus may be hindered. Vitamins and minerals are needed for growing new organs, for both their structure and their size and function. Micronutrients are about the long game. They shape the health of the baby before conception, during fetal development, during childhood, and into adulthood.

For most of evolutionary history, plants grew without the help of the industrial chemical industry. Likewise, people grew babies without the input of conventional nutrition recommendations, instead consuming traditional foods celebrated by their culture. Our plant and human ancestors have a lot to

# Methylation Matters

Methylation is a biochemical process where four atoms (one carbon and three hydrogen) are transferred from one substance to another. This process impacts biochemical reactions in the body, including liver, eye, reproductive, neurological, and cardiovascular health; DNA production, neurotransmitter production, detoxification, and fat metabolism. Methylation impacts how our bodies function and affects gene expression in both our body and our baby's body.

For optimal methylation, we must have adequate active folate (also known as methylfolate or 5-MTHF). When we take folic acid, our bodies must convert folic acid into its active form. Upward of 60% of the population has a genetic mutation that makes it hard for their bodies to do this conversion or create enough 5-MTHF.

When there isn't enough 5-MTHF to support the methylation cycle, many other molecules also can't be made efficiently in the body.

What you can do:

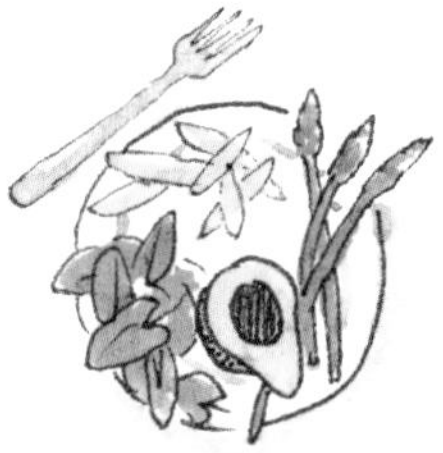

**1.** Eat healthy, whole, real foods that are rich in folate, like asparagus, brussels sprouts, leafy greens, avocado, beans, legumes, spinach, beef liver, and eggs.

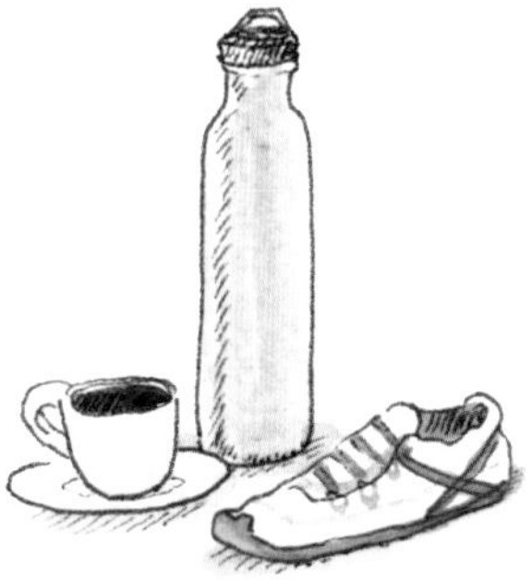

**2.** Move often, avoid tobacco and alcohol, and limit caffeine intake.

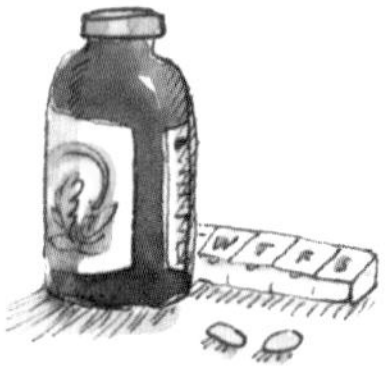

**3.** Continue taking a high quality prenatal vitamin.

teach us about how to support new life that our conventional guidelines miss out on. In her book *Real Food for Pregnancy*, Lily Nichols looks at the types of foods that build optimally healthy babies and examines the foods conventional nutrition recommends for pregnant people. She has found that the low-fat, carbohydrate- and grain-rich diets celebrated by conventional nutrition don't line up with what we actually need to grow and develop our babies with optimal health. Foods like eggs, pasture-raised meats, bone broth, full-fat dairy, and organ meats are key baby-building, traditional foods that conventional nutrition fails to include in its recommendations. In response to this outdated and truly unsatisfactory nutrition advice, Nichols writes, "I respectfully disagree with the conventional prenatal nutrition guidelines, and I cannot, in good conscience, recommend their sample meal plan to pregnant women."

## NAUSEA, A WEIRD COMPANION

My favorite foods during my first trimester were eggs and sourdough bread. I wasn't thrilled at the sight of a salad, and some of my favorite foods, like curry and spicy food, sounded good in theory but failed in practice. I would prepare a meal that I had previously enjoyed featuring these strong flavors, and then I wouldn't be able to take a single bite. Not only that, I needed the smell of the food out of my house. When Max ate the very flavorful food I made, I begged him to brush his teeth. Then I suggested he might consider taking a shower and changing his clothes. The memory of his garlic and onion breath still haunts me.

Eggs maintained their neutrality as a simple, easy-to-prepare meal I could eat immediately in the morning. This last bit turned out to be the key. If I didn't eat eggs immediately upon waking—as in, I rolled out of bed, went pee, then lit up the stove to heat my cast iron—I felt sick and threw up. Until I actually ingested the eggs, I balked at the idea of eating in general. Nausea was a weird companion. It stuck with me until I forced myself to eat, and then it was gone.

Nausea and vomiting during the first trimester (and sometimes beyond) are experienced by most pregnant people, but the cause is not fully understood. There are a few theories to explain why we feel sick during this initial period of gestation. One theory is that nausea protects babies from foodborne toxins that we might ingest. Our nausea stops us from eating certain foods, especially bitter ones, that, if consumed in excess, can be toxic and cause birth defects. We can probably blame hormones to some degree. The hormonal shifts in the body, including heightened hCG and the ovarian hormones estrogen and progesterone, slow gastric emptying and cause a disruption in gastric wave rhythms that may contribute to nausea and vomiting.

The list of potential nausea-inducing culprits goes on and on. Studies have identified a thorough list of risk factors for nausea and vomiting during pregnancy. If you have a history of motion sickness, if your corpus luteum is located in the right ovary, or if you have any imbalance in any of your hormones, you are at a higher risk for nausea and vomiting. Your psychological, economic, cultural, and social status potentially impact your level of sickness.

There is evidence that diet, both before and during pregnancy, impacts how sick we feel. Eggs in the morning probably helped me thwart feeling sick because they are rich in protein, vitamins, and minerals. Rich, orange-hued, pastured yolks are full of choline, which is as crucial as folate for growing baby's brain and preventing neural tube defects. The balance of fat and protein in the perfectly composed whole egg helps balance blood sugar levels and keep our energy stable. Blood sugar spikes and crashes, and the insulin response can lend itself to heightened nausea and vomiting, so choosing foods that promote energy stability and balance cortisol and insulin improves our resilience.

If reading this section made you feel sick, or thinking about eggs actually causes you to vomit, first, I apologize. Eggs aren't a cure-all for nausea and vomiting because we are all different. I experimented with different foods until I found something that worked, and then I stuck to it. You might have to go through this same trial and error, and on some days, it feels like nothing works and you just feel sick and tired. Second, you might be worrying about feeding your growing baby while simultaneously struggling to eat. A diverse and healthy prenatal diet helps build up your reserves of micronutrients for

# Tactics for Nausea

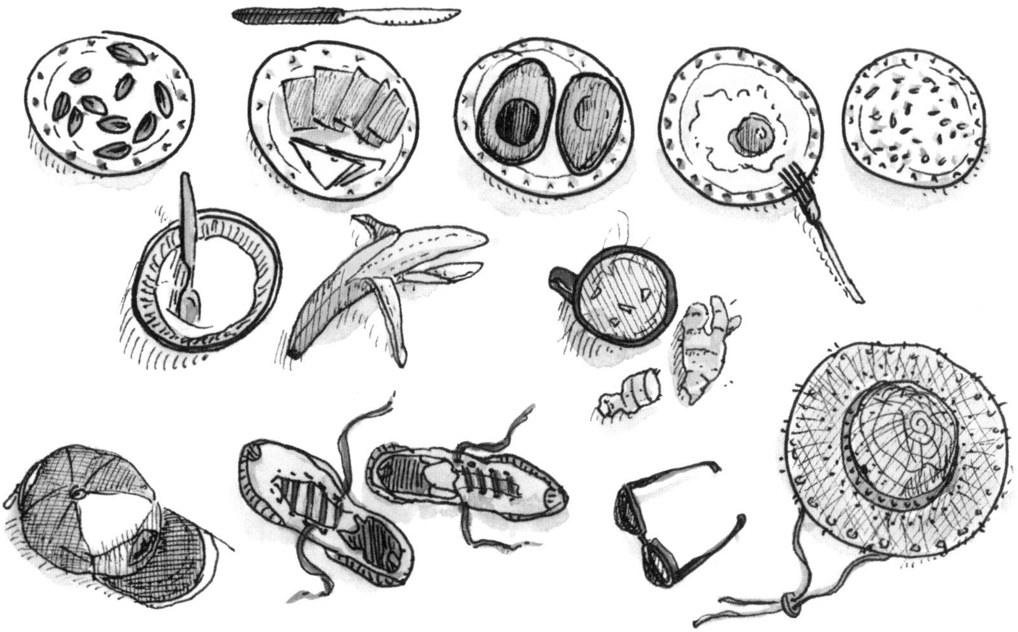

**1.** Eat small, frequent meals and drink liquids between meals. Focus on foods like fruits, sweet potatoes, nuts, cheese, avocado, yogurt, and scrambled eggs. Protein- and fat-containing foods help stabilize blood sugar, are easy to digest, and provide nutrition.

**2.** Consume $B_6$-containing foods, including avocado, banana, pistachios, sunflower seeds, meat, fish, and poultry.

**3.** Try drinking ginger tea and eating ginger candies, like ginger chews or crystallized ginger.

**4.** Smell good smells. Lavender and peppermint are especially soothing for nausea.

**5.** Try a magnesium supplement or Epsom salt baths.

**6.** Enjoy plenty of activity outside in fresh air.

the baby to pull from in your body. A quality prenatal vitamin and other supplements can pick up the slack in your diet and help manage queasiness. In general, but not as a rule, the waves of distressing nausea subside by the end of the first trimester and rarely persist past twenty weeks.

For one terrible, exhausting, queasy month during my first trimester, I worked nights. The nausea I experienced at night was ten times worse than during the day. One night, I was taking care of a sick patient who was vomiting profusely. The smells of the hospital were enough to make me feel sick and miserable, but this night forced me to really retreat into myself. While I was cleaning up this patient after another bout of vomiting, my friend and coworker, who was helping, looked at me with surprise and concern in her face. "Are you OK?" she asked. "You don't look OK." We finished and I went to the bathroom, where I noticed that my face was stark white and my eyes were sunken and dead-looking. I wasn't OK.

I knew I didn't want to work nights and that it was harming me physically and emotionally. Working nights impacts metabolic and hormonal activity, two crucial systems that mediate and maintain pregnancy. I spent time learning about the dysregulatory effects of night-shift working and how working nights carries an increased risk of miscarriage, low birth weight, preterm delivery, and reduced breastfeeding.

Presenting this information to my boss, I made a case against night-shift work for myself and gently begged her to allow me to work days while I grew my baby. She conceded, and I was grateful. I know many pregnant people who worked nights through their whole pregnancy. They were OK with night-shift working, but I wasn't. Information, empowerment, and self-advocacy are indispensable tools, especially while we grow new life. It is crucial for you to identify circumstances and situations that increase stress and discomfort and use information to advocate for yourself and your baby.

## READING YOUR LANDSCAPE

Plants that grow in pastures tell a story about the composition and health of the soil. In his book *The Third Plate*, chef Dan Barber writes how "the presence of chicory or wild carrot or the lovely Queen Anne's lace means the soil is low in fertility, a classic problem that arises when you harvest crops without returning nutrients to the soil. Milkweed is a sign that the soil lacks zinc, wild garlic means low sulfur."

While my belly never sprouted milkweed or wild garlic, stress sprouted and flourished when I needed to move more and spend time in the sunshine. Nausea erupted like an invasive weed when I required the steadying ingestion of protein or when I lacked adequate sleep. Regarding my body as its own ecological system allowed me to understand that the disparate parts are in fact a whole. Instead of thinking about how to subtract the signs of ill health, I wondered what I could add to my internal pasture that would improve deficiencies and balance the entire interactive system.

We are perhaps inexperienced at reading the story the plants tell us about a landscape, or the story our physical and emotional signs tell us about what our body and mind need. We need not be horticulturists or biologists to begin observing and learning about what nourishes, replenishes, and cultivates our inner landscape. The first step is understanding that we are composed of what we can and cannot see, and we live by the same principles and interconnectedness as the animals and plants around us.

The first trimester is a critical period of growth and development. The zygote becomes a blastocyst, which becomes an embryo, which becomes a fetus. Eyes, ears, nose, spine, and digestive tract spiral and twist into existence. All the organs, with their unique anatomy and function, form and develop. The heart starts beating a quick fluttering *thumpthumpthump*, distributing blood through tiny vessels and carrying nutrients and oxygen to, and waste from, the rapidly growing baby. Bones begin to form, and immature kidneys start secreting urine into the bladder.

Your baby starts to move as the amniotic cavity fills with amniotic fluid. This fluid, composed of the water we drink, becomes blood plasma that permeates the amniotic sac and bathes the baby who drinks the fluid. Of the water that eventually composes amniotic fluid, ecologist and author Sandra Steingraber writes,

> Before it is drinking water, amniotic fluid is the creeks and rivers that fill reservoirs. It is the underground water that fills wells. And before it is the creeks and rivers and groundwater, amniotic fluid is rain. . . . Amniotic fluid is also the juice of oranges that I had for breakfast, and the milk that I poured over my cereal, and the honey I stirred into my tea. It is inside the green cells of spinach leaves and the damp flesh of apples. It is the yolk of an egg.

The placenta, the umbilical cord, our enlarging mammary glands, and our expanding uterus are also made from the water around us and the food it grows. In this way, we are also made of sunshine.

Like trees with their fungal networks connecting their roots, we, too, are a network of connections. When we think like this, it becomes easier to read the signs our bodies are giving us and make choices that support our overall health. We have a voice box to grow, tiny delicate eyelids to form, and fingernails and toenails to compose. These structures are built by the foods we ingest, which were once living plants and animals. These plants and animals spent time drinking water and growing in fields and pastures. Were the fields fertile or did they sprout chicory and Queen Anne's lace? Was the rootstock able to dive deep, accumulate fertile micronutrients, and grow a healthy plant?

We are inextricably intertwined with the life around and within us. The bacteria, soil, plants, animals, and water—essential sources of sustenance and survival—become us and become our babies.

# TAKE ACTION

Imagine your origin story, the story of your conception, as a dialogue between sperm and egg that is interactive. This story of mutuality disrupts sexist notions of conception and values the essential roles of both the sperm and the egg in the process of making a person.

Embrace the physiological shifts and power of growing a person in your body. The first trimester is a time of great transition. You might feel tired and nauseous, anxious about the future, or creative and connected to your body and the world in a new way. Learn about your body and how you want to navigate your pregnancy so you can feel confident through the changes and in the conversations you have with your care provider.

Support your developing embryo and placenta with high-quality foods. What we eat directly impacts the composition, function, and efficiency of the placenta, and the nutrients from these foods pass through the placenta to grow our babies. Pastured eggs and organ meats, bone broth, slow-cooked meat, leafy greens and vegetables, fermented foods, cultured, full-fat dairy, and wild fish and seafood are traditional baby-building foods that also help balance our blood sugar and keep our energy levels stable, which can help reduce nausea and vomiting.

Listen to the signs your body gives you about what it needs. You might need more movement, more sleep and rest, or more water or protein, or maybe you need a massage, a bath, time with your partner, or meditation. Take care of your body with food and movement and understand that we are interconnected with our environment. Our choices truly matter.

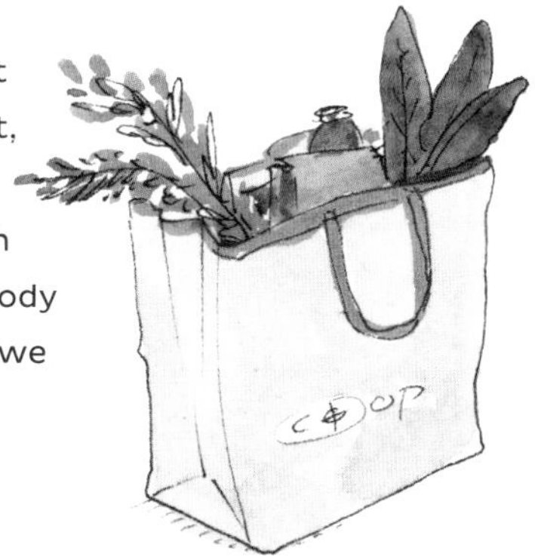

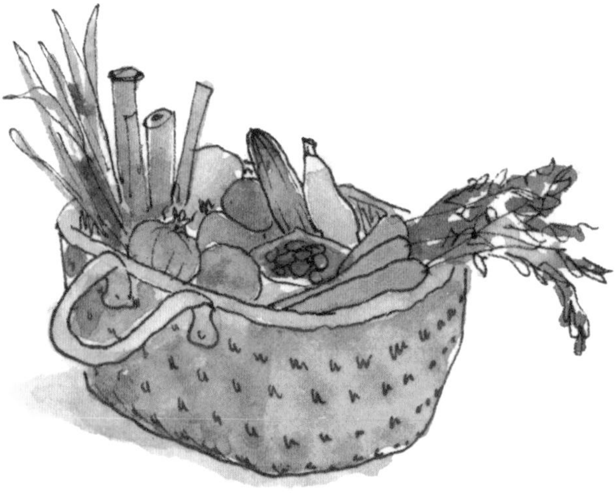

CHAPTER SIX

# Endocrine Changes & Avoiding Toxins

WHEN YOUR FUTURE BABY IS A BLASTOCYST, it contains precursor cells that allow it to become an embryo. The embryo, with its limb buds, eyes, head, trunk, and beating heart, morphs into a form we recognize as rudimentarily human over eight weeks. Precursor cells extend the limbs into their fully functioning form on the fetus—limbs that can kick you and fingers and toes that extend and grab and explore. The form becomes a person. This person might have your nose, your partner's eyes, your dad's ears. These precursor cells that take the baby on a morphological journey from one form to the next are susceptible to disruption by chemicals or agents, known as teratogens, that impact the formation and development of the baby.

The ability of the precursor cells to survive, differentiate, function, migrate, and proliferate is impacted by what we come into contact with in the world.

The timing of exposure to teratogens can have drastically different consequences. Early on, during fertilization and just after, the consequence might be miscarriage. Later, during organogenesis, when major body organs are differentiating and forming, disruption in development from exposure may cause a structural abnormality or birth defect like neural tube or heart defects or cleft lip or palate. Even later, during fetal development, the disruption might cause hearing loss, cognitive impairments, or lung immaturity.

Fortunately, we know the major teratogens to avoid: drugs like cocaine, alcohol, narcotics, and smoking. Each of these has different effects in the body and particularly on the function and anatomy of the placenta. Cocaine and narcotics cause problems with the uptake of protein, alcohol impedes nutrient transport, and smoking comes with a whole host of chemicals that decrease placental use of glucose and decrease protein uptake. Add artificial fragrances and oxybenzone, which is found in many sunscreens, to the list of chemicals to avoid, and minimize exposure to the conventionally grown and processed food that is wrapped in plastic and sprayed with pesticides, and you'll be off to a good start.

Because we don't know everything and growing life is inherently complex, it helps to return to the foundations of ecology and the principles that shape our home here in the world. All living things in the environment are in contact and conversation with each other, and the interrelationships thrive on diversity. Nothing is separate. This applies to the food we eat and the way we move, the products we put on our food and in our water, and the chemicals we use in our homes and put on our bodies.

Learning about the threats we face while we grow our babies is overwhelming and scary. When I turn toward fear, I'm reminded of a quote by writer and poet Gary Snyder:

> I have a friend who feels sometimes that the world is hostile to human life—he says it chills us and it kills us. But how could we be were it not for this planet that provided our very shape? Two conditions—gravity and a livable temperature range between freezing and boiling—have given us fluids and flesh. The trees we climb and the ground we walk on have given

> us five fingers and toes. The "place" (from the root *plat*, broad, spreading, flat) gave us far-seeing eyes, the streams and breezes gave us versatile tongues and whorly ears. The land gave us a stride, and the lake a dive. The amazement gave us our kind of mind. We should be thankful for that, and take nature's stricter lessons with some grace.

I feel at times like the friend Snyder described when I worry about the world, but thankful and in awe when I experience it. There is a balance, always, between how much we can take in and worry and the necessity of climbing trees, hiking trails, cooking over a hot fire, and swimming in cool water. The balance of these two parts of life—anxiety and joy—allows us to make conscious decisions about how to live, what to eat, and how to move, and then to enjoy the experience of those decisions.

## TWO WORLDS

Many pregnancy resources briefly mention, or gloss over, the real and serious risks we face from the chemicals surrounding us. Of one pregnancy book that quotes Voltaire's statement "In ignorance, abstain," Sandra Steingraber writes, "The same book that quotes Voltaire on alcohol, recreational drugs, and tobacco contains not a single mention of toxic chemicals in food, air, or water. And the rare book or magazine article that does choose to mention them surrounds the topic with tranquilizing reassurances and downplaying qualifiers."

This is generally the point where I might offer "tranquilizing reassurances and downplaying qualifiers." Instead, I can't help but think of the parallel worlds we occupy fully while growing a baby. In one world, there is pure terror. Of the unknown future, of birth defects, of environmental toxins and chemicals that disrupt our endocrine and reproductive systems. In the other, there's fascination and wonder. Of the anatomical and physiological changes in our bodies that support life, picturing tiny toenails forming on toes, and pondering what it will feel like to meet the person we grew in our body. Who will they be?

# *Healthy Alternatives*

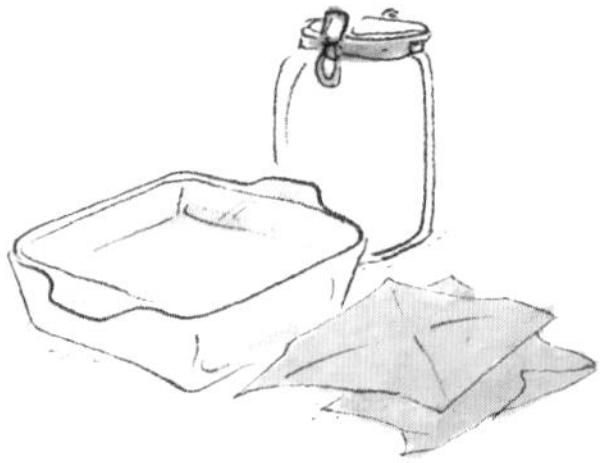

Store food in glass, stainless steel, or lead-free ceramic, and use beeswax wrap or parchment paper.

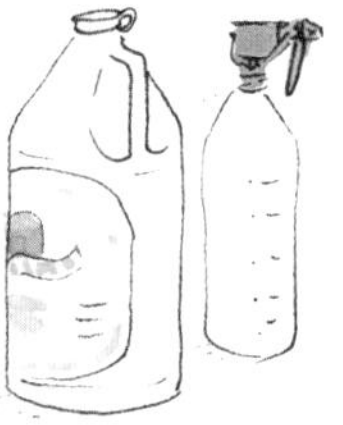

Use white vinegar diluted with water for cleaning.

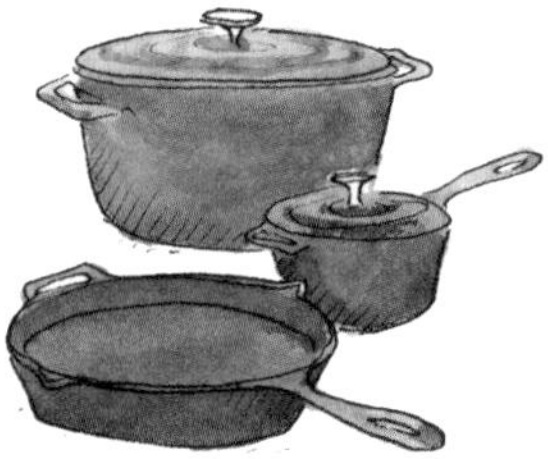

Cook with cast iron, stainless steel, or safe ceramic cookware.

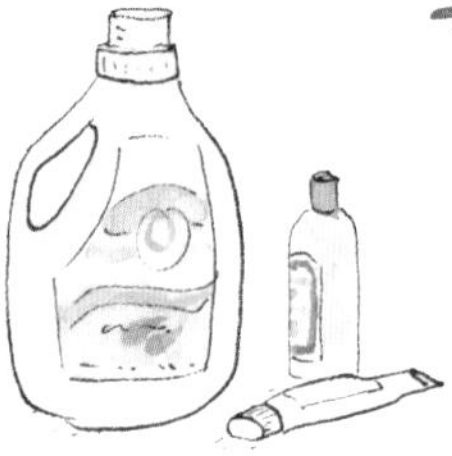

Use unscented, fragrance-free products.

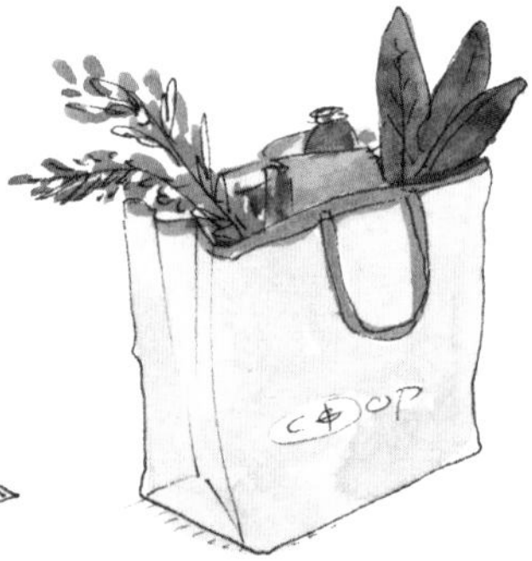

Buy food grown without the use of pesticides and that is organic and local when possible.

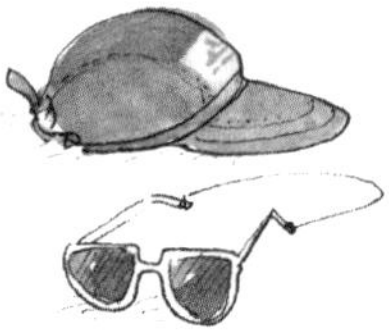

Wear protective clothes in the sun and use nontoxic sunscreen.

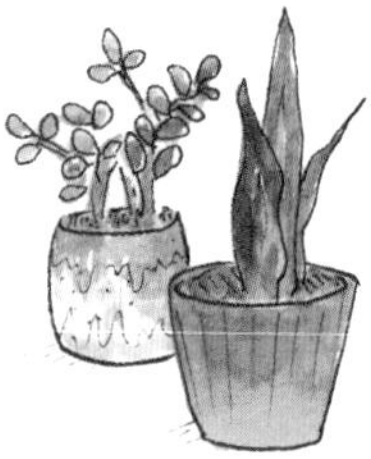

Open the windows and grow houseplants.

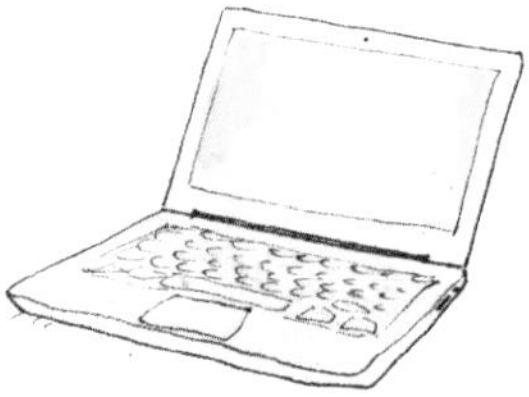

Research personal care and cleaning products (see EWG's Skin Deep cosmetics database).

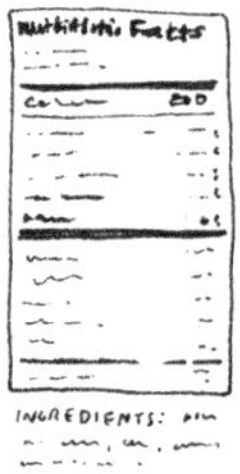


Simplify and read ingredient lists

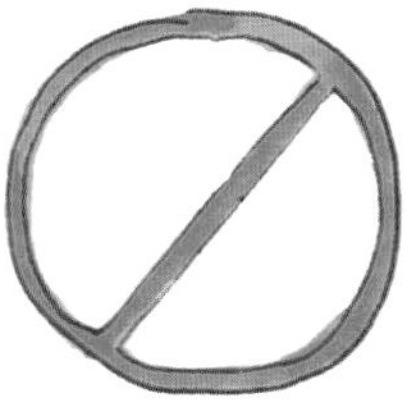

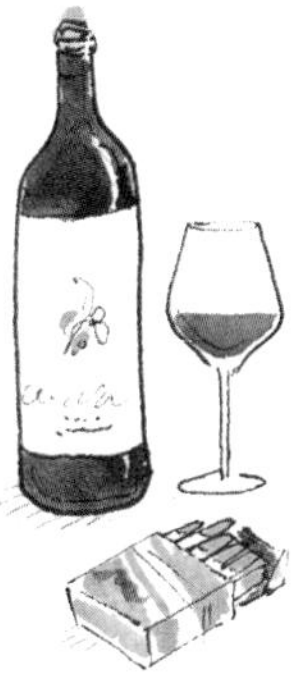

Avoid alcohol, tobacco, and other drugs. Avoid taking unnecessary medication.

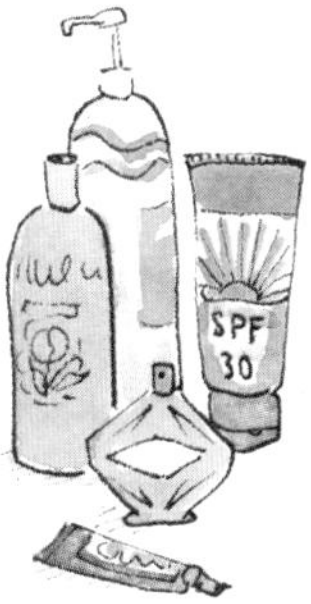


Avoid artificial fragrances, phthalates, and parabens. Avoid sunscreens with oxybenzone and added fragrance.

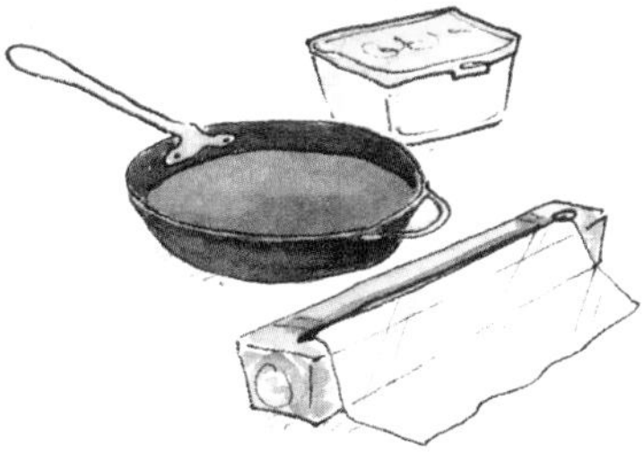

Avoid nonstick pans, reheating food in plastic containers, aluminum foil, and plastic wrap.

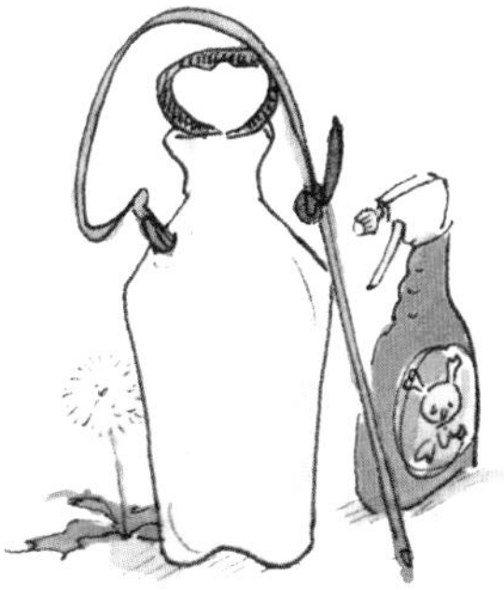

Avoid antibacterial products, pesticides, insecticides, and chemical bug sprays.

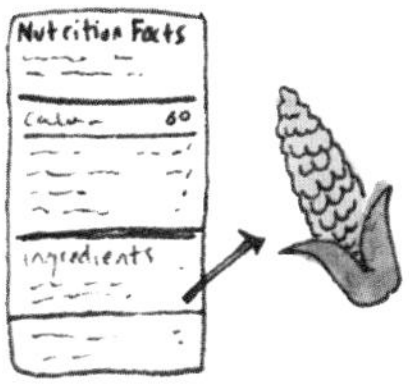


Avoid trans fats and vegetable oils like corn, soy, and canola.

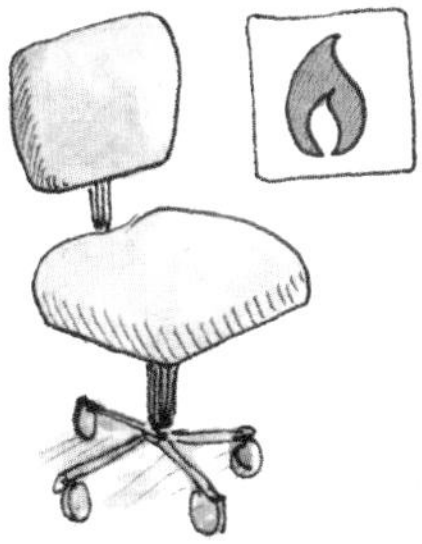

Avoid flame retardants—look for labels on furniture, foam products, and electronics. Call the manufacturer when in doubt.

In our bellies, at the boundary where our body interfaces with the baby, endocrine and metabolic changes shape the physical alterations we experience during pregnancy. Hormones and proteins originate here that affect every organ system in our bodies.

Starting with our cardiovascular system, the dynamic shift in our life-promoting hormone levels increases cardiac output by 20 percent by eight weeks' gestation. Cardiac output is the amount of blood pumped by the heart each minute, or the amount of work the heart must perform to meet the body's need for oxygen. Every tissue in the body requires blood flow for sustenance and nourishment, and these needs increase when you grow new life.

By twenty to twenty-eight weeks, cardiac output is up 40 percent and heart rate increases by ten to twenty beats per minute. This need for the heart to deliver more blood faster to the tissues in the body explains why it's important to rest and sleep on our sides as our bellies grow. Moving from a side-lying position to your back can drop cardiac output by 25 percent, restricting circulation and placental blood flow.

Blood and plasma volume increase. The rivers that run through our bodies change shape in a way that changes the ratio of red blood cells to plasma. Plasma is the yellow, liquid component of our blood that carries proteins and cells. The increased quantity of this golden fluid dilutes our blood so that we enter a transitory state of anemia. Making more blood means our iron and $B_{12}$ requirements go up two- to threefold and our folate needs increase ten- to twentyfold. These nutrients build our red blood cells, play a part in the production of certain enzymes, and are required by the growing baby. The components of our blood that promote coagulation increase by 50 percent so that we're in a pro-clotting state.

In case you thought your cardiac output couldn't go up any more, the first stage of labor increases it by another 15 percent and then another 50 percent in the second stage. Contractions elevate blood pressure, heart rate, and cardiac output, literally pushing more blood through our body, urging us to go on. At its peak, right after delivery, cardiac output jumps up 60 to 80 percent above normal and then rapidly declines about two weeks after delivery to the cardiac output you had before your body housed another person.

Our kidneys experience this increased blood flow, so much so that they increase in length by 1.5 centimeters by midpregnancy. The amount of blood that passes through the kidneys each minute increases 50 percent, and we may retain up to 1.6 liters of water. The kidneys, once quietly filtering our blood like a gentle background hum, become an orchestra, working hard to respond to the changes, adjusting with signals from hormones, balancing our electrolytes and fluids, all so that we can maintain pregnancy and keep growing the baby in the best environment.

As the heart beats faster and circulating blood volume increases, our oxygen demand and metabolic rate also rise. We tend to hyperventilate slightly and may feel breathless while we're resting or talking, but less so when we're moving. Each endocrine gland experiences dynamic changes. The thyroid requires more iodine, as this essential element is transported to the growing baby, and the adrenals produce cortisol levels that are three times higher at the end of pregnancy. The pituitary gland enlarges, prolactin-producing cells proliferate, and oxytocin levels steadily climb, peaking at term.

Alterations in glucose metabolism promote shunting of glucose to the baby. Early on, insulin levels increase, as does insulin sensitivity. Later we develop progressive insulin resistance that peaks in the third trimester. Increased use of glucose by the baby means that in a healthy pregnancy, fasting blood glucose levels drop, but after eating, glucose levels may be higher because of our decreased insulin sensitivity. Cells that secrete insulin in our pancreas adapt to these changes to maintain normal blood glucose; however, the overall picture of our blood sugar, and whether or not we develop gestational diabetes, is more complicated. Pancreatic and endocrine function, genetics and family history of diabetes, diet and body weight, age, and race all impact how our body adjusts and adapts to its altered metabolic landscape.

Our transformed metabolism impacts blood sugar and insulin levels and influences the way we metabolize other key nutrients like fats, protein, and calcium. LDL, the cholesterol that's been called "bad" by nutrition and medicine for decades, increases during pregnancy because the placenta uses LDL cholesterol to form biologically active steroid hormones that maintain pregnancy. We need more protein in our diet, much more, because of the transport of amino acids across the placenta to support the growth and development of the baby. Our bodies adapt to the fetus's need for calcium by increasing intestinal absorption of the mineral.

There is constant movement, adaptation, and compensation, almost like we're doubly alive. Some of the changes are more tangible because we can see, hear, and feel them.

When I was pregnant, I could hear my heart pounding all the time. It was like a drum in my ears and it throbbed in my wrists. I could close my eyes and feel blood flow through the vasculature in my eyes and feel the pulse in my neck. When my hips hurt at night and woke me up from a deep sleep, I could feel my whole body move rhythmically to my internal, nonstop *lub dub lub dub lub dub*. The feeling of blood pumping was a constant reminder of the work my body was doing. Every day, constantly, blood was formed by my body and distributed to all my tissues and pumped back and forth across the placenta.

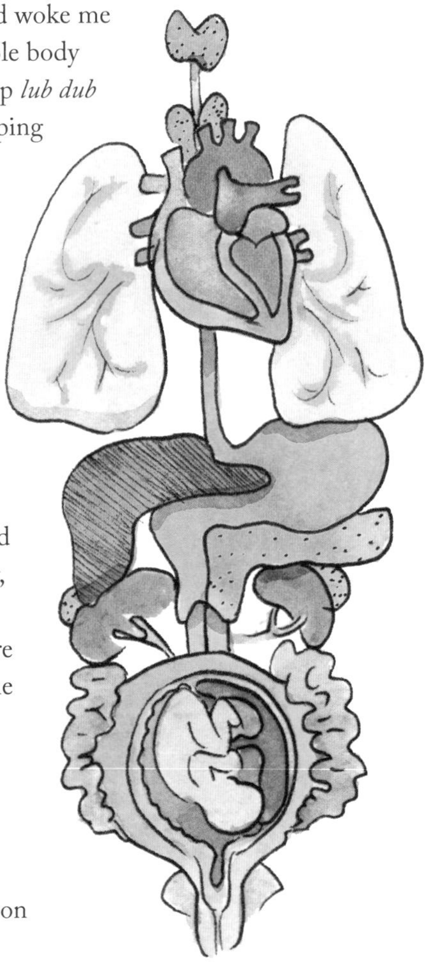

When the baby is in our womb, we can't hold them any closer, or protect them with our bodies any more thoroughly, but they still have a relationship with the world around us. They are impacted by the pesticides, pollutants, and industrial chemicals that we spray, scatter, and spread across the landscapes of our homes, farms, and waterways. But they are also impacted by our hikes in the sunshine and our delight at swimming in rivers, lakes, and oceans. They get the nutrition they need when we make a meal loaded with vegetables from the farmers' market and pastured meats from local ranchers. They are benefited by our barefoot walks on the beach and our hands digging in soil.

# The Changing Body

**FIRST TRIMESTER**

- By 8 weeks, cardiac output increases by 20%.
- Blood pressure decreases.
- Blood flow to the kidneys increases, as does kidney size.
- The hormone relaxin peaks at the end of the first trimester. It "relaxes" blood vessels, which increases blood flow to the placenta and kidneys. Relaxin also helps prevent preterm delivery by inhibiting uterine contractions.
- Breast sensitivity and volume increases.
- Insulin sensitivity increases.

**SECOND TRIMESTER**

- Cardiac output continues to increase.
- Insulin resistance increases.
- The first fetal movements are felt.

**THIRD TRIMESTER**

- Plasma volume increases 50% by 34 weeks.
- Blood pressure increases to pre-pregnant levels.
- Maternal blood volume increases.
- You may feel breathless at rest but able to breathe better while moving.
- Relaxin plays a role in facilitating birth by relaxing the pelvic ligaments, increasing the elasticity of the symphysis pubis joint, and dilating the cervix during labor.

**THROUGHOUT PREGNANCY**

- Iron needs double or triple.
- Folate needs increase ten- to twentyfold.
- $B_{12}$ needs double.
- Iodine needs increase.
- Metabolic rate and use of oxygen increase.
- The pituitary gland enlarges.
- Total cholesterol and triglycerides increase to meet the needs of the growing fetus and hormone production.
- Fasting blood glucose levels are lower during pregnancy, with an average of 71 ± 8 mg/dL, while postprandial glucose levels are slightly higher.
- Leukorrhea (thin, milky white vaginal discharge) increases.

This is what Gary Snyder means by taking nature's stricter lessons with grace. There are dangers and delights that surround us. We create the fluids and flesh, the five fingers and toes and whorly ears in our babies in the planet that is our body. Then the world we live in takes over. It's up to us to choose how we live in it and how it shapes us.

## THE SCALE

When I think about the scale of the problem with environmental toxins and chemicals versus the simple, actionable steps we often implement into our daily lives, I'm reminded of another Sandra Steingraber essay. She wrote a masterful book called *Living Downstream* that links chemical exposure to cancer. For four years she conducted research for the book, spending time in cancer labs and studying tumor growth in animals. In her essay "Household Tips from Warrior Mom!" she tells a story about her author press tour after her book came out.

She went on a talk show and the host asked her to come up with a list of cancer prevention tips. Tip one: "Identify corporate polluters in your community." Tip two: "Confront them." The host of the show balked and had her change her tips into things like "Avoid dry-cleaning solvents." Her message started big, with a call to arms, an upheaval, a revolution, and it was watered down into a laundry recommendation.

She discussed how, in her experience, when people feel that they can avoid environmental harm, they feel less urgency about pushing for environmental reform or confronting the polluters in our communities. There is a perceived safety when we have the advantage of choice. We are soothed into believing we live upstream, able to avoid the dangers that threaten our health, even though we are all truly living downstream.

I relate to needing tangible action steps and recommendations about the best products to use for practical everyday cleaning, laundry, and living. I sometimes feel overwhelmed by information that turns into inaction, a phenomenon known as "well-informed futility." I feel the same discomfort with the tragedy of the pollution in our water and the pesticides used in food production as I feel in the company of people who are grieving. I want to run away from the feeling. I want to work in my garden and turn the volume down to the world's problems. I do this and I think, I'm failing. My impulse for flight, for choosing to walk alone in the quiet hills instead of fighting a loud fight in my community, is the form of my futility.

But these walks of retreat lead directly to a refreshed sense of purpose and a desire to continue to live in a way that promotes the health of my home. These walks and the time I spend in my place connect me to the spirit of my place. Gary Snyder said, "To know the spirit of a place is to realize that you are a part of a part and that the whole is made of parts, each of which is whole. You start with the part you are whole in." We can start only with parts, and then slowly recognize that each part makes up the whole, meaning each part is essential.

Steingraber writes inspiring call-to-action books, and reporters continue to ask her about her lightbulb recommendations. They want diet tips and ideas for bathroom cleaners. She writes about how fracking for natural gas releases reproductive toxins, and her words that should spark outrage and revolution get reduced and repackaged into something that can hopefully be bought and sold.

There is a balance between outrage and the practical needs of the day. Often, practicality outweighs revolution. In learning about the dangers of our industrialized world, the threatening chemicals and injustice, we must still eat, move, drink water, go to the bathroom, and get caught off guard by the hoot of an owl at night. When I was pregnant I felt both outraged about and detached from the reality that the world we live in is dangerous for our health. How do we balance big-picture grief and outrage with moment-to-moment living?

In his book *Consolations*, David Whyte describes anger as "the deepest form of compassion." He says the feeling we call anger is

> actually only the incoherent physical incapacity to sustain this deep form of care in our outer daily life; the unwillingness to be large enough and generous enough to hold what we love helplessly in our bodies or our mind with the clarity and breadth of our whole being.

I am angry that our food and water and air are subject to our damaging indifference. I'm angry, and anger is useful and powerful. It's a feeling worth feeling. But we can't feel it all the time because we don't always have the energy to sustain this purposeful, warranted outrage.

I close this chapter on endocrine changes and environmental toxins this way because I want to acknowledge two truths.

1. You are growing new life and it's incredible, meaningful, transformative, and powerful.

2. You are growing new life and it is threatened by the products your neighbors spray on their bodies and lawns, the diesel fumes on the highway, and the poisons we put on and in our food and water.

These two truths held together in your body are both remarkable and enraging, and we have to figure out how to live with them without slipping into apathy or despair.

During pregnancy we are at once more powerful and protective, yet more vulnerable, than at any other time in our life. I hope while you make choices to minimize your exposure to dangerous chemicals and toxins that you can feel the intentions of Steingraber. She urges us not only to improve our diet with local and organic food but also to reconsider and reform the entire food system. To not just choose sunscreen and other products without artificial fragrance and oxybenzone but to also confront the chemical companies that still put these dangerous chemicals into our products and the environment.

As we make the moment-to-moment choices, we can hold our anger and use it to guide future confrontations against polluters. We can understand that anger is the deepest form of care and still take deep steadying breaths and continue to grow our babies.

# TAKE ACTION

Assess and reassess your environment for dangerous chemicals that hide in common everyday products like sunscreens and cleaning and personal care products. The first step we can take to reduce our exposure to environmental toxins and endocrine disruptors is to look at our living space and identify what products cause harm. Dispose of the bad stuff responsibly. EWG's Skin Deep cosmetic database is a good place to research the safety of specific products.

Remember that we have an interactive relationship with everything in our environment. Avoid drugs, alcohol, tobacco, artificial fragrances, perfumes, phthalates, and parabens. Replace nonstick pans with satisfyingly heavy cast-iron skillets. Store food in glass or stainless steel containers and, when possible, choose sustainably grown and raised food.

Maintain your wonder and appreciation for the world. There are scary threats to our health and irresponsible industrial practices we need to be aware of and fight against if we can. But don't let your fear or your righteous anger prevent you from seeing and enjoying the world's beauty.

Acknowledge the two truths: you are growing new life and you are tremendously powerful, and you are growing new life and you are tremendously vulnerable. You cannot control every part of your ecosystem, but you can make choices about the products you use and the food you eat that protect you and your growing baby.

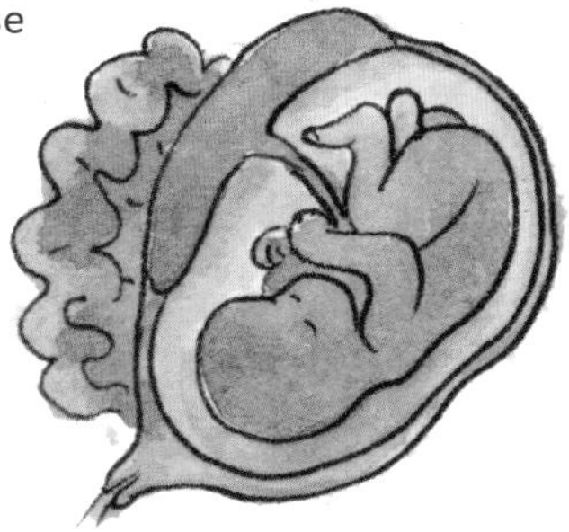

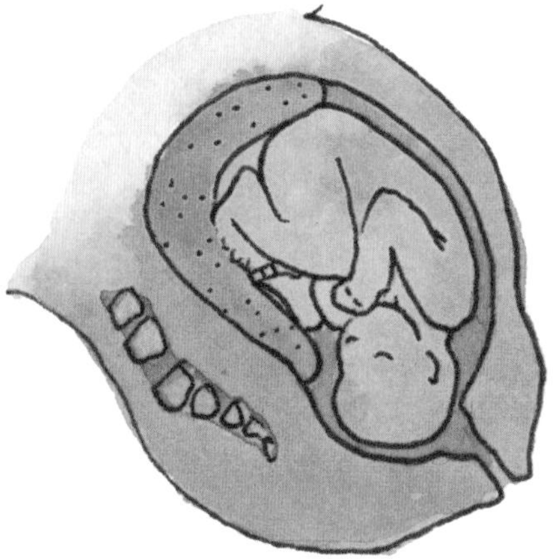

CHAPTER SEVEN

# The Second & Third Trimesters

I GLANCED AT THE CLOCK. It was 6:40. Five minutes, just five more minutes, and the night-shift nurse would be here, I'd give him my report, and then I'd be able to go home, take a bath, and go to sleep. 6:45 arrived, and then it was gone with no sign of my replacement. At what we call 1900 in the hospital, I got a call that a patient was transferring to one of my open rooms. This is basically the equivalent of stripping off your clothes to start a bath, then someone calling you and saying you actually need to go to the dentist for a root canal. It's not the call you want at 1900. Nineteen hundred is when the day should gently and gracefully transition into evening.

I looked around at my coworkers, happily handing off the patients they took care of for the last twelve hours, loading up their bags and water bottles, and cruising down the hall away from this place. I yearned to follow them.

Instead, I prepped my room for the incoming patient, looking hopefully around every few minutes, and then I went pee, probably for the fifteenth time that day. When the patient arrived, he was brought in by a flurry of nurses, doctors, respiratory therapists, and pharmacists. This patient was very old, over ninety, and he looked small. His body appeared hollow and pale, and I sighed with sadness.

The day and night crews were all there because the day was crashing into night and we were all trying to transition, some of us eager to get home, others to begin their day. So many people meant the patient was in critical condition, and the small room was packed with more than twenty health-care professionals. When we hooked the patient up to the monitors, his blood pressure was too low to read. Within five minutes he lost his pulse, a code blue was called, and he was intubated.

I helped record the code, writing down times and medications, and felt a strong kick in my side. I looked around, wondering who had hit me, briefly forgetting about the person who always kicked me in times like these. Another strong kick shifted my scrubs slightly. I instinctively put my hand on my belly, feeling for his kicks, my mind escaping the current situation for a moment, delighting in feeling his little reminder. I'm in here and I'm good, he seemed to tell me.

I wrote down more times and medications, and he kicked again. He kicked with a cadence, and then there was a new feeling: his hiccups. Hiccup. Kick. Hiccup. Kick. I recorded his movements in my mind. *Kick, kick, hiccup*, I wrote in my mind. *Epinephrine*, I wrote down with my pen. His movements centered and calmed me like they always did. I could feel the importance of staying in the moment. That was the reminder he gave me every day, whether or not I was in the middle of a crisis at work, walking, or resting. *Relax, I'm in here*. Kick. Kick. Hiccup.

Babies start moving long before we can feel them. Throughout pregnancy, your baby will move their head, hands, tongue, arms, legs, and jaw, bend sideways, suck and swallow, yawn, stretch, touch their face, and grimace.

We feel remarkably little for how much the baby moves, usually feeling the first little motion around sixteen to twenty-four weeks. Many movements are fluid, performed like a training program with different speeds and bursts. Not all movements are planned. While the womb is safe and protected, babies still get startled. They hiccup and twitch and flex. Hiccups shake their head and trunk, sending a wave through your internal ocean. I imagine hiccups rippling across amniotic fluid, a little jolt in the salty sea.

At around twenty weeks, I felt whispers of motion. The first flutters felt like they were crafted in my mind, fed by my desire to feel my baby move, and I wondered if they were real. Then they became strong and definite, like an announcement: *I'm here!* I felt my son hiccup most often at work and move his body in the afternoon and as I lay down to sleep. Sometimes, when he wasn't moving around, I'd press gently on my stomach. Then I'd give him a little poke, and finally, after a few prods, he'd give me what I imagined to be a tiny fist bump. I wondered if I was bugging him too much and imagined him saying, *I'm trying to sleep*, as he rolled away from my hands. Maybe he didn't mind and got used to my hands communicating with him over the landscape of my belly.

We're encouraged to pay attention to fetal movements because they are linked to fetal health. Too little movement might mean the baby is in danger. Noticing movements is a matter of your perception, and perception can change from one pregnancy to the next and is not the same for everyone. While variability exists, pregnant people do tend to feel stronger, more vigorous movements as the baby gets bigger, and these movements are most often felt at night, since babies follow a diurnal rhythm. Babies tend to have longer periods of quiescence, or movement-free times, as pregnancy progresses, and these quiet moments tend to happen in the morning. If these quiet periods increase at night, we have more reason to worry and need to let our care providers know. More often than not, dynamic and exuberant movements pick up right as you lie down and close your eyes, as if the baby is saying, *Wake up, I'm ready to play now!*

Moving around in the womb helps support the development of a functional skeleton and supports joint and cartilage formation and bone development. Our skeletons are constructed to protect and support us, and they form and adapt in response to physical stimuli—that is, movement. The formation of the baby's skeleton, in all its functional glory, requires a full range of movements by the baby in the womb. Baby kicks generate forces that stimulate the skeleton. Through stress and strain, skeletal tissues are urged to respond and develop. Babies who don't move, or who move abnormally, can develop neuromuscular disorders such as hypomineralized bones and malformations of the skeleton. This is because the skeleton, and each cell in the body, is formed by an architect of loads, adaptations, stresses, and strains.

From twenty to thirty weeks, fetal leg bones morph and change geometry in response to the stimulation from stress and kicking the uterine wall. At twenty weeks, the baby's legs can kick you at a force of about six pounds. At thirty weeks, they can kick you with ten pounds of force. As the baby grows, the baby gets stronger, but the living quarters get more cramped. The arrangement of the baby in relationship to the space in the womb alters such that the force of those kicks decreases, but the baby continues gaining strength.

## ANIMAL COUNTERPART

Throughout my pregnancy, I wanted to know if there was anything I could do to increase my chances of having an unmedicated vaginal birth. I recognize now that I felt apprehensive and fearful about birth. I didn't fear pain as much as I feared an epidural and the loss of control. Our fears, and how we navigate them, build our path and shape the choices we make.

My fear set me on a path to figure out how my body alignment, posture, and movements impacted my baby's position. I knew there was a chance, always a chance, that I could do everything "right" and still struggle with my labor, or my baby could be in a physiological state or position that required a C-section. We all live with the very real possibility that things might not turn out how we want, no matter what we do. But if there was a chance that my choices about how to move could make a difference, I wanted to take that chance.

# Movement and Development

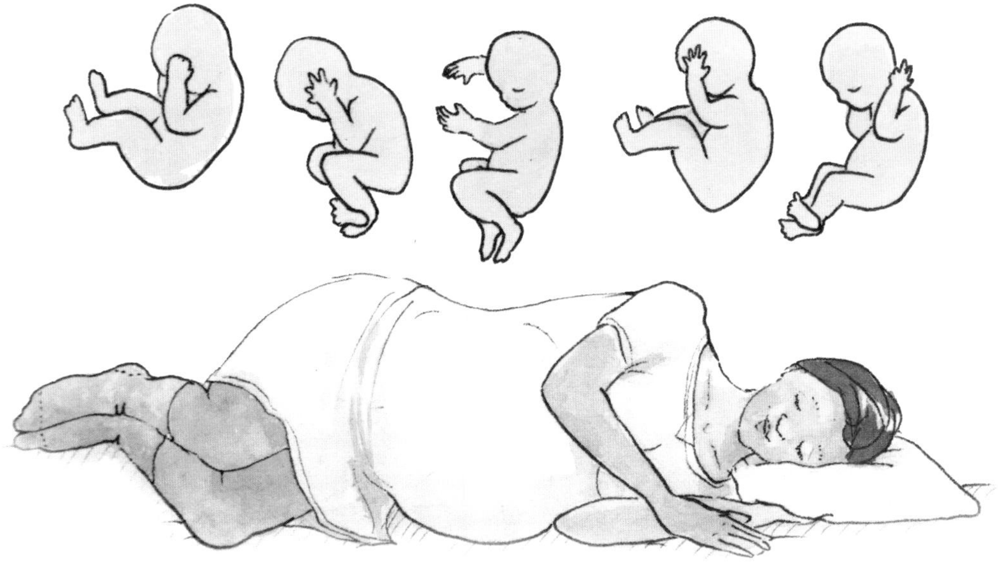

- Fetal movement begins as rhythmic bursts as motor neurons in the brain differentiate and innervate the skeletal muscles. These bursts of movement increase the amount of calcium in the neurons and influence gene expression.
- Movement allows the fetus to feel the space surrounding it and to feel its body in that space. This process is known as "body mapping," wherein the fetus experiences sensory stimulation and develops motor control.
- As the fetus develops, it responds to the external environment (touch, voice, light, sound) and moves its body toward the stimulus.
- A fetus is like an astronaut exploring its body in space: it can't understand how to move and the consequences of movement without first exploring through movement.
- Both in the womb and out, babies move their bodies to understand themselves and the world through action. This impacts brain and musculoskeletal development and allows them to try out new behaviors like curiosity, which ultimately serves to prepare them for life in the real world.

This quest to understand how my body shape, strength, alignment, and motion impact my baby's position, which impacts birth, led me again to Katy Bowman. Her words reframed my understanding of what it means to birth babies in the context of our modern world. Bowman says "we need to train for delivery" because, even if we believe birthing is a natural event, the way we live isn't exactly natural and is "completely foreign to our animal counterpart." When I first read this, I had a vision of my animal counterpart. She was undoubtedly outside, moving around all day gathering food, resting here and there in shady spots under trees, and dipping into the river to cool off. She was strong and resilient. Her connection to her landscape was not some ideological aspiration; it was physical and essential to survival.

As I thought more about my animal counterpart, I noticed the distance between us was greater than I imagined. She did not work on a computer, sleep on a mattress in a house, or spend too much money on clothes and shoes. She rarely even wore shoes. I had to reckon with the reality that, even after training my whole life as an athlete and moving a lot, I had a long way to go.

I could not be my exact animal counterpart, but I could start somewhere. That starting point came in the form of walking long distances and pulling up all the carpet in my home. My partner ripped the carpet out, and I pulled up the carpet staples. My animal counterpart had never even seen carpet, but here I was, working on my hands and knees, squatting, pulling, lifting, crawling, and moving all over in my environment.

I ripped up thousands of staples out of the plywood subfloor. After I pulled all the staples out, one by one, with pliers, I learned that a tool called a sharp-bladed floor scraper exists that does the job much faster. But if I had used the sharp-bladed floor scraper, I would have missed out on thousands of movements. This choice between pliers and the sharp-bladed floor scraper became the metaphor I thought of each day when I chose between convenience and more movement. Choosing more movement isn't always possible because our circumstances and time sometimes steer us toward convenience, but the benefit of hand-pulling carpet staples with pliers came in the form of many squats, which contribute to strong glutes and thighs, which help strengthen and balance the pelvic floor and contribute to a movable sacrum and muscular body that hopefully, possibly, contributes to an unmedicated, vaginal birth.

## ALIGNING OUR EQUIPMENT

While vaginal delivery is "natural," Katy Bowman says we "no longer have naturally aligned equipment." Our equipment is impacted by our sitting, movement habits, stress, the way we breathe, how much we squat and walk, how we hold our bodies, and the shoes and clothes we wear. The differences between me and my animal counterpart represent the monumental shift in the way humans live, move, and birth. The decrease in biological movements like walking long distances in minimal shoes and squatting to go to the bathroom compromises the health of our bodies and, Bowman writes, puts the process of vaginal delivery at risk.

Biological movements impact the physics of birthing. The mobility and position of the sacrum in relation to the pelvis and tension in the pelvic floor are shaped by the habits of our daily motion. The uterus also plays a crucial role in maintaining the function and structure of the pelvic floor, and these parts have to work together in a specific and coordinated way during the birth of a baby. For the uterus to generate its full mechanical force, a force necessary during birth, it needs to work with other body parts that are aligned, strong, and preferably not holding chronic tension. When the uterus is working with chronically tight and misaligned hips, psoas muscles, quads, inner thighs, hamstrings, piriformis, and pelvic floor muscles, the forces it generates are hindered by the restrictions imposed on it by these structures.

We're told to exercise consistently throughout pregnancy, but our movements are generally not tailored to the process and action of birth. Some exercises don't prepare us adequately for birth, while others can create more tension in the body and exacerbate imbalances. The overall effect of our decreased movement and the way we think about moving is a body that is shaped by a different external environment than our ancestors and thus experiences birth differently.

While I stress over geometry and the mobility of my sacrum, my animal counterpart trains for birth by squatting when she pees and poops. She walks more than five miles a day and squats often to gather and process food. She sits on the ground and walks barefoot along the river. She doesn't keep track of any of these movements or call them "training." Her legs are strong from hiking up hills and walking long distances, which improves her strength-to-weight ratio during pregnancy more than biking, swimming, or running.

She's been performing full-body movement her whole life, so her uterus is in balance and stabilized adequately by the ligaments that support it. Her ligaments and fascia, which act like a suspension bridge for the bladder, urethra, vagina, and uterus, are able to contract and relax. They are elastic yet strong. Because she's been walking often and far in minimal or no shoes and not sitting in a chair all day, she doesn't have as many imbalances in her body that show up as round ligament or sacroiliac pain.

Her aligned body and symmetrical uterus promote an optimal environment for the baby, with adequate space to move. Her psoas muscles are not overly tight or spasmodic from chronic sitting, cycling, or running, and they are not hypermobile from too much stretching. They are supple and able to stabilize her pelvis, which is aligned and promotes optimal fetal positioning.

The benefit of imagining this other me who lives in the world fully and moves her body wholly is that I can find her and become her daily. At the beginning of a walk, I'm still the person who thinks about responding to texts, calls, and emails. I worry about my eye health after looking at the computer screen all morning, and my body feels a little lost in the space of the outside world. Transformation, as it's prone to do, sneaks up on me when my mind has released control and worry. Walking across streams, panting uphill, jumping in an alpine lake, searching for an adequate bush to pee behind, getting down low to examine a plant or flower, I find the part of me who doesn't live inside and wouldn't even think of calling this adventure exercise.

I also like to imagine that my animal counterpart is spared from a sexist culture that shapes our minds and bodies in negative ways. In the supportive, idyllic, and egalitarian world of my imagination, people listen to and respect each other. They understand that equilibrium and interconnection are essential to survival. The shared intentionality of my animal counterpart's culture, the culture I want to cultivate, fosters powerful and embodied birth experiences and values mothers and all forms of mothering, fathers and all forms of fathering, parents of all genders and their parenting.

# The Psychology of Support

**TYPES OF SUPPORT**

**Giving:** Gestures of caring like making or bringing home favorite foods and giving free time without distractions

**Acknowledgment:** Recognizing how hard someone is working; speaking words of affirmation, gratitude, and/or love

**Acts of service:** Filling up the water bottle, cleaning the house, doing the laundry, grocery shopping—doing what needs to be done without being asked

**Physical touch:** Embracing, massage, sex, and/or cuddling.

**Information support:** Learning about the body and what to expect during pregnancy, labor, delivery, and postpartum.

**Network support:** Create a team that includes, for example, your partner, family, friends, midwife/OB, doula, lactation consultant, other parents, therapists, etc.

**BENEFITS OF RECEIVING MATERNAL SUPPORT**

- Smoother progression of labor
- Reduced stress
- Lower rates of depression
- Higher quality of life
- Improved communication and relationships

Just as the uterus functions at its best when the body parts around it move the way they were meant to move, supportive communities, families, and partners impact the experience of birthing people. Greater social support increases the odds that we'll experience empowering births and better health outcomes for our babies. Lack of support increases the risk of depression and poor quality of life. Feelings of well-being and personal control, which are encouraged by supportive relationships, lower stress, which has biochemical consequences for you and your baby. Because support is psychological in nature, meaning our degree of satisfaction with our support affects the impact it has on us, it's worth defining what type of support we need and value. When we receive the kind of support we need and value, research shows that we progress more smoothly during labor and deliver healthier babies with higher birth weights.

Our physical and psychological health share a beating heart with our surroundings, and the more we nurture that which surrounds us, or our entire ecosystem, the greater the benefit to us, our families, and the babies we grow.

## THREE PRINCIPLES

Spinning Babies, one of my favorite pregnancy resources created by Gail Tully, cites three central principles that guide preparation for birth: balance, gravity, and movement. The goal is to follow these principles throughout pregnancy so that the baby is gently urged, by our physiology, alignment, and anatomy, to find the best position for birth.

There are a few fetal positions that are considered ideal. The most famous is left occiput anterior (LOA), in which the baby is head down, facing toward your back, and their back is on your left side. This position appears to help babies tuck their chin and make their way into the pelvic brim at the end of pregnancy. Often, but not always, babies facing posteriorly have more trouble tucking their chin, so their head circumference is larger than anterior babies. Fetal position affects labor duration and progress, but it is not the only detail that matters in the story of birth. The tightness or mobility of the muscles in the pelvic floor as well as the psoas muscles, round and broad ligaments, the symmetry of the uterus, and the shape of the pelvis are also central to the birth experience.

The first principle, balance, refers to symmetry and alignment of the pelvis, uterus, and supporting structures. When we feel pain or discomfort, we're receiving a cue that our body is out of balance. Imbalance is fed by our sedentarism and chronic tension or weaknesses held in muscles and ligaments. The sports we played growing up, injuries, and car accidents can create imbalances in our bodies that impact fetal position and birth. Movements during pregnancy can promote greater balance or imbalance. Poor fetal positioning can also contribute to discomfort and pain.

Since most of us didn't grow up living a hunter-gatherer lifestyle, we have imbalances that can be challenging to address on our own. Bodyworkers who specialize in prenatal care, including pelvic floor physical therapists, prenatal chiropractors, craniosacral therapists, and other movement professionals who understand how our bodies impact the baby's space and our birthing experience, can help us achieve greater balance and symmetry.

I saw a pelvic floor physical therapist twice during my pregnancy: once during my second trimester and once during my third trimester. Visiting a pelvic floor PT a few times helped in several ways. First, it put me in touch with the muscles and fascia in my pelvic floor. My experience with my pelvic floor muscles, as for most of us, was limited to sex, masturbation, and menstruation with little consideration for symmetry, tension, and balance. Second, I was able to visualize my vagina, cervix, and uterus and for the first time truly understand, but perhaps not fathom, that a baby was going to pass through these structures.

The second principle, gravity, joins forces with the balance and symmetry of our bodies. Gravity is with us always. While we walk and stand, our relationship to gravity encourages babies to settle with their heads down. One of my favorite movements from Spinning Babies, the forward-leaning inversion, played with my relationship to gravity. By placing my knees up on a chair and my forearms on the ground, I was able to gently lengthen my uterine and cervical ligaments in a way that promoted symmetrical alignment.

This movement helped relieve pain in my back and hips, and it can help the baby's head shift into a position that encourages the cervix to dilate more easily during labor. I took three long, deep breaths and imagined my baby's head settling into an optimal position. I imagined my cervix dilating fully and efficiently during birth. This move is contraindicated for pregnant people with high blood pressure, heartburn, and high-risk pregnancies.

The changes in our bodies during pregnancy, especially increased weight and altered alignment, can impact body stability and lead to pain and discomfort. Because of our increased weight, existing malalignment and structural imbalances cause greater pain and stress on our bodies. I noticed, as my belly grew rounder, that I had a tendency to push my pelvis and chest forward. This position, where you feel like you're standing up really straight and practicing good posture, changes the way the force of gravity pulls on your weight. The loads from this position create more compression in our lumbar spine, which can cause pain and long-term damage in multiple places in our bodies.

To counteract this habit, Katy Bowman recommends backing up our hips so they line up over our knees. Another way to think of this is sticking out your butt and dropping your ribs, or, as Bowman describes it, placing the contents of your abdomen over the contents of your pelvis and lining up your ribs with the front of the pelvis. This adjustment in our positioning allows us to load our weight vertically, which works better for us when it comes to gravity and the forces it places on our bodies. Vertical alignment places appropriate tension on the pelvic floor so that it is both relaxed and strong. It places loads on our very strong, and growing stronger, glutes, which also balance out the pelvic floor.

Look at yourself sideways in a mirror. How are you standing? My brain grappled with how I thought I was moving in space versus how the mirror told me I was moving in space. Sometimes it felt like my head wasn't on my body right, or I'd catch myself fidgeting with the position of my ribs and belly like I was a puppet whose master couldn't quite figure out the strings.

Because I have a tendency to get stuck in my head, the best way for me to figure out where to put my body parts was to escape the questions and doubts of my mind. I did this, naturally, through movement. I'd go on walks and swing my arms. I'd skip and jump and climb trees. I'd hang from the monkey

# Three Principles

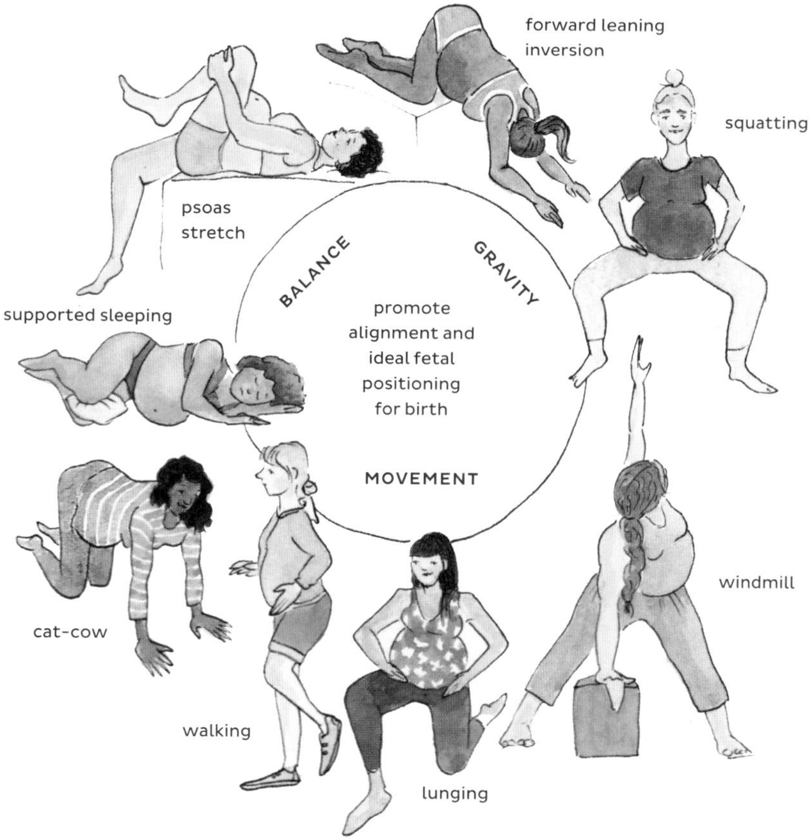
forward leaning
inversion
squatting
psoas
stretch
BALANCE
GRAVITY
supported sleeping
promote
alignment and
ideal fetal
positioning
for birth
MOVEMENT
windmill
cat-cow
walking
lunging

- Walk daily (build up to 3+ miles).
- Sit less, but when you do, sit on your sit bones (ischial tuberosities).
- Untuck your pelvis.
- Wear shoes with a negative or zero-drop heel, and walk barefoot when you can.
- Take deep, diaphragmatic breaths.
- Get a Squatty Potty for your bathroom.
- Address imbalances and pain with professionals who understand how alignment impacts fetal position and birth (pelvic floor PTs, prenatal chiropractors, Spinning Babies educators).

bars and engage my shoulders, noticing how heavy my belly was getting. I'd turn on music and dance and move all the parts of my body. I'd notice each step and how my body was moving together as a whole. In other words, when I was stressed about how my body parts were aligned, I'd play. I'd play and then I'd stretch gently, releasing tension in my arms, neck, and back.

Moving, the third principle, got me away from stasis in my body and mind and helped me feel a sense of dynamic stability. I was a diligent everyday walker and mover. Movement is as essential as food and water for the health of our own bodies and our babies. It creates the loads, stresses, and tensions that form us, the space in the uterus the baby kicks and bends and hiccups in, and the dynamic structures of the ligaments that are able to contract and relax, both elastic and strong. Movement is the action we must choose every day.

## AN ESSENTIAL ENVIRONMENT

The second trimester is the time when your baby's body parts move closer to where they belong. Eyes that sense changes in light, with eyelids that open and close, gently move forward. The ears move to a satisfying position on the sides of the head and begin to hear, allowing your baby to start responding to sounds. From around four and a half inches long and four ounces at the beginning of the second trimester, to around thirteen to sixteen inches long and two to three pounds by the end, the creature within us becomes something we recognize and can imagine holding in the palms of our hands.

The bits and pieces that make your baby a unique human develop during this period of rapid growth. Eyelashes and eyebrows and fingerprints and fat stores start growing and shaping this person. Kidneys are functioning and producing urine, fingernails and toenails lengthen, and the gallbladder produces bile. If your baby is female, eggs have formed in her ovaries between weeks seventeen and twenty. Within you is the future, like a Russian doll nestled neatly together: eggs within her ovaries within your womb.

At fourteen weeks blood begins to form in bone marrow, and at sixteen weeks a fine hair called lanugo starts to grow and cover your baby. At twenty weeks oil glands in the skin start to work, and your baby may suck its thumb. Babies start working on swallowing and sucking in the womb. The baby's ability to nurse and receive breast milk once they leave the womb requires coordination between breathing, swallowing, and suckling. Swallowing amniotic fluid strengthens their muscles. The central nervous system must mature so that the breathing and suckling occur independently but in concert.

The development of the lungs starts during the first trimester and continues after birth. The lungs, with their differentiated cells and unique structure, prepare to keep the baby alive and functioning via gas exchange. During late pregnancy, just before birth, the lungs mature. A complex substance composed of fats, proteins, and carbohydrates called surfactant allows the baby to breathe as it decreases surface tension where alveoli, the tiny air sacs that allow the lungs to rapidly exchange carbon dioxide and oxygen, interface with air. Each day of lung maturity matters. At birth, 50 to 150 million alveoli are present in the baby's lungs. By the time we're adults, our lungs contain over 500 million alveoli.

Vernix caseosa is a creamy, white, lipid-rich biofilm that covers the skin of your growing baby during the second and third trimesters. Both in the womb and out, this yogurt-like substance helps prevent excess water loss, regulates temperature, and protects the baby's skin from infection. The interaction between vernix and surfactant from the baby's lungs plays an essential role in preparing the lungs for their transition from in utero to ex utero. As surfactant levels increase, the proteins in this essential substance cause vernix to detach from the baby's skin. Your baby swallows this mixed substance and amniotic fluid becomes turbid, or cloudy, which is a key indicator of lung maturity.

The vernix barrier essentially waterproofs fetal skin so that it can fully develop without too much exposure to amniotic fluid, and it protects the fetus from the loss of fluid and electrolytes. During birth, vernix helps minimize friction. Both antimicrobial and insulating, this biofilm protects babies from dangerous microbes and oxidative stress. If we could apply vernix caseosa like a serum, we'd find our skin supple and moisturized, our wounds healed, and our skin surface clean and intact.

Like the lungs, brain development starts early and continues long after birth. For a brain to form, ridges rise and fold and fuse, segments divide and subdivide, regions and patterns emerge that specify and refine certain locations. The dramatic changes in anatomy represent the changes being made at the cellular level as neuron production and migration ensues. The cerebral cortex, the gray matter that covers each brain hemisphere, becomes organized. Communication between the hemispheres develops, and the building blocks of the nervous system, or synapses, form connections.

## Supporting Fetal Brain Development

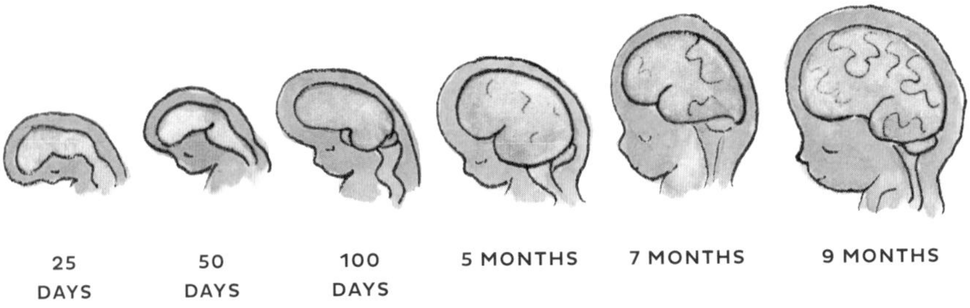


- Take care of your overall health, which impacts baby's overall health.
- Increase foods rich in omega-3 and DHA, such as wild fish (salmon, anchovies), cod liver oil, eggs, walnuts, chia seeds, flaxseeds, and avocado.
- Move your body, as physical activity during pregnancy leads to advanced motor and coordination skills for baby.
- Manage stress, as stress impacts fetal brain development and functioning.
- Take a high-quality prenatal vitamin.
- Avoid environmental toxins, alcohol, cat feces, and medications, if possible.

Looking at images of fetal brain growth is like watching a caterpillar become a butterfly, which then transforms and divides a million more times to become something that contains multitudes. The development is dynamic and orderly, and it depends on the right things happening at the right time. At each point of development, genes and interaction with the external environment play a critical role in providing the directions that shape the developing brain. While genes provide the template for development, the environment provides the essential input that shapes the emerging neural networks in the brain.

You are an essential environment. Simple but still profound, it is worth continually remembering that our bodies, the food we eat, and the choices we make create the environment that provides essential information to the cells of our developing babies. The food we eat becomes nutrient molecules that pass through the placenta to help form the fissures, sulci, and gyri of our babies' brains. Who they will become depends on this absurdly complex web of connections that is fed and molded by our interaction with the world.

The third trimester is about bulking up, maturing, and settling. This period of growth is also about sensory input, electrical impulses and signals that start traveling through our babies' bodies more efficiently. During these months, babies transform from scrawny, wrinkled creatures into slightly plump baby animals as fat stores develop under their skin and smooth it out. Densely vascularized and mitochondria-rich brown fat accumulates during the third trimester. This special, metabolically active fat is able to generate and spread heat as blood passes through it. Newborns, who cannot shiver to generate heat, rely on brown fat to protect them from the cold and to maintain core body temperature.

Around week twenty-five, myelination, a process in which an insulating sheath surrounds nerves to allow electrical impulses to travel rapidly, begins and continues after birth and into adulthood. Babies start to grow hair on their heads. Their head bones remain pliable for birth while the rest of the bones begin to harden. Between weeks twenty-eight and forty, neurons that proliferated rather exuberantly during early brain development are pruned. This scheduled, necessary cell death helps protect the remaining cells in the developing brain.

Our circadian rhythm and melatonin impact our baby's maturation and physiology. During the last trimester, it is crucial to avoid night-shift work and bright lights before bed. These disruptors of our circadian rhythm can be detrimental to baby's long-term metabolic function and behavior. Other steps we can take to support our circadian biology include wearing blue light–blocking glasses when we look at screens, turning off our screens an hour before bedtime, and using softer lighting like salt lamps or beeswax or unscented candles.

Interruptions in the natural rhythm of light and dark disrupt and suppress our normal circadian-melatonin rhythm. Every part of our biology depends on this rhythm. Melatonin protects the placenta from free radical damage and thus the baby from the deleterious impact of these compounds. Blood pressure is mediated by melatonin, with the lowest pressures occurring at night. Some research has shown that gestational hypertension and preeclampsia may be linked to a disruption in our circadian rhythm. Melatonin works with oxytocin to increase the strength of uterine contractions during birth, and the melatonin content in breast milk ebbs and flows, rising higher at night than during the day.

We are our baby's master biological clock and microbial inoculation center. From the first to third trimesters, the sheer quantity and diversity of bacteria in our gut increase dramatically. The critters that live here in their chosen niche of our temperate bodies impact our health, immunity, and hormones. They also have a huge effect on our baby's long-term health, body composition, and likelihood of developing chronic diseases. Imagine the trillion dancing, twirling viruses, fungi, archaea, and bacteria that make up your unique microbiome and interact with your human cells. These bugs and the way they communicate with your body while growing your baby influence whether your children are overweight or obese and whether they develop asthma, allergies, or autoimmune diseases. No matter how many new studies I read about our resident bugs, I am still filled with wonder at their role in determining how well we live in our bodies and how our babies will live in this world.

## PREGNANT LADY

In my memory, there is a wide separation in time between the first three-quarters or so of the third trimester and the final days leading up to birth. During the third trimester I still went to work, but during the last two weeks I was done taking care of other people. I wanted quiet space and time with my body and my belly that felt undeniably huge and heavy. I'd go outside in my underwear on a sunny day in the winter and imagine my baby squinting in the sunshine.

As much as I walked and moved, my hips hurt and woke me up at night during the last few months of growing my baby. I was never cold, even when we visited Jackson Hole in the middle of winter, where it regularly dips below freezing. My baby was radiating body heat, and I felt it warm me from the inside out. At work and when I lay down to sleep, I had frequent Braxton Hicks contractions. My whole abdomen felt like it was made out of elastic fabric that was suddenly pulled tight. I'd pause, observing the sensation. It wasn't painful, and these contractions were nothing like the contractions I felt during labor.

Around week thirty-seven, people started asking me if I was ready to pop, a verb I learned to hate during pregnancy, since the word "pop" elicited fear in my whole body. I didn't want anything popping. People asked me if I was sick of being pregnant. I wasn't. In fact, I told them, this baby can cook until he is nice and done. They said my belly was too small or too big. I was told I was tiny and that I needed to eat more. A few people told me I was huge.

I learned that when you're a woman who has become pregnant, you become a "pregnant lady." This designation made me feel quaint, homely, and not especially vibrant. I also discovered, like every other pregnant person, that growing a baby in your body gives other people, both family and perfect strangers, newfound confidence to comment on your changing body. It seemed like people felt compelled to say *something, anything* about my appearance. These nonstop comments became part of my daily life. As unwelcome as some of these comments can be, I think they come up because people feel connected to your experience and can't help but offer their unsolicited observations and advice on your pregnancy and parenting.

Pregnancy is a private experience going on in your body, and it's your business. Unfortunately, we have to navigate the reality that our private business is undeniably public. Our bellies give us away, inviting hands and appraising looks, comments and stories. I found it crucial to collect good stories and birth experiences. I was told so many horror stories about birth and raising babies that the few good ones I heard planted in my mind, where I repeated them and made them shade out the horror stories. I learned the importance of creating boundaries. The combination of boundaries and good stories created something like a little garden in my mind where I could protect myself from fear and doubt and instead cultivate calm and a quiet kind of belief that, no matter what happened, things would be OK.

## THE ESSENTIALS

I entered my second trimester during my favorite time of year: persimmon season. As the leaves turned vividly yellow, orange, and red and crunched under my shoes on my walks, I felt more at home in my changing body. I filled my basket with persimmons, my favorite cheese, and walnuts and ate them with great joy and future nostalgia, already lamenting their passing. The second trimester is a short season in life that is usually sweet and balanced like my favorite fruit. I wrote to my baby that the food he was tasting with his developing palate was mostly persimmons and figs, goat gouda and funky blue cheese, sweet cherry tomatoes, spicy peppers, and greens from the garden. He had his daily yogurt with fruit, fried eggs and bacon, some grass-fed beef liver, and bone broth. That bitter taste was a cup of coffee and some dark chocolate.

The foods we eat flavor the fluid our baby swims in. Our babies can taste these flavors in utero because their taste buds and olfactory systems develop and allow them to experience the sensation that will urge them to eat and keep eating their whole lives. The baby lives in this taste. It bathes their bodies, flowing into nasal passages and building taste preferences and memories that last long after they exit this swimming pool of flavors.

In the same way that we breathe in and imagine the taste of cookies as they bake in the oven, babies in the womb inhale odors and swallow flavors and tastes that shape their experiences with food. I love the idea that food is something we experience in utero. The food we consume is not simply growing essential parts like brains and bones, it is shaping perception and preferences that last through childhood and beyond. Flavor is one of the first lessons about culture. While your baby can't see the world on the outside or smell the air after a rainstorm, they are part of your food story and desires. Exposure to a diverse array of foods and flavors in the womb increases the likelihood that your baby will like and accept these foods later.

During pregnancy, certain types of food are needed in our diets in greater quantities. One of these is the amino acid glycine. In her book *Real Food for Pregnancy*, Lily Nichols writes that prior to pregnancy, our bodies easily make glycine from other amino acids. But the requirements increase when we're growing new life. Glycine plays a crucial role in helping build the blocks that make a baby. It serves as fuel for the parts of our body that are expanding, like our skin and uterus, and helps build important parts of the baby, like blood vessels, organs, skin, and bones.

In addition to these essential functions, glycine supports healthy management of stress, digestion, relaxation, toxin elimination, and central nervous system health and function. Collagen and gelatin are rich in glycine. When we boil bones, tendons, and ligaments to make bone broth, eat the skin on roasted chicken, consume liver and other organ meats, and cook tough, grass-fed or pastured meats low and slow until they are tender and flavor-packed, we nourish our body with this amino acid. Dairy products, pastured eggs, and wild fish are also rich in glycine and other essential nutrients like omega-3s and the B vitamins, especially $B_{12}$, folate, and choline.

There is an overlap between what we need from the food we eat and what makes sense based on how we used to live as humans. Eating the whole animal, from head to tail, provides us with the pieces we need to grow new life. Even if we didn't taste these foods in the sea of our own amniotic fluid as we grew, we are able to pass on the taste and benefits to our babies. That these foods are also delicious and deeply satisfying is yet another benefit.

On my long walks, especially in the winter when it was snowy and cold, I'd bring a big thermos full of bone broth with me. On the top of the mountain, looking out at the sagebrush, I'd sip the warm, nourishing liquid and feel it settle into me. The sensation of calm was immediate. I could feel the broth becoming part of me as it swirled around the space in my uterus, warming us up just enough to take the sting out of the air.

Occasionally, we bought bone broth. More often, my mom made us some or we made big batches of it, simmering the golden liquid for a few days until it was packed with enormous flavor. I found it more delightful to eat the foods I needed when they were attached to a pleasurable ritual and narrative. Eating eggs gathered from our chickens or sipping bone broth that my mom made seemed to contain greater nourishment. I needed the story of the foods as much as I needed the actual foods.

Stories, especially about food, can either connect or disconnect us from food. My mom taught me by her example that liver is a delicious treat, organ meats are to be savored, and no part of any given food, plant or animal, should ever go to waste. In her cooking, thrift, creativity, and appreciation live together in dishes that fill me all the way up and give me exactly what I need.

More than anything, my mom's example and my own beliefs make me determined to figure out how to cook animal parts like beef liver. When I first ate grass-fed beef liver, I was overwhelmed by the flavor and size of this monstrous organ. I learned that if I keep it frozen and slice it paper-thin, it tastes incredible fried quickly in bacon fat with a bit of sea salt and served with thinly sliced apples (also fried in bacon fat). It is too easy to assume that we don't like something because it's weird, or looks gross, or we didn't grow up eating it. While learning about food outside the narrow cultural stories we're used to is challenging, it is endlessly intriguing and rewarding. Like so many important parts of life, trying something new and figuring out how to incorporate it into your life in a meaningful way takes imagination and an open mind.

Glycine is not the only pregnancy-specific compound we require in abundance. Vitamin D is another essential, which is, in fact, not a vitamin at all. Instead, it's a prohormone steroid that is fat soluble. We get vitamin D from three sources: the sun, vitamin D–rich foods, and supplements. When the sun shines down on our skin, vitamin D is synthesized and enters our circulation, where it is converted by our liver and kidneys into the active form that is measured in our blood during routine lab tests.

Food sources rich in vitamin D are limited, but they include cheese, egg yolks, salmon, beef liver, and cod liver oil. It is difficult to get enough vitamin D from food alone, and multiple factors impact our vitamin D levels. The amount of vitamin D synthesized by our skin is impacted by latitude, season, time of day, air pollution, surface reflection, and cloudiness. Our age, our skin thickness, whether or not we're overweight or obese, our skin color, our clothing, our workplace, our lifestyle, and the sunscreen we use further impact our vitamin D levels.

While we are taught to fear the sun because of the threat of skin cancer, we learn less about how vitamin D supports our skin health and immune function, allowing us to protect against, and fight, infections. Too much sun exposure can be damaging, but vitamin D is photoprotective for our skin and may protect us against many different types of cancer. This sunlight hormone protects against preeclampsia and infections. It decreases the risk of preterm birth, asthma, and gestational diabetes, is essential for neurodevelopment and placental function, and may protect against autism and attention disorders.

Vitamin D requirements are personal. The best way to figure out how much you need is to have your blood levels drawn before pregnancy and a few times while you're pregnant. The current recommendation for vitamin D intake is 400 to 600 international units (IU) per day for pregnant women. If you are a sunbather or a lifeguard living at a sun-rich latitude, a field-worker or landscaper, or an indigenous woman living in a traditional, native environment, this might be adequate. But most of us don't live this way. Depending on your serum vitamin D levels, you might take a vitamin $D_3$ supplement in the 4,000 to 6,000 IU/day range. In fact, recent studies recommend supplementing with 4,000 IU/day because of the way we live, the differences in our vitamin D binding proteins, and other factors.

I developed a few habits that I enjoyed and that helped me get what I needed while I was pregnant. One was sipping bone broth in the sunshine on my long walks when I had a day off from work, which helped meet my glycine and vitamin D needs. Another ritual that caught and stuck during my pregnancy was my two-breakfast habit. I'd eat my eggs with greens and cheese, enjoying each savory bite, then a few hours later I'd eat unsweetened, full-fat plain or Greek yogurt with seasonal fruit, unsweetened coconut flakes, cacao nibs, cinnamon, and nuts. Sometimes I'd add a date or two. I love breakfast dessert. Having it helps me cope with the mourning feeling I get when I finish my last sip of coffee and last bite of eggs. The main ingredient in breakfast dessert—full-fat grass-fed yogurt or kefir—is loaded with probiotics and vitamin $K_2$. Vitamin $K_2$ is crucial for bone health and may help normalize blood sugar. Fermented foods like yogurt, kefir, sauerkraut, and kimchi represent an amazing relationship between humans and microbes. Creating environments for microbes to improve the taste and nutrition of our food is a testament to our interdependence and to the potential for cooperative benefits when we nurture environments for beneficial microbes.

When dairy is fermented (a process in which milk becomes something healthier and more digestible through microbial action), two of the main health benefits are metabolic and immune health. These two realms of health are crucial for pregnant people to nurture since our immune and metabolic functions undergo dynamic shifts while growing a baby. Like fermented dairy products, nondairy sources of fermented foods are rich in beneficial bacteria and also appear to improve insulin sensitivity and glucose tolerance.

The nourishing food we require in abundance while growing babies has the potential to fill us up with nutrients and satisfaction. I imagined my baby inhaling the flavors of each season, experiencing the diverse tactile and sensory delights. Pastured pork chops with kale, broccolini, and sauerkraut one night, and wild salmon with sweet potatoes, avocado, bok choy, and kimchi another. I wanted him to learn, through a full-body sensory experience, that good food is both nourishment and pleasure, and it acts as a perfect introduction to the world.

| | |
|---|---|
| **GLYCINE**<br>slow-cooked bone-in meat, bone broth, eggs, dairy products | builds connective tissue; helps with stress; supports expanding uterus, placental development, methylation, and neurotransmitter production |
| **VITAMIN D**<br>sunshine, vitamin $D_3$ supplements, wild fish, beef liver, cheese, eggs | protects against preeclampsia and infections; decreases risk of preterm birth, asthma, and gestational diabetes; supports neurotransmitter and placental function |
| **B VITAMINS & CHOLINE**<br>eggs, liver, pastured meats, leafy greens, seafood, poultry | supports normal brain development; protects against neural tube defects and maternal anemia; aids in fetal vision development and methylation; appears to protect baby from mental health problems |
| **ANTIOXIDANTS & MINERALS**<br>leafy greens, vegetables, fruits, seaweed, dark chocolate | supports maternal and fetal tissue development, normalizes blood pressure, promotes normal blood clotting, balances oxidative stress in maternal and placental circulation |
| **CALCIUM & $K_2$**<br>full-fat and fermented dairy, aged cheese, eggs, butter, fermented foods, yogurt, kefir, animal livers, sardines, duck fat, natto, collard greens | $K_2$ maintains both maternal and fetal bone health and skeletal and nervous system formation. Calcium supports fetal and maternal bone health and is protective against preeclampsia and preterm delivery. |
| **PROBIOTICS**<br>sauerkraut, kimchi, lacto-fermented vegetables, miso, yogurt, kefir, kombucha | improves immune defense against infection by improving intestinal bacterial flora, supports the development of the baby's brain, immune system, and long-term health. Reduces risk of preterm delivery, preeclampsia, and gestational diabetes. |

## THE NECESSITY OF LIMITS

To the best of my ability, I trained for birth and ate nourishing food. I didn't start living outside and assume the life of my animal counterpart. I wanted to emulate this other me within the context of my culture, breaking the pattern of modern Western culture without totally leaving it behind. When we were ripping up carpet and working on our home, I fantasized about hiring professionals to do all the work. Then we could hike, climb, and play more. Our inability to do so taught me about the value of limits—the importance of how we navigate them and how essential they are to living well in the world. We are so used to hearing that we are limitless, that everything is possible, but what I find truly fascinating is that there is incredible potential and creativity when we learn to thrive with what we have. In an essay about the necessity of limits, Wendell Berry writes,

> As earthly creatures, we live, because we must, within natural limits, which we may describe by such names as "earth" or "ecosystem" or "watershed" or "place." . . . We must learn again to ask how we can make the most of what we are, what we have, what we have been given.

Limits, then, are not a wall or a stop sign; they are an invitation for creativity, resourcefulness, and imagination. I thank the limits of our finances for my increased movement and for Max's basic education in the inner working of toilets, door installation, and other house-related troubleshooting. Working within our limits encourages us to find solutions to challenging situations, like figuring out how to move more if we work at a desk all day, how to walk more if we work long hours, and how to eat nourishing food if we feel constricted by money or time or ingrained habits and tastes.

Limits are a pathway to abundance and opportunity. When we learn that the home we have is the only one we get, and that our actions matter, we take better care of our place. This place is our bodies and the rounded bellies that house our growing babies. It includes our backyards, communities, and greater ecosystem. Limits are not bad; they are necessary. For, as Berry said, "Nothing can take form except within limits."

# TAKE ACTION

Train for labor and delivery. Choosing more full-body movement, squatting for elimination, and walking long distances in minimal shoes help our bodies find strength and balance, which helps encourage our babies into more ideal positions for birth. When in doubt, imagine your animal counterpart living wildly and become that animal daily. Remember the three principles—gravity, balance, and movement—and practice them throughout your pregnancy to support the physiological process of birth.

Define what support looks like for you. People who receive the kind of quality support they need and value experience more empowering births, better health outcomes for themselves and their babies, increased feelings of well-being and personal control, and lower stress. They progress more smoothly during labor and tend to deliver babies with higher birth weights. Support is essential and personal. Spend time defining what you need and take steps to cultivate your supportive environment.

Devour abundant essential foods for growing your baby. The nutrients we need during pregnancy are found in grass-fed and slow-cooked pastured meats, organs (such as liver), bone broth, wild-caught fish, fermented foods like yogurt and sauerkraut, vegetables, and leafy greens. Check your vitamin D levels and supplement with vitamin $D_3$.

Live within natural limits. We all face certain, essential limitations because we live on earth in an ecosystem. Learn to live well within your ecosystem by making the most of what you have and by creatively discovering how to move more, eat better food, and create a more supportive community. Limits are opportunities to take better care of ourselves and our place.

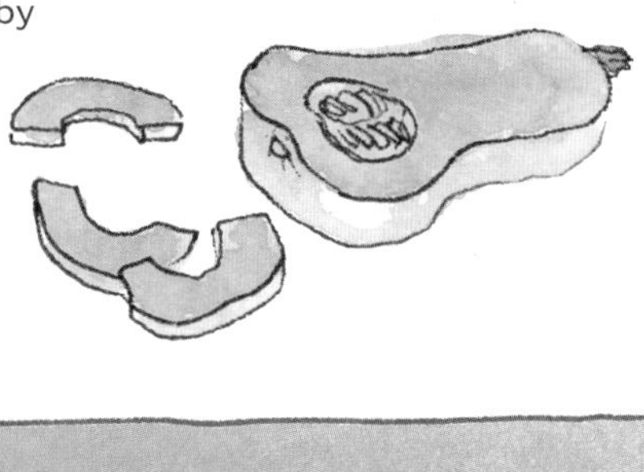

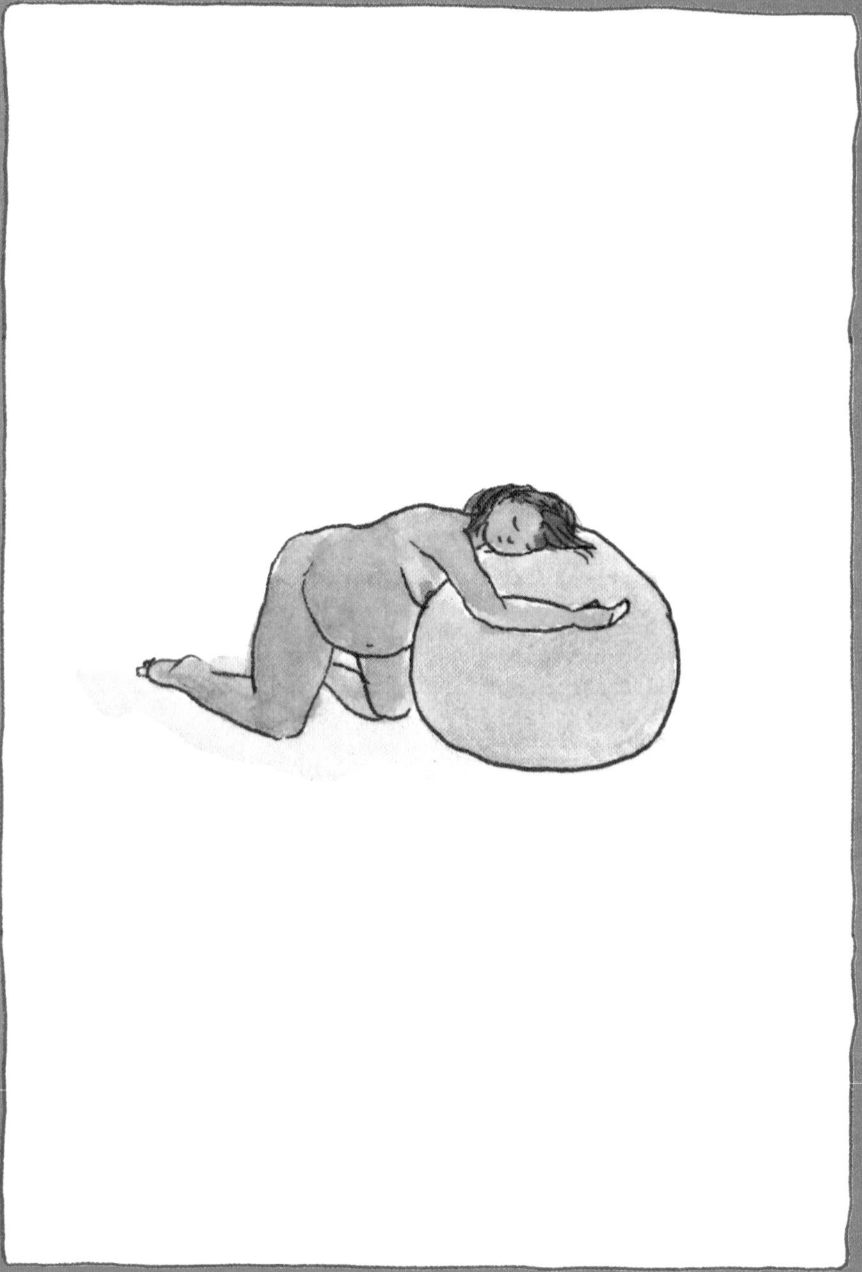

CHAPTER EIGHT

# Birth!

**JUST AFTER 9 P.M.** on March 7, 2018, I googled a question that, apparently, many others had also googled based on the number of results that popped up. Like so many questions I have for Google, I knew the answer to this one and typed the question anyway. Google, did my water just break or did I pee (a lot)? I was lying on my side in bed, one day before my due date, and Max was rubbing my feet and legs. I felt a sensation of rushing, like a dam opening in my body, and I jumped up just in time to let the water rush out of me into the toilet.

Contractions started soon after. I timed them for around two hours before I texted my midwife, Amanda. My mom showed up at my house around midnight. My contractions had picked up, and we thought maybe this baby would come during the early morning hours. I learned later that these early labor contractions were incredibly gentle. I was listening to a hypnobirthing soundtrack and breathing peacefully through the contractions while leaning on my yoga ball. I thought, I can totally handle this; look at me breathing and managing this pain. As dawn approached, my contractions slowed down. I lay down in bed, trying to rest.

Amanda listened to my baby's heart rate and rhythm at around nine that morning and told me that my labor would probably pick up again that night. I rested, and my mom, who is not the kind of person to sit around and wait, cleaned all the windows in my house and rearranged furniture. Max, too, cleaned with uncharacteristic enthusiasm. It was as if we all had an unspoken agreement that everything should be as beautiful and clean as possible for the new life entering this space. We walked in the sun in the afternoon and I lunged up and down stairs. I paused during contractions, bracing myself against trees because they felt sturdy and capable of handling my powerful, full-body tightening. I came home and rested. We went for another walk. We waited.

Amanda came back at seven that night to listen again. She said she thought my contractions, which were much stronger now, would pick up around nine or ten and I'd probably have my baby soon after. She told Max to call her when he and my mom noticed a shift in me. Max asked what she meant. She said, "You'll know," and it was true. I know now that she was referring to the moment when "thinking Amy" became "animal Amy." This change, Max explained, was clear when he looked at my eyes and body. I took a shower. I moved from my yoga ball into my bathroom where I laid my head on the cool granite countertop and yelled and groaned a deep primal sound that felt like it came up through the ground, through me. I groaned and moaned through the pain, then my body gave me breaks. I relished these breaks. Thank you, I thought as I gained enough energy and resolve to continue. Thank you for this moment of pause.

Max told Amanda it was time to come over, and she showed up with the other midwives. They set up their equipment, checked my son's heart rate, and held space in my living room while I labored in the bathroom. Max talked to me. He reminded me to relax my jaw and yell deep and low because when I screamed at a high pitch, I felt out of control and the pain felt like too much. My mom sat just outside the bathroom, a calm, knowing presence.

I showered again, I labored on my bed on all fours, I went back into my bathroom and squatted over my toilet. Pushing started to happen, not willfully by me but reflexively by my body. I felt my baby's head. After so many birth stories, I expected to think, Oh great, here he is, just a little to go. Instead, I thought, Oh my, that's just the top of his head, I need to open up so much more! My body gave me breaks, and then it would resume pushing. Amanda told me, in response to my searching look, that it was OK to go slow, that my tissue was stretching. My tissue was stretching, I thought. My brain wanted to escape. Max told me to yell lower and deeper, he told me "good job," he told me to breathe, he told me all of this over and over again, all so quietly, and right next to me the whole time. Oddly, my cat rubbed against me during contractions, and even though I was in my animal body, I had some space in my mind to consider how weird this scene was.

When it was time to really push my baby out, that last monumental heave-ho in which the effort of my body combined with my mind's determination, everyone cheered me on. Max, my mom, and the midwives rallied around me. I was in a half squat over the toilet, and I watched wide-eyed in pain and disbelief as his head and then his body came out of my body, and then he was in my arms. It was just surprising beyond anything.

When he came out he sneezed first, then cried and settled onto my chest. I looked at him, quietly. My arms had never felt so full and my body had never felt so empty. It was a dichotomous moment of abundance and vacancy, as my arms were filled with more love than I could imagine and my body was left freezing and empty. I delivered my placenta and got back into bed and lay there with my son on my chest, where he latched and nursed a little on each of my breasts. My mom turned up the heat and layered blankets over me.

After the midwives left, Max and my mom took turns holding the now-sleeping Holden, enamored with his newness and surprisingly cone-shaped head, while I showered my sore, cold body in hot, soothing water. After my shower, around 4 a.m., I asked Max to heat up a cast-iron panful of my mom's premade lasagna. He filled the whole pan, imagining we might share it as a celebratory meal after the birth of our little creation, but instead, I devoured it whole, letting it warm and fill me. My mom knew what I would need after this tremendous effort, and her lasagna filled some of the space in my body with her love, and lots of cheese.

## THE POWER OF "WHAT IF"

As much as I learned about the events that scientists believe trigger the beginning of labor, I lived in a state of anticipation and trepidation for the last few days of my pregnancy. Would labor start on a walk? Would it start at night? What would it feel like? Where would I be? OK, deep breaths, keep walking, wait with grace. But what if it doesn't start for two more weeks? I've never been a person who waits gracefully. My body was so full. I felt hazy, but I also felt fully alive. This period of time before things went down was the weirdest pretransition of my life. I knew something was coming, but when and how? I think this time period, with its mental somersaults, tricks, questions, and wondering, is necessary because when labor actually starts, you think, *Finally!* Finally, I'm ready to move beyond this in-between. Without those days that are characterized by a sense of purposeful waiting, almost like meditating with the weight of the future on your whole being, maybe it's harder to be prepared to welcome the moment when life changes forever.

While I learned that internal hormonal and physiological events led to my labor starting, I had no way to look inside my own body and see that my estrogen levels were higher than my progesterone levels, which causes the smooth muscles of the uterus to become more sensitive to stimuli that cause contractions. I understood that birth requires synchrony between me, my baby, and the placenta, each party throwing hormones into the proverbial punch bowl, urging the uterus to squeeze with more force and strength to get the baby out. I knew that my body, through a cascade of internal events, would go from tightly closed to wide open. The question was when and how?

In the quintessential birthing book, *Ina May's Guide to Childbirth*, Ina May Gaskin writes,

> The physical changes that take place in a woman's body during labor are perhaps the most dramatic that occur in humans. They involve more movement, more shape-changing of various organs, more prolonged physical sensation, and considerably more effort than do other physiological functions of the body such as yawning, swallowing, burping, sneezing, coughing, laughing, crying, digesting, breathing, peeing, vomiting, pooping, farting, and coming—the functions we experience on a more regular basis. Birth—as experienced by the mother—is the Mount Everest of physical functions in any mammal.

When I read this I thought, I haven't climbed Mount Everest, but I've climbed other big mountains. What did I need for those adventures? I needed a high base of fitness and endurance. I needed snacks and water. I needed to be present and aware but not afraid. I needed an attitude that allowed me to wake up at 3 a.m. and start walking, not knowing exactly what the day would bring, but knowing that I could make it to the top. I needed the ability to keep going through discomfort like wind, extreme cold, and exhaustion. I needed a partner to climb with. I needed to understand that the top was only halfway, and I needed to stay focused and determined all the way down. And finally, I needed enough humility to recognize when I needed help.

Even if you're not a mountain climber, the metaphor holds. Not only because you need a strong butt and legs for mountain climbing and birth, but also because our attitude toward the action shapes the outcome and our perception of the experience. I chose to do my Mount Everest birth at home because it felt right for me, not because I thought my choice was superior or because I believed with blind faith that everything would be fine. Instead I felt a quiet kind of hope that things would work out.

I remember reading a paper over a decade ago about language, attitudes, motivation, and outcomes. The paper compared the language people use to

# Packing List

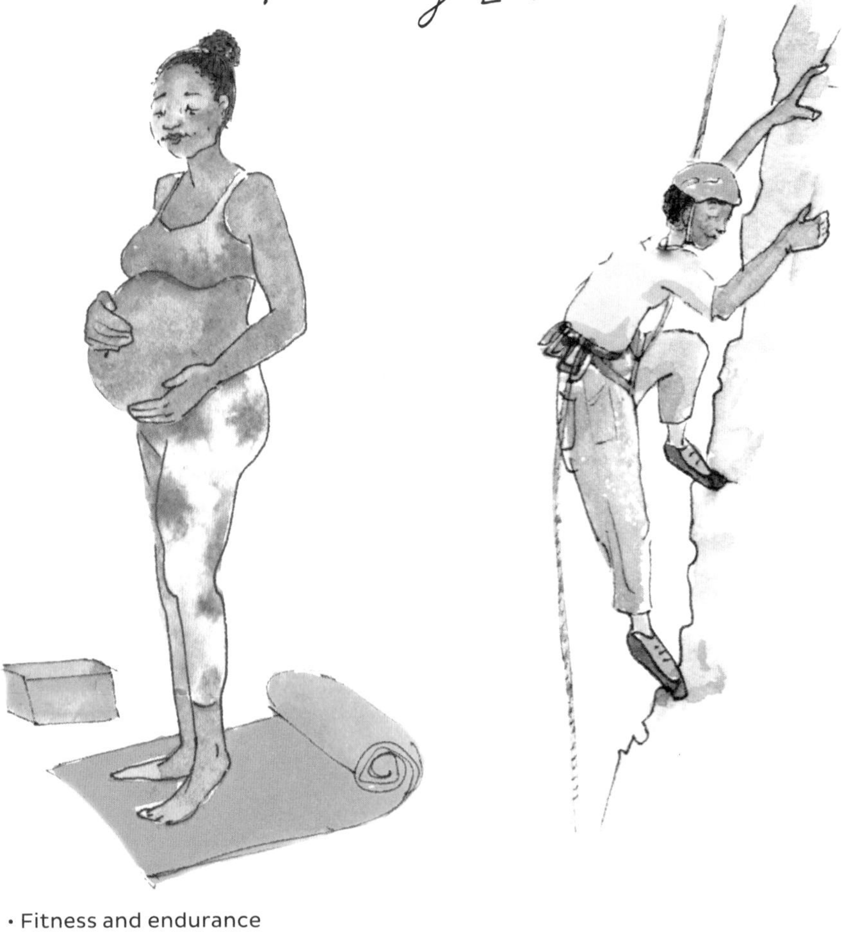

- Fitness and endurance
- Snacks and water
- A state of being present and aware but not afraid
- Movement and breathing through pain and discomfort
- Continuous support and feeling of safety
- Moments of rest
- Knowledge that the top is only halfway
- Humility to recognize when help is needed

motivate themselves during exercise or other objectives. Some people said with conviction, "I can do this." Others said, "What if I try this?" One statement is declarative, while the other is a pondering question. The first time I tried this language was on a run, years before I got pregnant. What if I run another mile? I immediately felt a sense of freedom, of giddiness, like I had entered a game with myself that was free of pressure. I ran farther and enjoyed it more than I ever had before.

When my birth expectations started to feel heavy, I used the question "What if?" This question, instead of the statement "I will," "I can," or "I must," softened my hardest edges. What if I have a home birth? What if I get transferred to the hospital? This question starter helped me more than any stubborn belief or declarative statement like "I can do it no matter what" or "I won't get transferred." The what-ifs encouraged a calm openness in me and helped me frame the questions and situations I couldn't control. It helped me remain aware of different outcomes and ponder them with curiosity instead of fear.

I moved away from superstition and toward answers to hard questions. For example, if I were to be transferred to the hospital, I would be supported by my whole birth team, and they would advocate for me. If I needed a C-section, I would turn down the immediate infant bath and request skin-to-skin contact right after delivery.

Originally when I thought of going to the hospital, I imagined myself putting on boxing gloves, preparing to fight against every intervention and recommendation. I was angry at imaginary nurses and doctors. I was a defensive, nightmare patient. But I took my boxing gloves off sometime during the third trimester and realized after my labor that it would have taken tremendous effort to put them on and fight with everyone. What made more sense was working together. I still had a strong sense of what I wanted, and I was prepared to advocate for myself, but I knew that coming in swinging probably wasn't the best way to enter through the automatic doors. I imagined myself, instead, coming in grateful but empowered with information. Even though I didn't experience this imagined event, I felt my attitude change. My attachment to outcome repurposed itself into a feeling that, no matter what, I was capable.

A lot of my questions during pregnancy were what-ifs, and the question helped me face my greatest desires and my greatest fears. What if I have my baby at home? What if I have my baby at the hospital? What if, instead of feeling fear, I felt like my mind and body were able to rise to the occasion? Wherever we decide to birth our babies—at home, in a hospital, or at a birthing center—we are in charge of our bodies, and we hold the power in our hands.

Asking "What if?" and feeling the lightness of this question sweep through my nervous system, centering and calming me, allowed me to detach from expectations. The question has a buoyancy about it that makes me shrug my shoulders as if to say, "Anything could happen, but let's hope for the very best."

## ACKNOWLEDGING AND RESHAPING FEAR

Most cisgender women I talk to who have either never been pregnant or are pregnant for the first time say they are terrified of giving birth. This fear has been reinforced by medical language, horror stories, movies, TV shows, our friends and family, and all the anxieties and worries about something going wrong. These negative experiences get shared with pregnant people and increase their anxiety, fear, and negative expectations related to childbirth. Heightened fear and negative expectations make the birthing experience harder and more painful. We learn not to trust our bodies, we accept that interventions are necessary, and then we have a negative experience with interventions. These experiences get shared with other pregnant people, and on and on it goes.

Fear during pregnancy and toward the process of birth has a negative effect on our emotional health. When we feel fear about our safety, pain, and lack of control during birth, we are more likely to have negative feelings about being pregnant and to feel less positive during the first weeks with our baby. Pain feels more intense when we're afraid, and anxiety during pregnancy is associated with an increased risk of postpartum depression. If you feel afraid, you're not alone, and you shouldn't feel ashamed.

Most of us didn't grow up watching people give birth, and without seeing this event, it can feel scary and impossible instead of common and doable.

Of all the births I observed in the hospital as a student, none were unmedicated vaginal births. I didn't have a model of what this could look like, so I started collecting stories and attempted to build one. First, I collected my mom's birth stories: Three unmedicated vaginal births in the hospital. Then I read birth stories in books and online. I listened to good stories and how people told them. Finally, I watched births online. I watched until my horror and discomfort shifted into familiarity. Most of us see one childbirth video in high school, or maybe college, and young men cover their eyes and shout and the event is dramatic and we're taught to see this event as unnatural and unfeminine.

## *Transforming Fear*

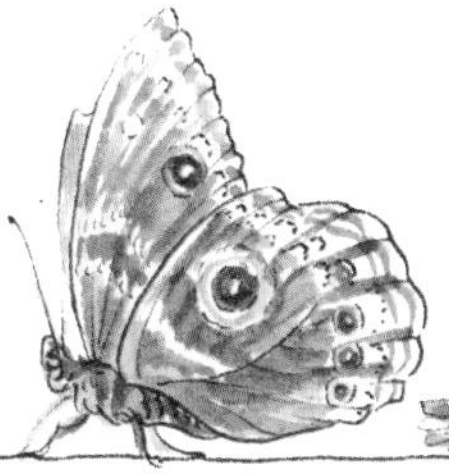

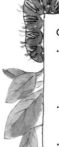

**COMMON FEARS**

- Unknown and unpredictable nature of birth
- Harm to baby and/or self
- Pain
- Loss of control
- Interventions
- Loss of agency in decision-making
- Being abandoned/alone

**ADDRESS AND TRANSFORM YOUR FEARS** →

**HELPFUL PRACTICES**

- Talk about fears with care providers early on
- Create a supportive environment and community
- Gather information and good stories that allow you to feel empowered and confident
- Practice positive daily mantras, meditation, and movement
- Trust in your body and your instincts

# The Hormones of Pregnancy & Labor

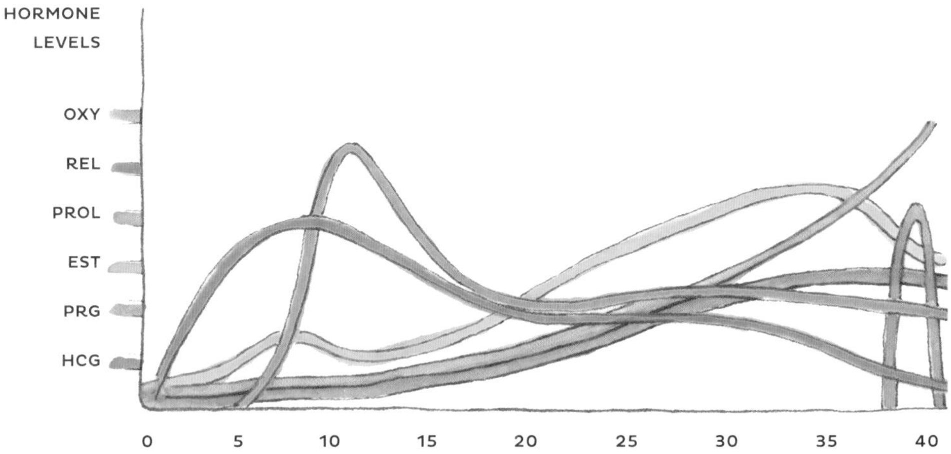


Progesterone climbs steadily throughout pregnancy, reaching its peak at 36 weeks. One of its many roles is to inhibit uterine contractions, protecting the fetus from preterm birth. As progesterone levels decrease in late gestation, the amount of estrogen becomes higher than the amount of progesterone, which causes the uterine smooth muscle to become sensitive to oxytocin. Oxytocin stimulates forceful and effective uterine contractions during labor and birth. Fetal cortisol and prostaglandins are also involved in the strength of uterine contractions. Notice that prolactin levels gradually climb during pregnancy. This hormone plays a role in developing the fetal lungs and brain, stimulates oxytocin release, and is required for enlarging mammary glands and for milk production.

When I had watched enough birth videos and read enough stories, I started to feel comfortable in my discomfort. One shift I felt distinctly was my ability to relate to the birthing people in the videos and stories. Before, they were "other" and their experience was unimaginable. They eventually became my connection point to possibility, and I was encouraged and supported by their stories. When you are told to face your fears, perhaps it means living them over and over and over again until they are no longer fears but possibilities for empowerment.

In one study, pregnant people who identified as "self-determiners" who were not afraid of childbirth, who believed birth is a natural process, and who had clear attitudes about their birth preferences, had the highest numbers of unmedicated vaginal births compared to those who were fearful and those from the "take it as it comes" group, who weren't necessarily afraid but didn't have a clear preference for vaginal or C-section birth. The presence of fear has the greatest negative impact on our feelings about pregnancy, our emotional health, our experience of birth, and our parenting. Our attitudes and beliefs, more than any other factor, shape our birth experience and outcomes.

## THE HORMONES OF LABOR

Giving birth is a coordinated event of transition that requires participation and harmony among you, your baby, and the placenta. For many months, your uterus has quietly held your growing baby, maybe practicing for birth here and there with Braxton Hicks contractions. When labor begins, the smooth muscle of the uterus wakes up and becomes a powerful, rhythmic contraction machine. These contractions synchronize with the changes in the cervix while hormonal, neuroendocrine, immune, and inflammatory mechanisms overlap and contribute to the onset of labor and its progression.

Your cervix structurally changes as you near the onset of labor and prostaglandins encourage it to soften and thin. Throughout pregnancy, the cervix is cinched closed, and its job is to keep the baby in your uterus so they can fully grow and develop. To do this, your cervix must be strong because the amniotic sac and growing baby are heavy and exerting immense pressure on this small structure. Then, as labor begins, the cervix gets the opposite job: soften, shorten, and dilate so that baby can emerge.

The cervix manages these two equally important but opposite roles through its unique structure. The composition of the cells in this sphincter give it the ability to change morphology, which it does before, during, and after birth, when it regains its nonpregnant structure. The mucus plug, an important but poorly named blockade in the cervical canal, sheds either before or throughout labor, and this shedding is described by medicine as the bloody show.

Labor is triggered by a complex series of hormonal and physiological changes. Progesterone levels gradually climb throughout pregnancy, reaching their peak at around thirty-six weeks, and then they start to decline. Progesterone's role is to relax the uterus, and it indirectly prevents uterine contractions. As progesterone levels fall, estrogen levels continue to climb. When the level of estrogen is higher than that of progesterone, uterine smooth muscle becomes more sensitive to stimuli that cause contractions.

Oxytocin, secreted by you and your baby's pituitary, stimulates contractions. Gradually, uterine smooth muscle becomes more sensitive to oxytocin, which results in stronger and more forceful contractions. Stronger contractions, as a result of higher oxytocin levels, tell the brain to keep sending down more oxytocin so that contractions remain effective and forceful. Our coping strategies, such as movement, touch, and moaning, encourage the continued release of oxytocin. Oxytocin is also produced by specific cells in the hypothalamus and bathes your brain. As the pain of labor intensifies, oxytocin increases as an adaptive and protective response to stress. Oxytocin, while cheering on and accelerating labor, also helps us cope with the process.

Beta-endorphins, our internal opiates that are released by the pituitary, increase our tolerance to pain and affect our experience with the present. As we labor more intensely, beta-endorphins rise, reaching their peak when the baby is born. They help us manage pain by altering our perception of discomfort. This is described as a dreamlike state, but my experience didn't feel removed; it felt like I was acting from a deeper place in myself. Another description of the role of beta-endorphins is that they allow us to go into ourselves and become more intuitive. Pain is instrumental and important for this process because it forces us to develop a rhythm and strategies to cope. If I focused on the pain as a thing that was separate from me, it felt too big and my mind started to fight against the feeling. The beta-endorphins seemed to alter my perception such that I knew the pain was purposeful. The pain wasn't bigger than me, the pain was me, and I needed to lean into it and keep going.

Catecholamines, which include epinephrine and norepinephrine, rise during labor and peak when the cervix fully dilates. At the end of my labor, during the final monumental contractions, I felt overwhelmed. The feeling was so big that when I think back on it, I can't even access the physical sensation or remember what I was seeing. This feeling of overwhelming pain with powerful contractions at the end of labor stimulates a generous release of catecholamines in both birthing parent and baby, giving us a boost of focus and extreme strength to push out the baby.

When we feel anxious or fearful or we perceive danger during early labor, catecholamines can inhibit uterine contractions and stop labor. This makes sense in the context of our evolution. These hormones allowed laboring people in danger to find a safer place to labor. Conversely, when catecholamines progressively increase and peak at the end of labor, this rise gives us an extra boost to push out the baby. These hormones also help babies during the birthing process and in their transition to life outside the womb. In her book *Gentle Birth, Gentle Mothering*, Sarah Buckley writes,

> High CA [catecholamine] levels at birth also ensure that the baby is wide eyed and alert at first contact with the mother. The baby's CA levels also drop steeply after an undisturbed birth, being soothed by contact with the mother, but norepinephrine levels remain elevated above normal for the first twelve hours. High newborn norepinephrine levels, triggered by a normal birth, have been shown to enhance olfactory learning during this period, helping the newborn learn the mother's smell.

This paragraph illustrates a few key concepts about the role of hormones in birth. First, they help facilitate the birth process. Second, our hormones fluctuate in a way that helps us build important relationships with each other

# Consider Your Senses

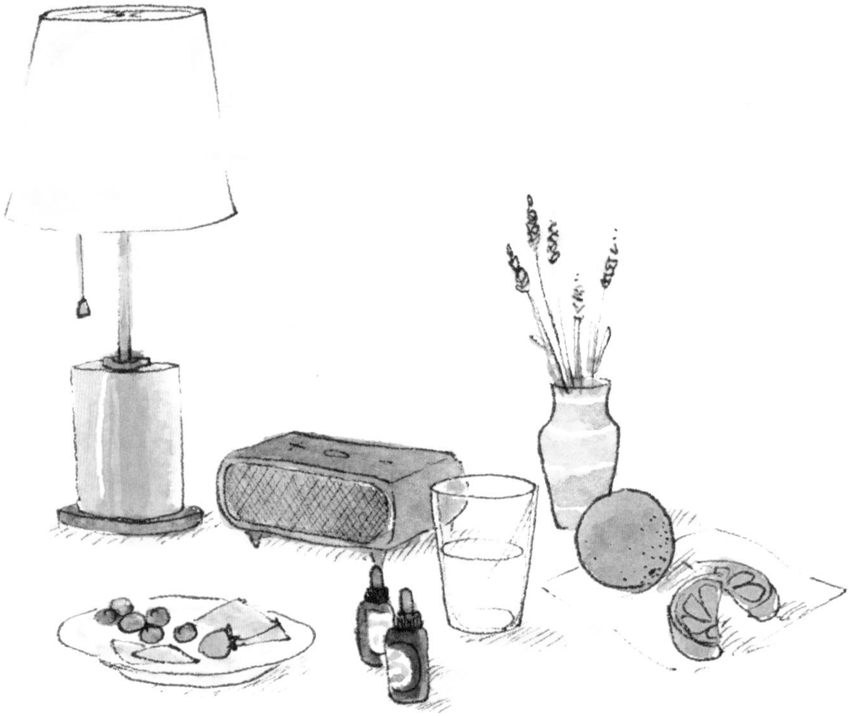

**SEE:** lights dimmed or off, light a candle or use battery-operated candles
**HEAR:** gentle music, nature sounds, mantras; turn off phones and ask people who are talking to step outside the birthing space
**SMELL:** aromatherapy, essential oils (e.g., peppermint, citrus, lavender, clary sage)
**TASTE:** light, easy, energizing foods, like nut butters and fruit, water, and coconut water
**FEEL:** soft fabrics; gentle, soothing touch; massage; counterpressure; skin-to-skin contact with baby and a warm, cozy blanket after birth

and the world. Third, the interaction and role of our hormones evolved for thousands of years when birth was undisturbed and unmedicated.

Each of the hormones that mediate birth are susceptible to disruption. As an exercise, imagine you are sitting next to a river with tall trees surrounding you. You can't hear cars, music, or machines. The river is soothing and the leaves are gently humming in the breeze, scattering warm sunshine onto your skin. You smell the forest and your shoulders relax and you understand what researchers mean when they write that physiological relaxation effects are caused by forest-derived olfactory stimuli.

Now imagine sitting on the side of a highway. You are rightfully scared. Your nostrils and eyes burn as you breathe in the unpleasant smell of exhaust. Cars and trucks rush past you, honking and swerving. Your stress hormones kick in to keep you alive. It is loud, uncomfortable, hot, and you feel out of control.

Go back to the forest. Our senses—what we see, hear, taste, smell, and feel—give our body information about how to function, and this information impacts hormonal secretion. Disruptions in the form of panic—by the birthing parent or team, painful or disruptive procedures, lack of support, or constant interruptions—can stall our labor as they increase catecholamines. We sense that this isn't a safe place to birth our baby, and our bodies respond in turn.

Oxytocin and beta-endorphin production are supported by feelings of calm and safety and are disturbed by unwelcome people and noise. Oxytocin works synergistically with melatonin. Regardless of age, labor most often peaks between midnight and 5 a.m. Turn down the lights. In early and active labor, catecholamine levels stay lower when we feel private and safe. When we trust our team, feel confident in our capabilities, and are informed, we can go into ourselves.

## THE PURPOSE OF PAIN

Wherever we decide to birth our babies, and whatever decisions we make about that process, it is essential to remember that our bodies feel safe and calm in a forest type of environment. The hospital can feel like a highway and interventions like swerving traffic. The medical model of birth views discomfort as something to be treated and it offers a hand to patients, saying, "Let me help you do this" instead of "You are fully capable." So much of this model is demonized, but it is actually based on a type of kindness.

The pain of labor, I've heard a few doctors say, is just like any other pain and should be treated the same way. They say that we have tools that treat pain and we should use them. Those tools are focused on interventions like epidurals and medicines, not necessarily environmental modulation, movement, and support. I used to fight against the idea that childbirth pain is just like other pain, but then I realized it both is and it isn't.

The pain of birthing a baby is like other pain in that it tells your brain to protect your body. In response to a painful sensation, you try to figure out how to make it more manageable. Moving, breathing, moaning, swaying, leaning against another person—all these actions are physiologically normal responses to pain. Just like we walk differently to protect a sprained ankle to prevent further injury, we move and change positions during labor. These movements help us cope and stay calm, which allows the hormones that progress labor to operate optimally, and they also encourage the baby to turn and move down through the birth canal. These movements we perform in response to pain help protect our birth canal and the baby who moves through it. Pain forces us to acknowledge and respond to pressure, and as we shift or lean forward and move in ways that are unrestricted, those movements facilitate birth. Pain is not an unfortunate side effect of labor; it is a facilitative and essential part of labor and birth.

Where labor pain differs from the pain of a sprained ankle is in how we manage and approach the pain. A sprained ankle is a problem and the solution is rest. If we treat labor like a problem and the solution as rest in the form of something like an epidural, we can't feel pain and we stop moving. This change can alter our hormonal response, and our inability to move changes how we birth and is less protective for our baby and birth canal. The standard of care for hospital birth includes continuous fetal heart rate monitoring, epidurals (restricted movement), restricted eating and drinking, and IVs. Again, these interventions come from a place of care and are sometimes essential to protect birthing people and babies. Unfortunately, they can also interfere with our instincts and with the physiological process of labor and birth.

## INTERVENTIONS AND CHOICE

There is no morality associated with how you birth your baby. You are not lesser or incapable if you choose an epidural or require a C-section. Epidurals can provide birthing people with essential rest and pain relief, and C-sections can save lives. The point of this discussion is that there can be a mismatch between how we as mammals have historically birthed and the environments where we give birth now. In all circumstances, you should feel empowered and able to create and promote the best possible environment for you and your baby no matter how or where your baby is born.

During the last four weeks of my pregnancy, I had appointments with my midwife, Amanda, once a week. "How are you doing?" she'd ask me. "Good, fine," I'd respond every time. Throughout my pregnancy, and especially during these weekly visits, we discussed her approach to interventions. When it came to inducing labor, for a healthy mom and baby with no complications, she said she wouldn't bring it up until around forty-one weeks. I was relieved that I didn't have to think about the possibility for a few more weeks. If a provider recommends or offers labor induction, we have the right to understand why, and we can ask if there's any way to wait until thirty-nine weeks to induce.

I'm the youngest of three in my family and the most stubborn. My oldest brother was born a week before his due date, and his labor was smooth. My mom went to the hospital in the morning, had him in the afternoon, and left that night. My other brother was born two weeks before his due date. When he came out my parents knew, immediately, that he was different from my oldest brother, and they learned he had Down syndrome pretty soon after he was born. When my mom was pregnant with me, she scheduled an amniocentesis, canceled it, then scheduled it again. The context of her decision-making changed based on her prior experience. She was part of a support group for parents who had children with disabilities. When I was a week overdue, she was worried about health problems for me. Her labor was induced with Pitocin, and I was born vaginally a few hours later. She said I was by far her most painful labor, but she was grateful I was healthy.

Inductions should be offered when medically necessary, such as when the birthing parent has a health problem like preeclampsia, if there is an infection in the uterus, or in other circumstances where the health of the birthing person or baby is threatened. The common interventions used to get labor started are synthetic prostaglandins (which thin and soften the cervix), artificial rupture of membranes, and membrane stripping, which can also release prostaglandins and encourage contractions to start. Pitocin, which is synthetic oxytocin, is often used when a birthing person gets an epidural and labor slows down or when a baby is past due.

The chemical structure of synthetic Pitocin is the same as our endogenous oxytocin. The difference between the two is the way it is delivered in the body. Oxytocin, as discussed earlier, is produced by the pituitary and hypothalamus. The pituitary releases oxytocin into the bloodstream through pulses. These pulses of oxytocin cause the uterus to contract rhythmically. The amount of oxytocin released gradually increases in a complex and interactive relationship with our bodies and with where we're at in the labor process. Our environment impacts our nervous system, which affects whether oxytocin is released or inhibited.

When we receive Pitocin through an IV, the dose is not tightly regulated by the brain and it's not delivered in pulses. The result is contractions that are longer, more forceful, and closer together with less pain relief, since Pitocin is unlikely to cross the blood-brain barrier to help us cope with the increased stress and pain. When contractions are longer and more forceful, babies are squeezed tighter and we worry more about their oxygenation and heart rate. Continuous heart rate monitoring tends to be standard fare, but some hospitals offer mobile or intermittent fetal monitoring, which allows for movement.

# Labor and Birth Positions

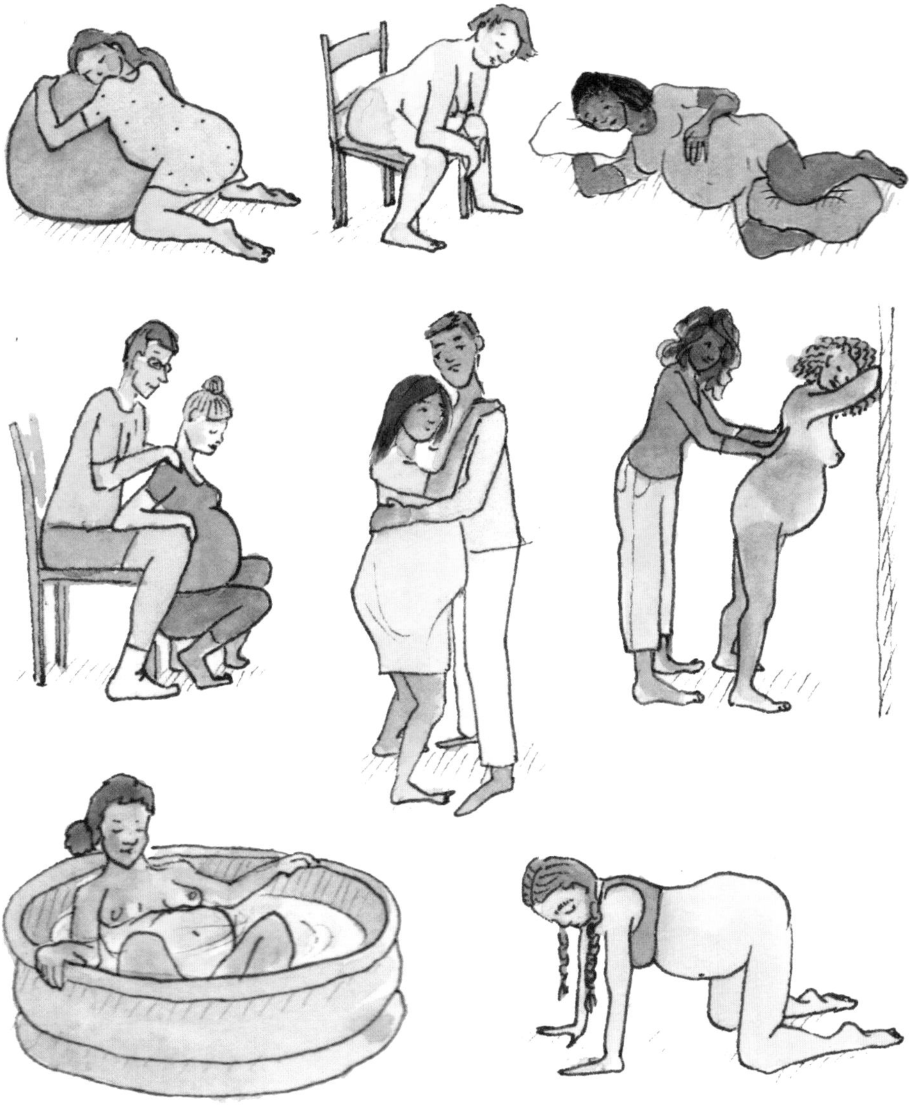

# The Four Stages of Labor

**SIGNS OF LABOR**

- "Bloody show" (mucus mixed with blood) expelled from the vagina.
- Contractions (generally intervals of less than 10 minutes).
- Rupture of membranes (water breaking).

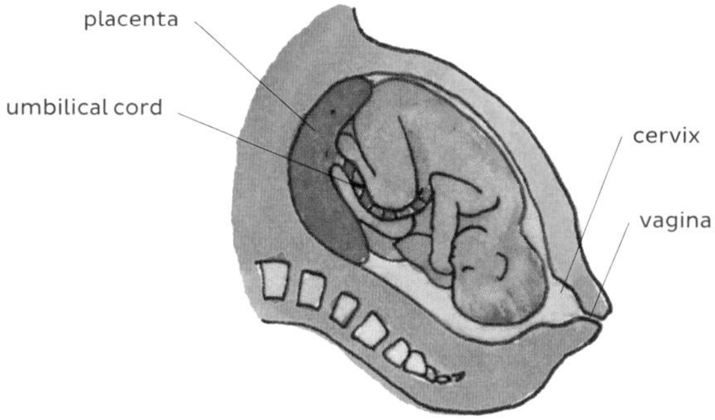


**STAGE 1**

**Early Labor/Latent Phase**

- The cervix opens to 4 cm.
- Contractions are generally 5–20 minutes apart (or all over the place!), becoming more frequent.
- This is usually the longest and least intense phase.

**Active Phase**

- The cervix opens to 4–7 cm.
- Contractions become stronger and are generally 3–4 minutes apart.

**Transition Phase**

- The cervix opens to 8–10 cm.
- Contractions are strong and last 60–90 seconds every few minutes, which is when you'll likely feel the urge to push.

### STAGE 2

- This stage begins when the cervix is completely dilated and ends with the birth of your baby.
- Pushing generally lasts 30 minutes to 2 hours.

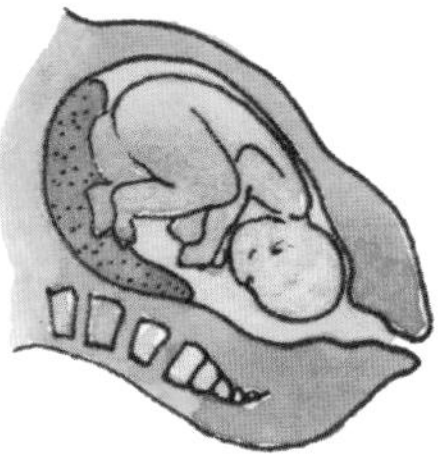

DESCENT, FLEXION

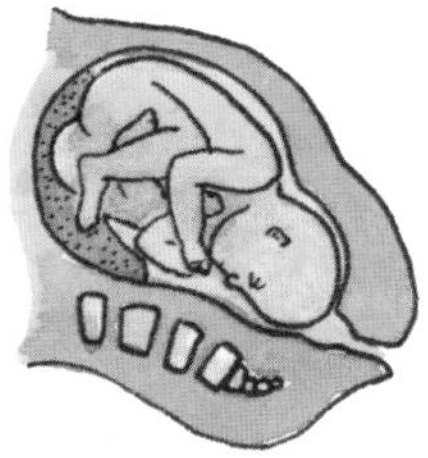

INTERNAL ROTATION

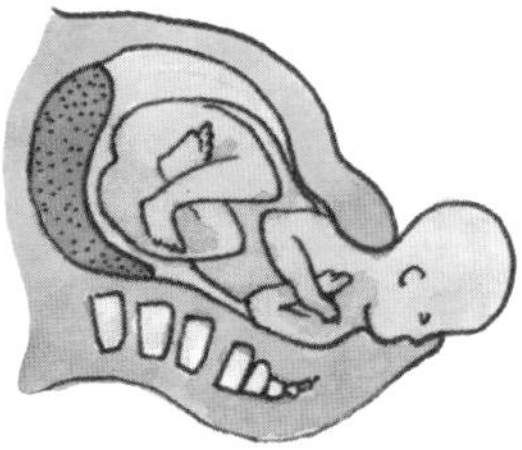

EXTENSION

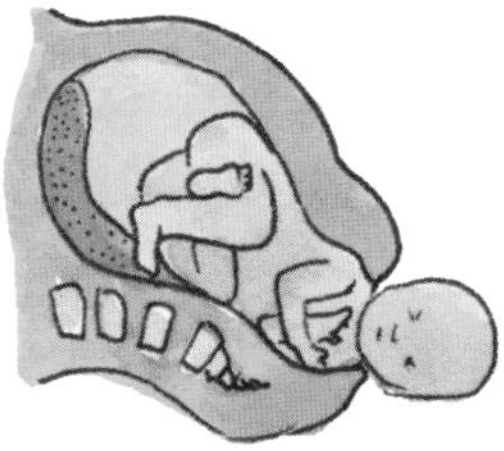

RESTITUTION

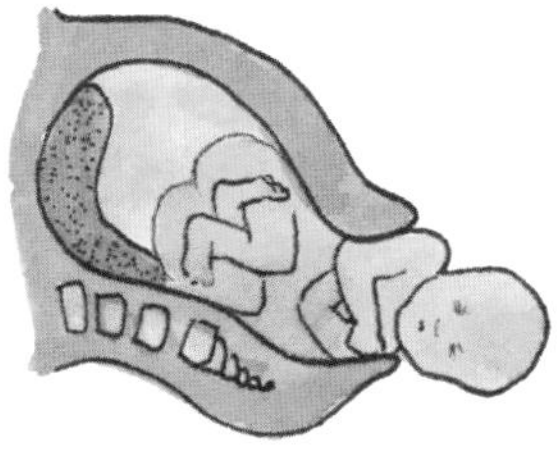

ANTERIOR SHOULDER DELIVERY

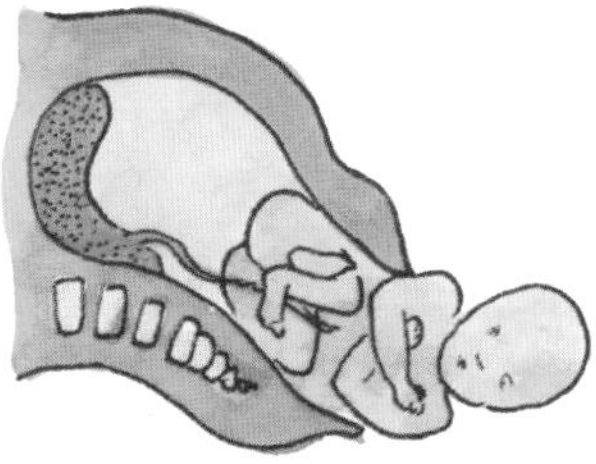

POSTERIOR SHOULDER DELIVERY

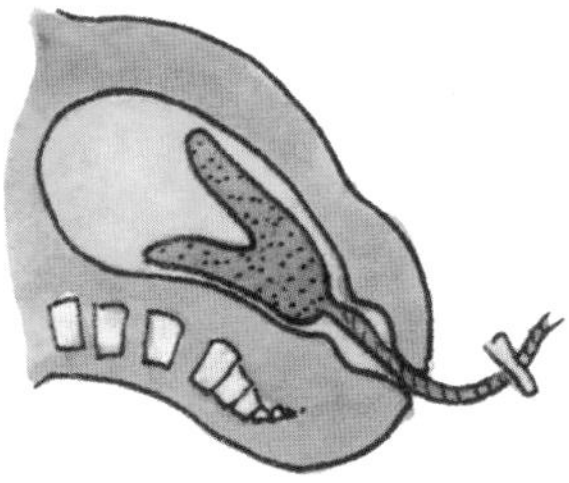

### STAGE 3

- The uterus continues to contract, and the placenta is usually delivered 5–15 minutes after the baby.

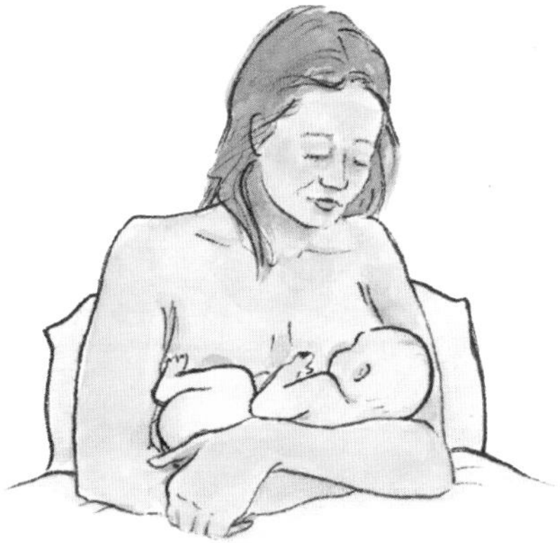

### STAGE 4

Recovery, bonding, and rest.

Pitocin and epidurals tend to go hand in hand. Epidurals are the most common, and normalized, intervention. According to a 2018 study from the journal *Anesthesiology*, 71 percent of birthing people in the US opt into epidurals or other spinal anesthesia. The word "intervention" refers to an intervention of the birth process, which means an intervention of our physiology. Epidurals interfere with the communication between our brain and our body, and this numbing of the lower body is one of most effective measures for pain relief. The risks include a dangerous drop in blood pressure, fever, headaches, itching, a prolonged second stage of labor, and a higher likelihood of the use of vacuum or forceps delivery.

Before I gave birth I had a hard time believing, or I didn't quite understand, what people meant when they talked about birth as a spiritual or transformative event. It was like everyone else had climbed to the top of the mountain where they experienced something that changed their life, and when they came back down and told me about their journey of transcendence, it was almost impossible for me to relate because I hadn't been there.

Unless we've lived the thing, we tend to meet the exuberance and conviction that follow transformation with derision and eyerolling. But when we go through our own transformation, or fall in love, we quickly become the people we so easily dismissed. Birth is like this. No matter how your baby is born, everyone gets a birth story, and it changes their whole life.

All interventions carry risks, and sometimes they happen even if we didn't want them or plan on them. Not all interventions like C-sections are bad experiences. They can be empowering, romantic, calm, and positive. They don't have to be lonely or scary. I know birthing people who have had C-sections, epidurals, and home births. There is no ranking or hierarchy connected to how we birth. What matters is that we feel empowered and that we're given every opportunity to bond with our babies.

## PROCESSING AND TELLING YOUR BIRTH STORY

I wrote down my birth story a few weeks after it happened. One reason I waited was because I needed to recover and care for my newborn. The other reason was that, right after birth, I thought, I don't want to do that again. That feeling took about a year to dissipate.

I noticed that my feelings toward birth changed with time. Right after, I felt sore all over. The experience of birth doesn't end when the baby and placenta come out. It persists with afterbirth as your uterus contracts and gradually returns to its prepregnancy size, a process called involution. I was ready for most parts of pregnancy, labor, and birth, but I wasn't ready for the pain of birth to persist. I thought that when it was over, it was over. Instead, for a few days, every time I fed my baby with my blistered nipples, my uterus was stimulated by oxytocin to contract and shrink. Those days were long.

Growing a baby, giving birth, and becoming a parent is a monumental transition. I had an innate desire to remember what happened and to integrate my experience into a narrative. In her book *Birth Your Story: Why Writing about Your Birth Matters*, Jaime Fleres writes,

> A birth story is the personal equivalent of the creation story that every civilization throughout time has constructed to make meaning of its collective experience. Consider the birth of Gaia in Greek mythology, Mary's birth of Jesus, and all the origin stories of cultures throughout time and space. We have a deep longing to know how we came to be and a deep need to share the incredible stories of bringing a child into this world.

After Holden was born, Max and I talked about the experience, recounting the story. I found it remarkable that we remembered parts of the process differently. We talked about the birth and ran into certain key moments where our realities diverged. "Then I lay down to birth the placenta," I said, nearing the end of the birth story. "You weren't lying down—you were sitting up, leaning against me," Max countered. I realized I wasn't a totally reliable narrator.

I had to gather some information and talk about the birth with Amanda, my mom, and Max, a process that helped me make meaning of my collective birth experience and see how a story was starting to take shape.

Writing has always helped me work through and understand important moments in my life. I figured out through writing my birth story that I felt more positive about the experience than I realized. Because I set out to write a story with a narrative arc, I examined the characters involved and felt more grateful for them. When I focused too much on pain, I searched for moments of humor and relief. I remembered details, like my cat rubbing against me during my contractions and blocking the doorway, so Amanda had to step over her to get to me. I remembered my mom bringing me breakfast the morning after Holden was born. She brought me three huge pieces of bacon and three eggs fried in bacon fat, and it was the best thing I ever tasted.

Writing about birth helps us process hard feelings like shame, embarrassment, and anger. Giving these feelings a name and exploring them frees them from repression so that we can begin to heal or see what we need to start healing. When trauma lives in the body, we suffer emotionally and physically. One reason trauma can harm our health so deeply is because our understanding of traumatic events is fragmented and doesn't make sense. In other words, the facts don't fit into a cohesive story, and as a result, we avoid thinking about them, but they beg our minds to resolve the fragments. In his article "Trauma and the Benefits of Writing about It," Art Markman writes,

> The mind is most settled when there is coherence to our thoughts. We seek to resolve conflicting thoughts by remembering them and processing them. So, a dangerous cycle can develop with traumatic events. Because they are fragmented, there are constant reminders of them. But, because they are painful, we do not process them deeply. And so, we suffer the stress of remembering a painful situation without resolving the incoherence.

One of the simplest and best therapies we have for processing trauma is writing. Writing allows us to explore connections and create a cohesive story. This process is not always enjoyable—it can be painful and emotional—but the long-term effects include better overall health and lower rates of depression.

The act of processing and telling our birth story allows us to choose how we want to remember the event. The form of sharing and who we share with is also our choice. We may want to share our stories with just ourselves, or an audience—we get to choose. Writing about birth is an act of agency. The story we craft gives us creative control over the narrative that shapes us and honors our experience through recollection and the process of writing, which requires immense care and attention to detail.

Writing is a recursive process. This means there are steps and stages that loop and bounce off one another, including invention, research, drafting, revision, and editing. These steps don't follow a specific order; they are alive and evolving. Long before I wrote down my story, these processes were happening naturally in my mind. When you feel ready to write your birth story, it helps to understand that the process isn't linear. We don't have to know where we're going or where we'll end up.

Our collective stories are powerful. Your story contains vital information that can ease other people's fears and anxiety. Your story can shape how others experience birth, decrease their pain, and improve their birth experience. Writing a story, like birth itself, is about the process. Each step, or word or contraction, leading to another and another, until you are holding a baby, or a story, in your hands, and it is more profound and meaningful than you could have ever imagined when you started.

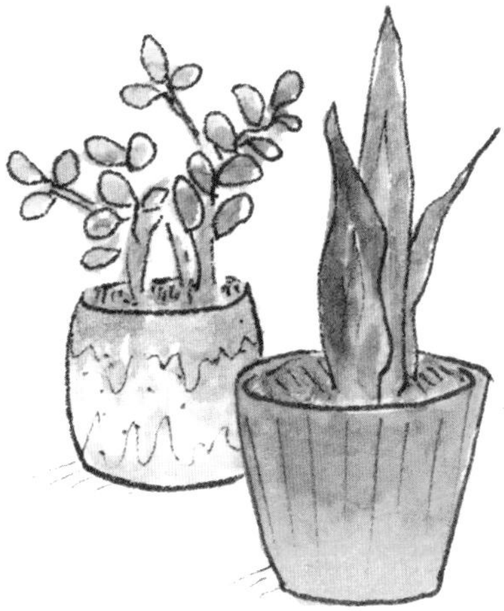

# Writing Your Birth Story

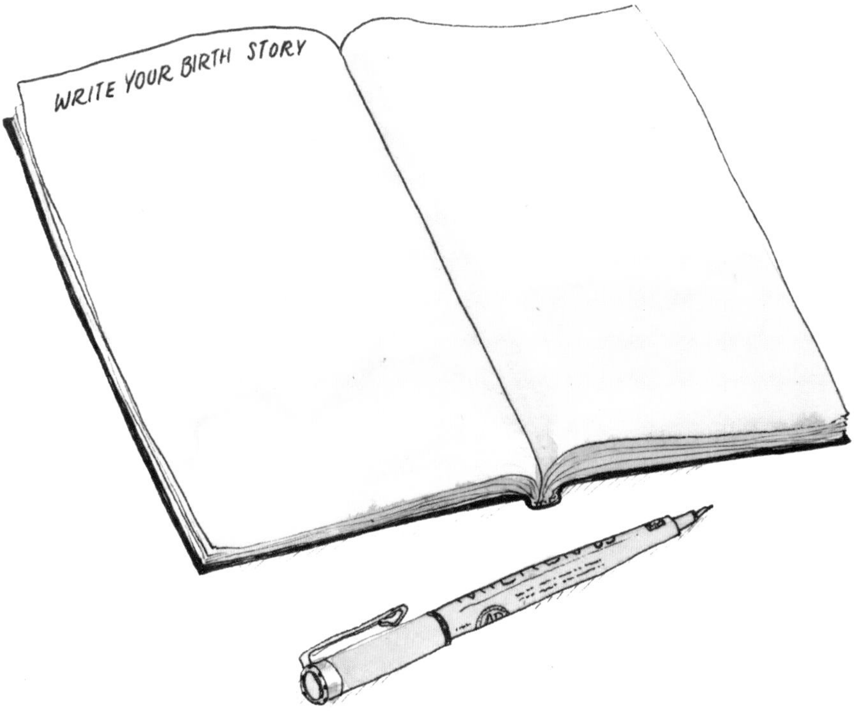


- Timeline of events: How did the birth begin? What events do you remember most? Least? What was unexpected, funny, scary, or beautiful? How do these events connect?
- Who was with you?
- Revisit your senses: What did you see, hear, smell, taste, and feel?
- If you're not ready to write the whole story, start with the small details.
- Integrate the details and reclaim your birth story so that it is healing and empowering for you and your baby.

# TAKE ACTION

Ask, "What if?" What if everything goes as planned? What if it doesn't? There are a lot of unknowns and what-ifs when it comes to birth. Asking yourself this question helps you face your greatest desires and fears and shapes your approach to labor and birth. Our attitude toward labor and birth impacts our perception of our experience. Remain open and aware that plans change and outcomes vary, but maintain a feeling of empowerment and know that you are capable.

Tend your senses and birth hormones. The hormones that facilitate the birth process are supported by feelings of calm and safety. They are disturbed by unwelcome people, noise, and feelings of fear. Consider each of your senses and create a birth environment that looks, smells, sounds, tastes, and feels nurturing and safe. Understand the role of pain in labor and birth and ensure you have the support you need.

Know that there is no morality associated with how you birth your baby. Your choice is paramount. Your unique physiology, personal history, and present situation come together to form your experience of becoming a parent. You deserve access to high-quality information, deep, unwavering support, and a feeling of focused empowerment.

Write your birth story. Processing and integrating your birth experience into a written story allows the mind to put fragments into a cohesive narrative. When you write your story, you explore connections and you choose how you want to remember the event. The writing, like birth itself, is a process. Be gentle and kind with yourself.

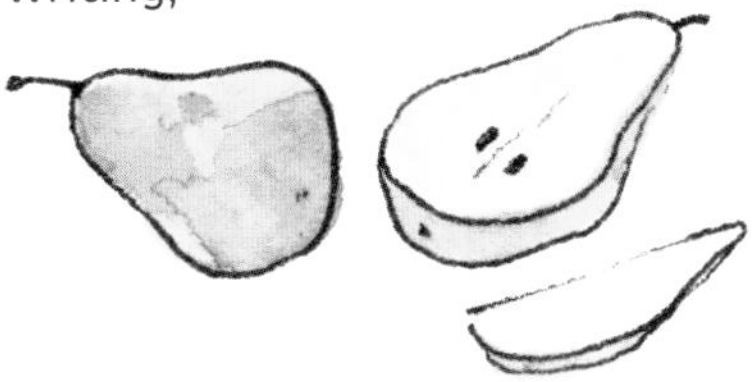

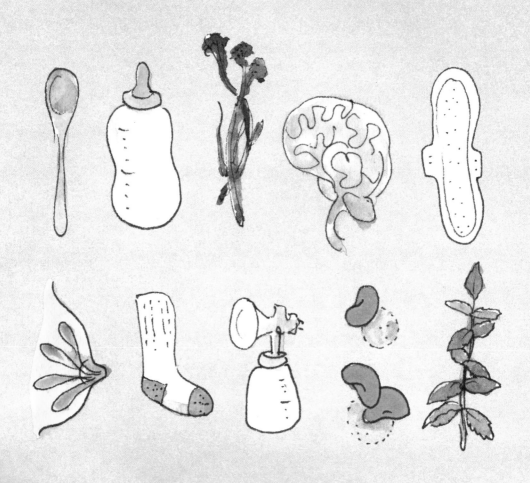

# Part Three

# GROWING YOUR BABY on the OUTSIDE

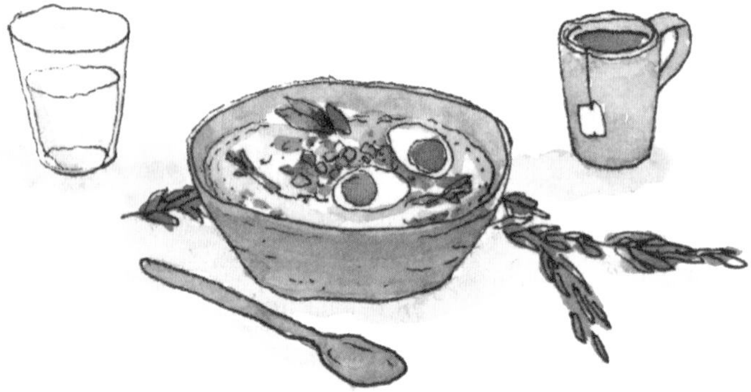

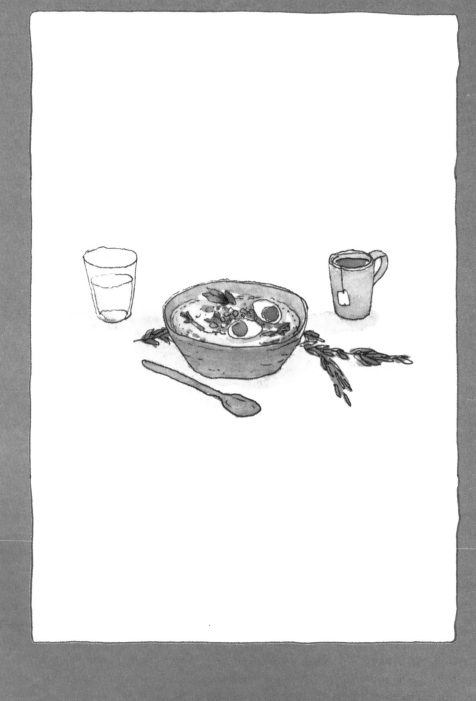

CHAPTER NINE

# Rest, Recovery & Gentle Movement

A WEEK OR TWO AFTER Holden was born, when winter was cascading into spring, I heard a sound around four in the morning that at first surprised me with delight and then suddenly and unexpectedly filled me with a sense of relief. The sound was one of hope and possibility. It seemed to fill my house and reverberate through my body like a cheering squad. The music of this sound urged the sun to come up and at the same time filled me with lightness. Because of the sound and the day it brought, I never missed watching a sunrise when Holden was a newborn. I watched the sun come up and light the faces of Max and Holden, who often slept in the same position with the same expression.

The birds' spring song was my beacon of hope. Their cheery, industrious music soothed my mind during my transition into motherhood. When I heard their song, I relaxed and understood that my new worries and anxieties were feelings I had to learn how to manage and live through. With the surge of new love I felt for Holden, I also felt an overwhelming feeling of worry and responsibility. Each day cycled like this for a while. I'd feel confident and capable during the day, especially when I was moving in the sun with my baby. Around dinnertime it occurred to me that the night was coming, and I felt a quiet kind of dread, and then the birds sang to me at dawn and the sun came up again. I'm not sure why the birds made such a difference. I just let the good feeling of their song sweep over me without question.

Routine beacons of hope, like birdsong and beautiful sunrises, centered and soothed me after Holden was born. When my tunnel vision widened, I could look outside and realize I was just like the other animal mothers, and we were all welcoming dawn together with relief.

## MATRESCENCE AND TRANSITION

The goal of anthropologist Dana Raphael was, through her writing and research, to support people during birth, breastfeeding, and the process of becoming parents. She coined the term "matrescence" to describe the transition birthing people experience when they have babies. Like adolescence, matrescence is a physiological-hormonal-emotional event. And, like puberty for adolescents, birthing and caring for a baby deeply and irrevocably changes us. In the literature, matrescence applies to the birthing parent and is understood as a uniquely maternal phenomenon; however, parents, regardless of gender, experience a state of transition with the arrival of a new baby.

The concept of matrescence has since been expanded and popularized by Dr. Alexandra Sacks, who describes matrescence as an "emotional tug-of-war." Just as pregnancy changes the shape of our bodies, caring for a baby changes the space we occupy in the world. We fit differently, not only into our clothes but also into the social structures we built around ourselves before we had a baby. Joy and tension, love and anxiety, hope and fear live together in our bodies like new roommates sharing a studio apartment. We may fight to hold on to our separateness or find ourselves intertwined so fully with our babies that we lose sight of ourselves. Figuring out the balance between our separate identity and our identity as parents who recognize and meet our babies' needs takes time and learning. Matrescence is a transitory journey, and there are many forms of normal within the process. Where one parent may feel love-struck and blissful with their newborn, another may feel lonely, overwhelmed, and detached. Or all these feelings may overlap.

The postpartum period, in Western culture, is defined as a period of six to eight weeks wherein your body returns to its prepregnant state. At the time of this writing, Holden is nearing his second birthday and my body has yet to return to its prepregnant state. My clothes from before all fit, but the shape of my pelvis feels different. My weight is the same as before pregnancy, but I wear it differently. My right breast is significantly larger than my left and produces twice as much milk. My brain, as I'll discuss in the chapter on brain changes and neuroplasticity, has changed since he was born. My wiring is different. You cannot, therefore, have a baby and then return to a prepregnant state.

Instead of expecting to return to a prepregnant state, many cultures around the world practice postpartum rituals and habits that nurture matrescence and the newborn. The postpartum period is about transitioning to a new reality, not returning to a past body. Traditional postpartum practices focus on a defined period of rest, a specific prescribed diet, and prearranged support.

## BREAKING THE RULES OF *ZUO YUE ZI*

Rest is vaguely prescribed to all new parents after giving birth. While I understood the idea and goal of rest, I wasn't sure what it would look like for me and what practices would allow me to feel truly rested. Before Holden's birth I read about how, in other cultures, the defined period of rest, confinement, or lying-in after birth generally ranges from thirty to forty days. I imagined the walls of my home growing thick, expanding like a fortress covered in impenetrable ivy that would protect us during our time of bonding and healing after birth. But then I imagined an open window that let in the sunlight and my garden full of winter greens and my chickens clucking in the spring air. From my imagination I learned that I needed to navigate a postpartum path that worked for me in my world and culture.

Traditionally, Chinese women "sit the month," a practice called *zuo yue zi* in Traditional Chinese Medicine. Warm and restorative food and drink promote the restoration of their vital energy and balance. A few of the traditional rules of *zuo yue zi* include avoiding contact with cold and wind, avoiding showers and baths, consuming warm, cooked, restorative foods and liquids, resting, sleeping, eating, and feeding your baby without distractions (like books and TV)—and no visitors. *Zuo yue zi* includes a caretaker for the full month that helps facilitate rest and focused newborn care. Even now, when I read about *zuo yue zi*, I feel the essential importance of caring for the new parent and new baby. But as I reflected on my postpartum period, which felt sacred, cocooned, and restorative, I realized that I broke almost every *zuo yue zi* rule.

The first rule I broke was the one about showering. During Holden's birth I experienced a small labial tear. While I lay there with my aching sore legs wide open, getting stitches, I learned that the labia is a weird place to tear and a challenging place to stitch. My legs were so heavy and achy from laboring in a squat that I needed help from the midwives to move them when they finished. When I tried to go pee, I felt a sense of fear and nothing came out.

When I carefully made my way into the shower, I felt each incredible, hot drop of water land on my skin and melt some of my pain away. The shower allowed me to relax enough to pee. I peed and kept peeing like I hadn't peed in months. Relief crashed into my aching body. Blood and birthing fluid washed away down the drain. I closed my eyes and felt water cascade over my head and face. When I washed my hair, I inhaled the uplifting, clean smell of my shampoo. My shower was my sensory renewal. It was my own baptism after becoming a mother.

# Traditional Postpartum Practices

**INFANT CARE:** Intentional and deep bonding between the birthing parent and new baby is prioritized. This bonding is intended to establish breast-milk supply and breast-feeding and nurture the relationship between parent and baby without stress and distractions.

**REST PERIOD:** A period of 30–40 days spent staying home, limiting visitors and media, and moving gently is crucial for emotional and physical healing and for bonding with baby. Many cultures believe this period of rest is essential for long-term well-being and that without it, parents are vulnerable to illnesses and imbalance.

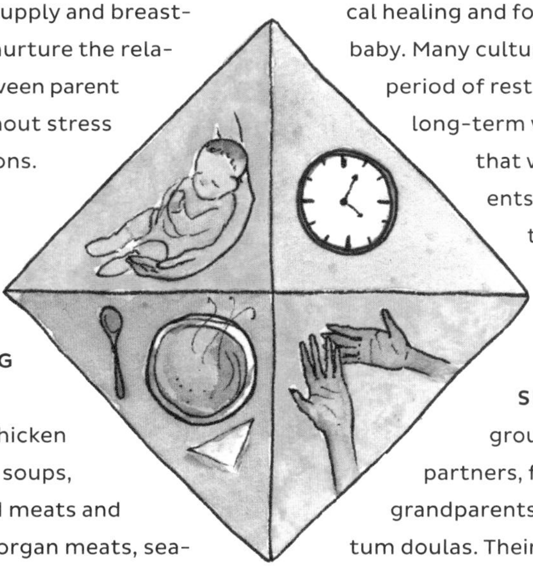

**NOURISHING FOOD AND WARMTH:** Chicken and seaweed soups, slow-roasted meats and stews, eggs, organ meats, seafood, bone broths, congee, ginger, cinnamon, curries, and herbal teas are examples of traditional postpartum foods that help tissues heal. These foods replenish nutrient stores, enrich milk, and offer a sense of well-being. Warm baths, hot massages, warm clothes, and hot wraps are believed to prevent illnesses and restore balance to the body after birth.

**ORGANIZED SUPPORT:** This group may include partners, family, friends, grandparents, and postpartum doulas. Their role is to take care of you so that you can rest, recover, and bond with your baby. Crucially, organized support helps relieve feelings of loneliness and isolation.

Breaking the rule about showering taught me a lesson about what I needed for my own rest and recovery. The shower taught me about sensory rituals. To be OK, I learned that I needed to get up in the morning, wash my face, and get dressed in clothes that weren't pajamas. When I washed my face, I massaged my cheeks and forehead, head and neck, and applied my face oil lovingly. I handled myself the same way I handled my baby—with supreme tenderness and care. Taking this time was a lesson in feeling whole. Each gentle motion put some pieces back together and connected me to myself. When I ate, I tasted each incredible bite of food. When I moved, I checked in with each part of my body. These sensory, ritual acts set my system such that my interaction with Holden was equally intentional.

The next rule I broke was the one about lying in and not going outside. Two days after Holden was born, it was a beautiful spring day. We put on warm clothes and took a slow-motion walk around our very small block. I checked in with my pelvic floor. I scolded myself for getting out of bed. I should be resting, I shouldn't be walking yet—but the sun was warm on my back and the air was fresh. Carrying my baby these first few steps felt like a ceremony. My lochia, or the vaginal bleeding and discharge after birth, didn't increase with my five-minute walk, so I felt OK with my decision to move.

Even as I believed wholly that I should be resting, I felt the pull of the sun and fresh air. Walking was important to me before birth, and it was my therapy after birth. Each day I walked carefully and paid attention to my breathing. I held my baby in my arms, noticing his weight slowly increasing and my arms growing stronger. I felt my uterus change and noticed the position and shape of my pelvis. Each day when I returned from my walk with Holden, my house looked a little brighter and I felt more comfortable sitting and nursing for hours. Being a parent was, and still is, easier when I'm outside. I sense a change in Holden's nervous system when we walk out the door. If he is unsettled inside, he finds his feet firmly planted on the earth and his whole body engaged when we go outside.

Distractions came next. Faithfully and full of dedicated integrity, I tried not to use my phone, read books, or watch any shows. Slowly, over the course of a few days, a pile of fourth-trimester and baby books started to travel with me around the house. I would turn the pages while Holden nursed or slept on my chest and feel comforted just by reading information about my present reality.

A few weeks after Holden's birth, during a marathon feed, I watched an episode of *Chef's Table* with the sound on low. It was the one about Jeong Kwan, the Korean Zen Buddhist nun. With stunning cinematography of the temple and the surrounding forests, the episode is one of the most beautiful and peaceful in the series. Kwan moves through the world with steady fluidity and playful curiosity. Wasn't this how I imagined myself as a mother? I believe deeply that my ability to be open, playful, and curious are as essential as my ability to provide stability. As a parent and a writer, my actions are led not by a feeling of superiority and ego but by fascination and caring. And I am deeply and unwaveringly appreciative of food and the nourishment it provides. We live in a world where the media we choose can offer us either quiet beauty and insight about life or the opposite.

Max and I rewatched each episode of *Chef's Table* over the course of a few weeks. Sometime around two months old or so, Holden became increasingly aware of his environment. Now I reflect on that period of time with a sort of aching nostalgia. It's been so long since I've watched a movie or a show that I can't remember the last one I saw. Whether you choose to completely eliminate distractions or to dabble in some light reading and binge-watching, the quiet, sleepy days of early postpartum go by slow minute by minute but fast in the grand scheme of time.

*Zuo yue zi* and other healing postpartum traditions gave me an ideal model of what my fourth-trimester life could look like and how sacred that time was. Without a guide, I could have fallen into traps where I expected too much of my body and paid too little attention to the moment. Just as I would translate a different language into one I understand, I needed to translate traditional postpartum practices into my life and culture. I didn't break all the rules. I ate bowls of congee, a traditional dish where rice is cooked into a porridge with bone broth, and other nourishing foods that helped me heal and supported my milk production and Holden's development. For around thirty days after birth, life slowed all the way down, allowing me to tune in to this new person and our new reality.

## INTERTWINED

Slowing down and taking care of yourself after birth helps support your physical recovery and facilitates bonding with your baby. This matters, both for your well-being and your baby's well-being, because the interrelated hormonal physiology that existed between you and your baby when you were pregnant continues after birth. In other words, the hormones in your body and in your baby's body are impacted by your relationship. After birth, our progesterone and estrogen drop rapidly. For people with increased risk factors, which include prenatal anxiety and a history of depression, inadequate support, low socioeconomic status, family history, and others we're still discovering, this drop can result in the baby blues or trigger the onset of postpartum depression.

### The Stages of Postpartum

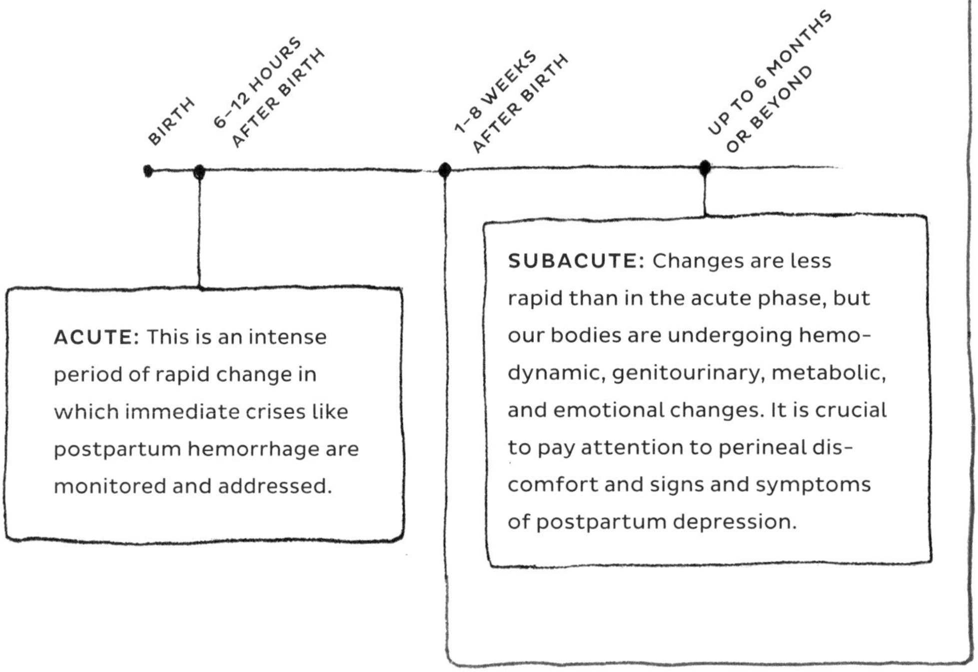

BIRTH
6–12 HOURS AFTER BIRTH
1–8 WEEKS AFTER BIRTH
UP TO 6 MONTHS OR BEYOND
ACUTE: This is an intense period of rapid change in which immediate crises like postpartum hemorrhage are monitored and addressed.
SUBACUTE: Changes are less rapid than in the acute phase, but our bodies are undergoing hemodynamic, genitourinary, metabolic, and emotional changes. It is crucial to pay attention to perineal discomfort and signs and symptoms of postpartum depression.

**Baby blues:** Baby blues are experienced by 50%–85% of birthing parents. The typical onset is 2–3 days postpartum, and symptoms such as mood swings, anxiety, sadness, irritability, crying, reduced concentration, and trouble sleeping last for up to 10 days and then tend to resolve. **What helps?:** Support from your partner, family, friends, or hired help; rest and nutrition; spending time outside; continuing to take vitamin D3 and prenatal vitamins; and being gentle with yourself and your expectations help alleviate the baby blues.

**Postpartum depression:** This condition usually presents within the first month postpartum but can happen anytime in the first year. Numbers vary, but some estimates state that 1 in 5 birthing parents experience postpartum depression, which is characterized by symptoms that last longer than 2 weeks, including severe mood swings and anxiety, a depressed mood, intense anger and irritability, insomnia or sleeping too much, reduced interest in previously enjoyed activities, feelings of guilt or inadequacy, and thoughts of harming yourself or baby. **What helps?:** Talk to your health-care provider and get a referral for a mental health professional. Treatments include different kinds of therapy and antidepressant medication. Social support in the form of partner support or parent support groups are essential for recovery. Checking your thyroid function, optimizing your rest, and eating nourishing foods (especially those rich in omega-3s) are important, as is movement (especially outside) and vitamin $D_3$.

**Postpartum psychosis:** Symptoms usually begin during the first 3 months postpartum and are characterized by a depressed mood, confusion, disorientation to place and time, obsessive thoughts about baby, hallucinations, paranoia, attempts to harm yourself or baby, and/or suicidal thoughts. **What helps?:** Postpartum psychosis is a medical emergency and requires immediate medical attention—that is, the ER or a crisis center. Treatment includes antipsychotics, mood stabilizers, and different forms of therapy.

**Delayed postpartum:** Technically this period lasts up to 6 months, but after you have a baby, you are in a postpartum period forever. The changes are gradual. You rebuild connective tissue and muscle tone, and you may feel shifts in your identity and relationship to your body, your partner, and your baby.

# The Hormones of Postpartum

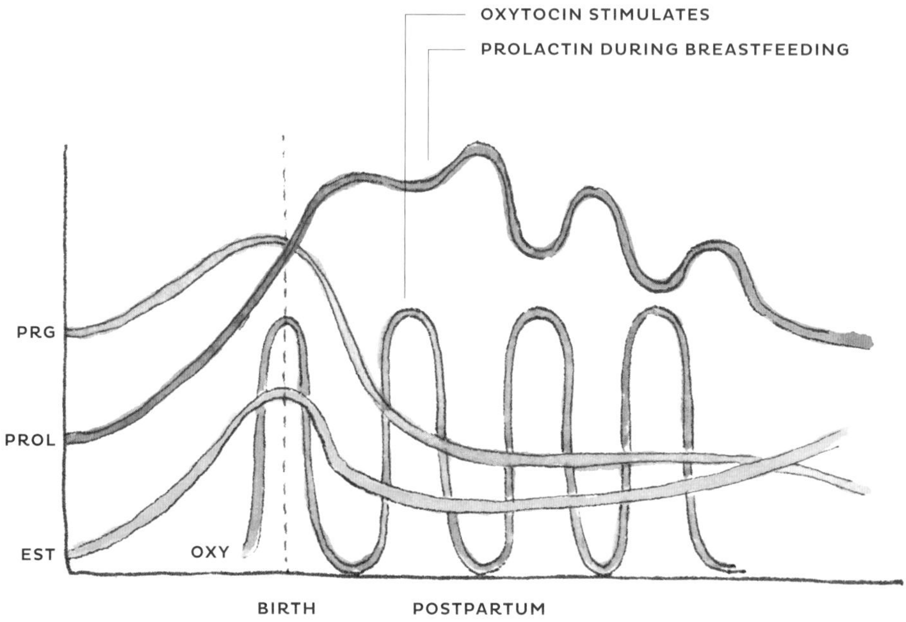


Birth is marked by profound hormonal changes in the birthing parent. Progesterone and estrogen peak at birth and then drop dramatically. Oxytocin and prolactin also surge at birth, and then levels ebb and flow with breastfeeding or chestfeeding. These four hormones interact in a complex dance that impacts mood, energy, anxiety levels, brain structure, breast size, and milk production. Oxytocin causes the uterus to contract and return to its normal size in about 6 weeks or so. Dynamic changes in hormones can also cause changes in your skin and hair loss and regrowth, and can impact the return of fertility.

While I didn't experience postpartum depression with Holden, I could feel it lingering nearby. Until I had him, I didn't understand why or how postpartum depression was so common. After his birth, I understood that any extra challenge—with nursing, birth interventions, medications, low birth weight, trouble with weight gain, sleep, behavior, lack of support—could easily invite anxiety, shame, and depression into the postpartum experience. Even in the absence of specific challenges and complications, the baseline requirements of caring for a newborn are demanding enough that anxiety and depression may still find their way into our bodies and impact our thoughts and behaviors. Each day after his birth I scanned my body and brain. Was I getting what I needed? Was I OK? Were we all safe? I ran through these questions with myself, answering them honestly, prepared to ask for help if I needed it.

Oxytocin is the great balancer to the hormonal transition we experience following birth. Nursing and skin-to-skin contact regulate newborns' and parents' oxytocin systems and physiology. When we experience challenges with breastfeeding or chestfeeding and lactation, postpartum depression is more common. The hormones prolactin and oxytocin regulate the synthesis and letdown of breast milk and regulate mood and behavior. Birth interventions like induction or C-sections can impact oxytocin and prolactin levels and receptors. Interventions and other challenges, such as low birth weight and preterm birth, can negatively impact how our bodies experience matrescence, or the transition into parenthood.

The way we process our labor and birth can impact our hormones, emotions, and healing. If our birth felt especially traumatic, or like a disappointment because it didn't go how we dreamed and planned, and we have nowhere to put these feelings, we can get stuck and our bodies and minds suffer. Processing the birth experience, through writing, talking, or working with a therapist, helps us process change and trauma. Positive social interactions that involve touch and emotional support increase our oxytocin levels, as do certain smells and foods. Our oxytocin system is continuously nurtured by a social environment where empathy, warmth, and support are abundant.

Quieting, settling, and calming are the postpartum practices that help our physiology recalibrate. No matter how your baby was born, there are ways to support your interrelated hormones. Parents are encouraged to practice sleep banking, or napping with baby during the day, to help mitigate the impact of sleepless nights. Newborns sleep a lot, and I am a bad napper. It wasn't realistic for me to always nap when Holden was napping. Instead, I would sleep for an extra hour in the morning while Max was on duty. For the first few months, Holden took most of his naps on me. Witnessing this practice, friends and family asked me if I could transfer him to a crib or bed so I could have freedom to get things done. The reality was that I struggled to rest enough, and when he slept on me I was forced to slow down. My increased oxytocin from skin-to-skin contact and breastfeeding allowed me to enjoy relaxing. Even if I didn't sleep, this forced rest allowed me to feel centered and connected.

When we're in a constant state of fatigue, cortisol, a stress hormone secreted by our adrenals, increases. When I'm exhausted, I am vulnerable to the suggestions of my elevated cortisol levels. Primarily, I crave and eat more sugar and then feel worse because eating sugar makes me feel more tired and crave even more sugar. When we lose sleep at night, we can't get it back, and our nervous system and immune function suffer. Chronic lack of sleep causes a loss of diversity in our gut bacteria. With that loss we become more vulnerable to immune system dysregulation and chronic inflammation. Adequate sleep, the kind that allows us not only to function but to thrive, is not a luxury; it is a requirement. Figuring out how much sleep you need to feel whole and capable is part of the postpartum process of discovery. Sleep builds our resilience, and sleep banking acts like a deposit of sleep into your bank to guard against exhaustion and disease.

In the spring, when Holden was born, the sun was still going down early and rising late. We followed its lead. By 7:30 p.m., we were usually in bed. During the short days of winter and early spring, fewer hours of sunlight signal our pineal gland to produce more melatonin, which allows us to feel sleepy earlier. As the sun started to set later in the evening, our bedtime shifted again. By the middle of summer, we were in bed around 9 p.m. and up early with the sunrise. Our circadian rhythms are shaped by our relationship to sunlight and are regulated by our internal biological clock, which is made up of genes and cells located throughout the body that have varying impacts on our behavior and physiology. Each day, our eyes send signals to our cells about the time of day. Our biological clock uses this information to adjust and sync to the earth's rotation. Instead of fighting for more daylight with bright lights and electronics, Max, Holden, and I kept the lights dimmed or used salt lamps or candles at night and spent as much time as possible outside or in natural light during the day. We still follow the lead of the sun. The result is a simplified routine where bedtimes and wake-ups are ideally set by the light/dark rhythms of the high desert.

Until about twelve to sixteen weeks, newborns' sleep is scattered throughout a twenty-four-hour period, and their circadian rhythms are still establishing. The circadian rhythm includes more than just our sleep and wake cycles. Blood pressure, cortisol, melatonin, digestion, deep sleep, and body temperature all fluctuate in relationship to light and dark. Newborns develop their rhythms the same way we do: through light exposure during the day and avoidance of light at night. When babies are exposed to bright light at night and minimal natural light during the day, their circadian rhythm is disrupted. This period of syncing to the sun and moon is crucial, as disruptions in the development of circadian rhythms during infancy cause long-term health problems and disease.

## THE FOOD THAT RESTORES

Of her approach to food and cooking, Jeong Kwan said, "With food we can share and communicate our emotions. It's that mindset of sharing that is really what you're eating." The potential of food to nourish and heal is profound after birth. My mom prepared soups, bone broth, and several lasagnas for us to keep in our refrigerator and freezer. She shared this food with us as a way to communicate her deep care, and we felt it in each delicious bite.

The food we eat impacts each cell in our body and each cell in our baby's body. Our hormones, healing, and physiology are supported when the foods we eat are nourishing. The same foods that build healthy babies—eggs, pastured

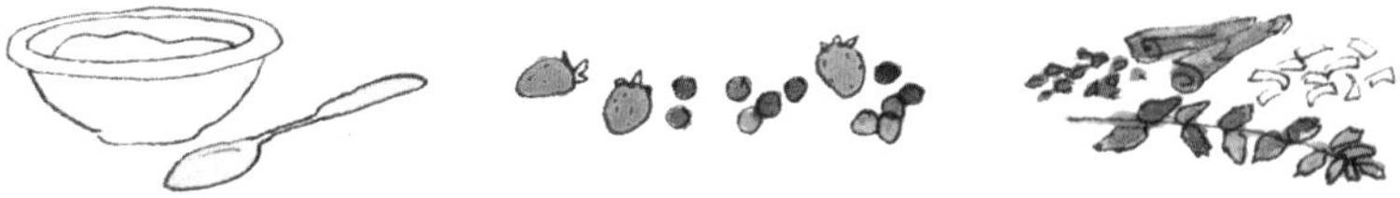

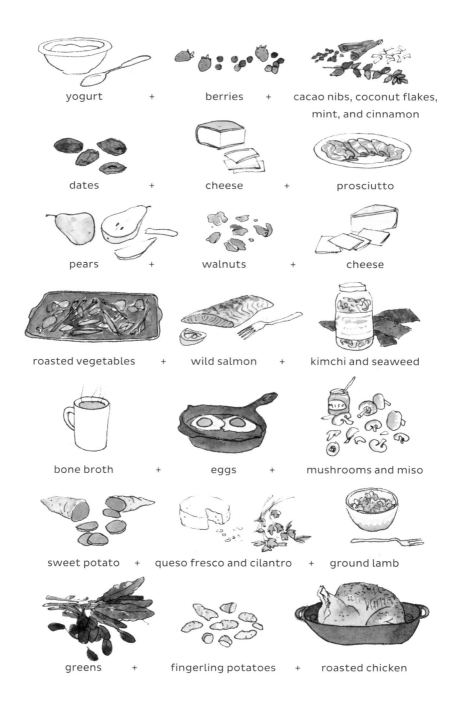

yogurt + berries + cacao nibs, coconut flakes, mint, and cinnamon

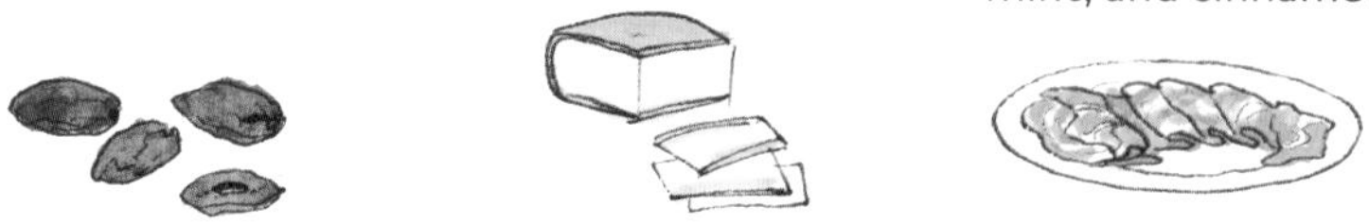

dates + cheese + prosciutto

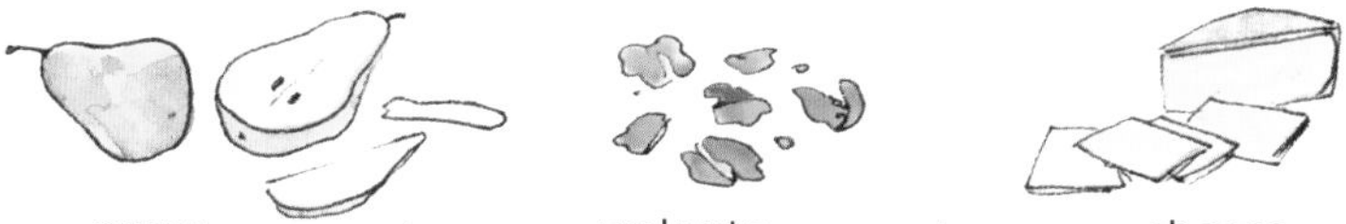

pears + walnuts + cheese

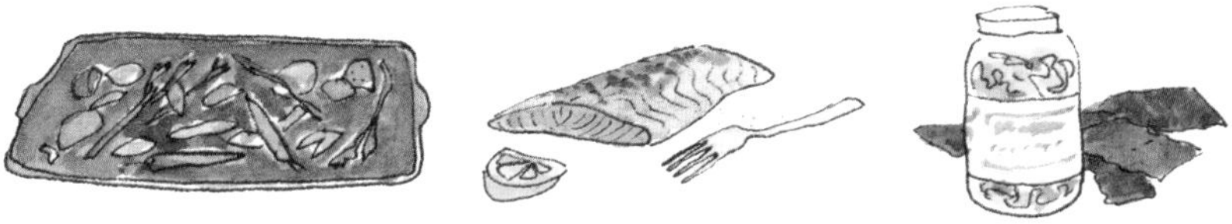



roasted vegetables + wild salmon + kimchi and seaweed

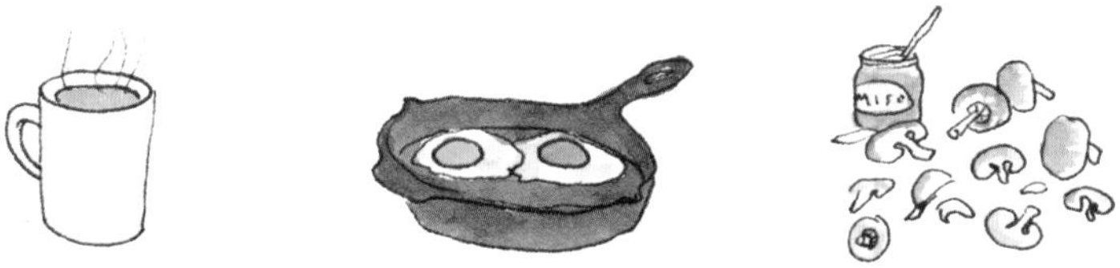

bone broth + eggs + mushrooms and miso

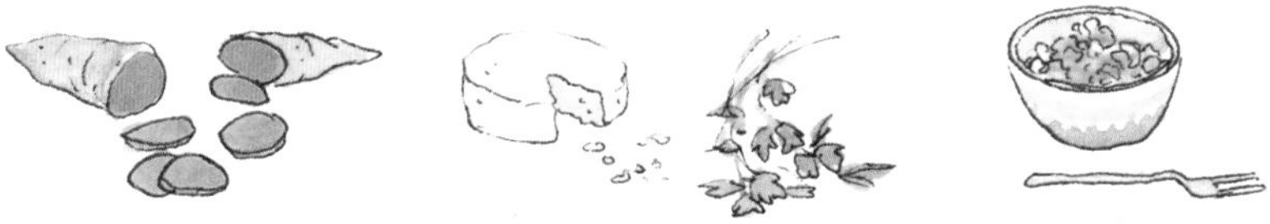

sweet potato + queso fresco and cilantro + ground lamb

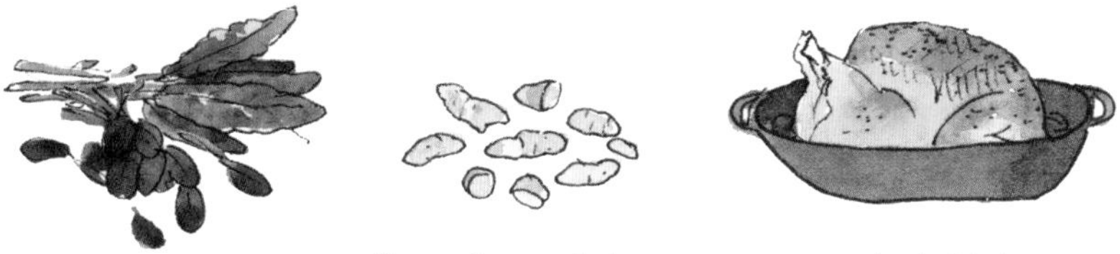

greens + fingerling potatoes + roasted chicken

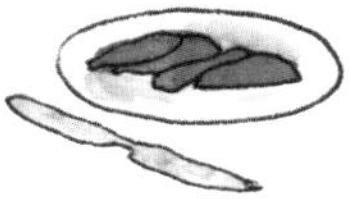
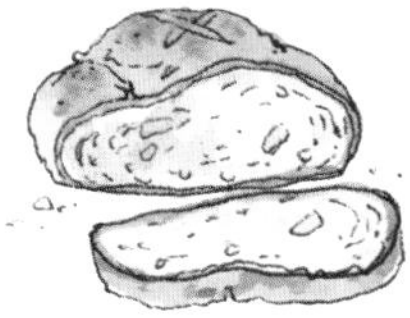
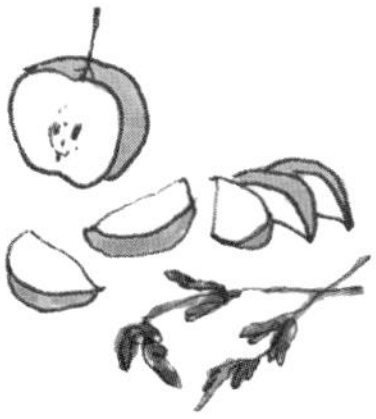

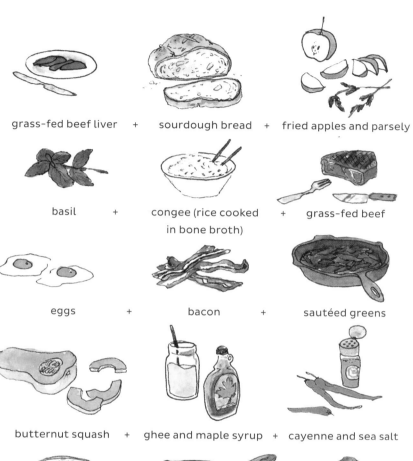

grass-fed beef liver + sourdough bread + fried apples and parsely

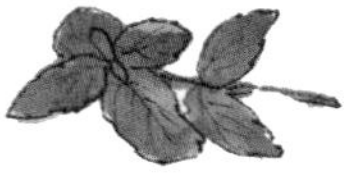
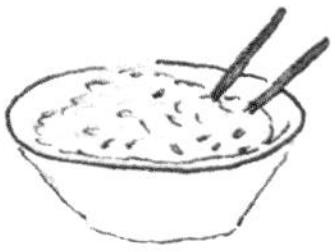
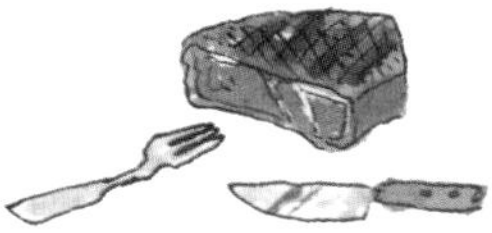

basil + congee (rice cooked in bone broth) + grass-fed beef

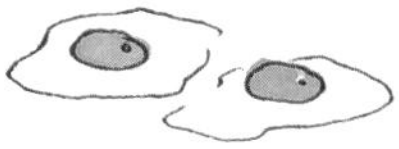
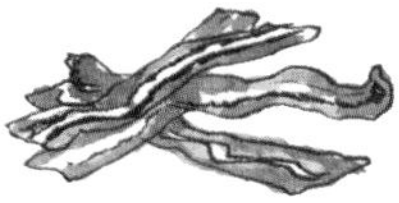
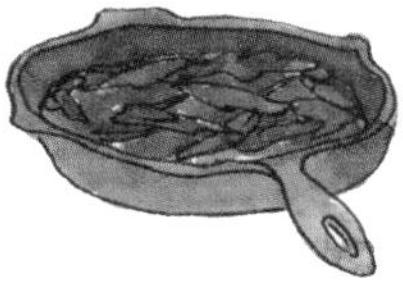

eggs + bacon + sautéed greens

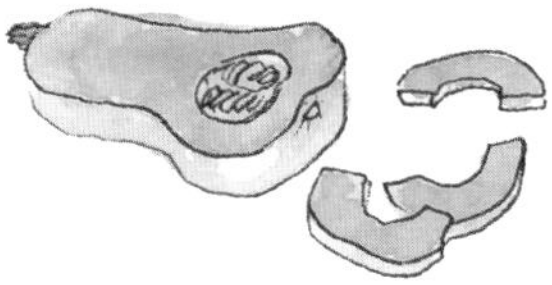
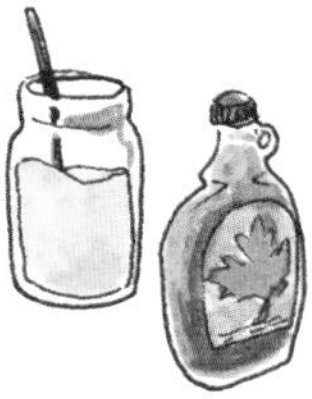
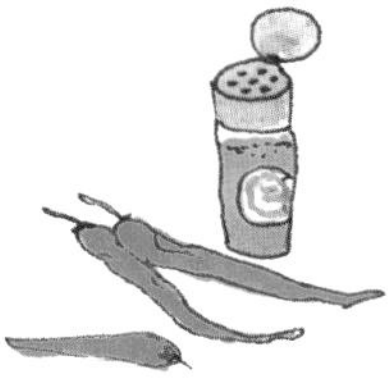

butternut squash + ghee and maple syrup + cayenne and sea salt

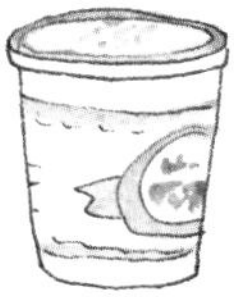
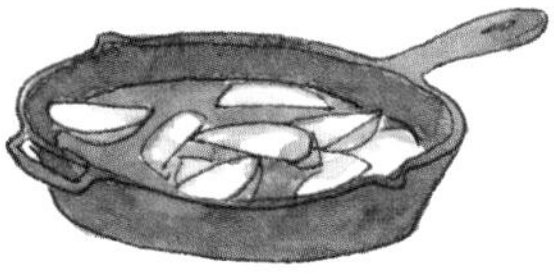
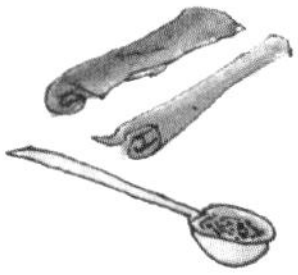

greek yogurt + apple slices fried in butter + cinnamon

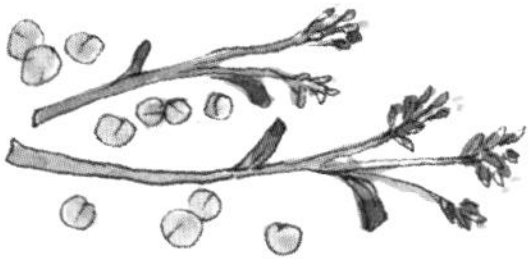
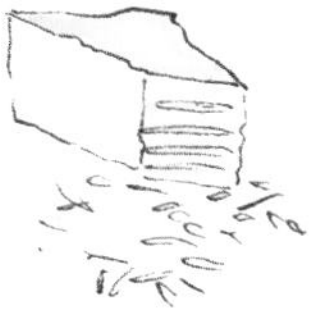
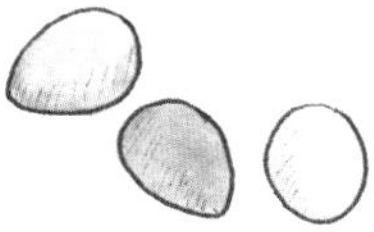

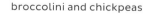

broccolini and chickpeas + parmesan + eggs

meats, organ meats, healthy fats, wild fish and seafood, fruits, vegetables, and fermented foods—restore and heal the body after birth. Food, as Kwan recognized, is powerful because it communicates with our bodies and gives us instructions about how to function. After birth, our need for nourishing food increases dramatically.

After giving birth, our bodies are in a state of healing and recovery. For those of us who choose to breastfeed or chestfeed, the amount of food we need is higher while we nurse than during pregnancy. Because growing a baby, birthing the baby, and keeping this baby alive is a full-time, energy-intensive job, our bodies understandably need nourishment from nutrient-dense food. During birth we lose blood and fluid and might experience tearing, or if we have a C-section, we have to recover from major abdominal surgery on top of caring for a newborn. Whether you decide to nurse or not, the mammary glands start producing milk, and the uterus shrinks. As our bodies recalibrate and continue to change, the food we eat helps facilitate healing, recovery, and skin elasticity and restores some of the energy and vitality we may have lost through the process of labor and birth.

The foods in the previous illustration provide some examples of nourishing meals and snacks. Some can be prepared with one hand, or you can show the illustration to your partner, parent, or friends to help guide them on how best to support your nutrient needs. For new parents, preparing some freezer meals before birth, setting up a meal train with friends and family, or hiring a postpartum doula if that is a financially viable option for your family can help keep you well fed and nourished while you care for your newborn. Many of the foods included in the illustration incorporate traditional healing foods, and I've included a few of my favorite postpartum treats, like apple slices fried in butter with Greek yogurt and cinnamon, and dates with cheese and prosciutto.

Remember that the hunger you're feeling is real and valid. You might be surprised to discover that you eat double the amount you usually do and that your need for water and other liquids is way higher than before. Your body is giving you a sign of what it wants and needs after giving birth. Listen to your hunger cues, eat food that is whole and nourishing, and accept meals and help from others when it is offered. Your body did a huge, incredible job and is in the process of recalibration and recovery. It deserves plentiful and healing food.

## GENTLE MOVEMENT

During labor and birth, the muscle cell organization in our uterus, cervix, and vagina changes so that a baby can come out. Pelvic floor muscles and ligaments support and stabilize these reproductive structures along with the rectum and urethra. For our parts to function—for example, the bladder, urethra, and supporting structures that enable urinary continence—we need structural and neurological integrity to stay intact. Pelvic floor disorders are common after vaginal birth because damage to both the shape and neurological function of ligaments, muscles, and nerves impacts how these parts work in relation to each other. The degree of our intactness determines whether or not we pee a little when we jump on trampolines or experience incontinence.

Hormones mediate physiological changes in the vagina and its surrounding structures. Increased collagen and elastin allow for more stretch and increased strength during birthing. After birth, our tissues undergo dramatic remodeling—again, through the synthesis of collagen and elastin. Trauma to the pelvic floor during birth, especially from forceps delivery, lacerations, or a prolonged second stage of labor, increases the risk of pelvic floor disorders. Despite how your baby was born, your reproductive organs and pelvic musculature are affected and in need of rest and healing.

In the immediate hours and days after birth, protecting the pelvic floor from stress and strain is essential. Carefully keeping the perineum clean through peri bottle rinsing and frequently changing pads helps protect the healing soft tissue. Drinking plenty of fluids keeps us peeing, and eating nutrient-rich, easy-to-digest foods and enough fiber keeps us from getting constipated. Straining to pee or poop is intensely uncomfortable for the pelvic floor, especially if damage or stitches are present.

For a few weeks, the only load I carried was my baby, nothing heavier. When I got out of bed in the morning, I carefully moved my legs to the side and pushed myself up with my arms so that I wasn't straining my core and pelvic musculature. My lactation consultant even recommended walking downstairs sideways to protect my pelvic floor from unnecessary strain.

# Healing the Pelvic Floor

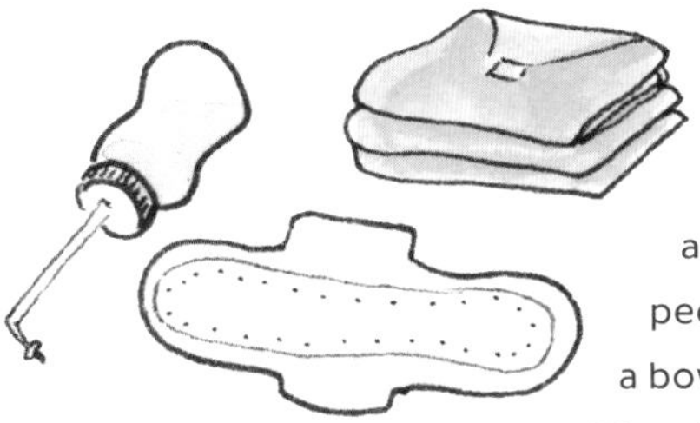

**HYGIENE:** Keep your perineum (the space between the anus and the vulva) clean and dry, changing your pad every 3–6 hours or as needed. Gently pat from front to back after peeing. Manually support your perineum during a bowel movement and rinse with a peri bottle. Wear loose, breathable clothing.

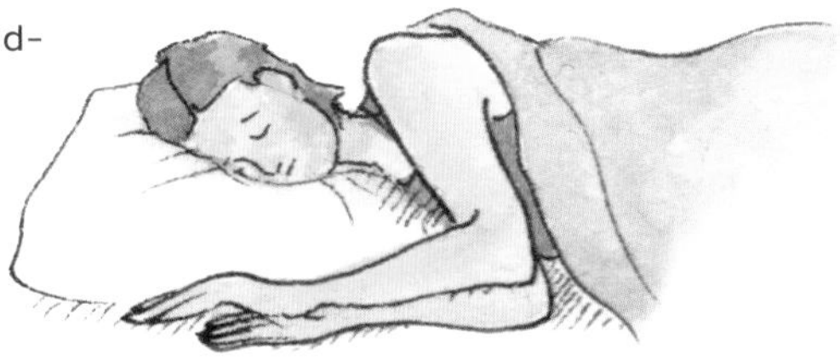

**REST:** Sleep, meditate, practice mindfulness, and nourish your emotional and physical health. Accept help from others, eat healthy food, and drink plenty of water to promote tissue healing and to prevent constipation. Learn to nurse in different positions, especially lying down. Treat yourself with the same gentle care as you treat your newborn.

**POSTURE:** Relax your shoulders, sit up straight, drop your ribs, and take deep breaths in and out of your nose. Notice whether you're holding tension while you nurse, and change positions frequently. Practice diaphragmatic breathing: Lie on your back with a pillow under your knees and place one hand on your chest and the other on your belly. Breathe in slowly through your nose, deep into your belly, then breathe out. Send healing energy to your pelvic floor.

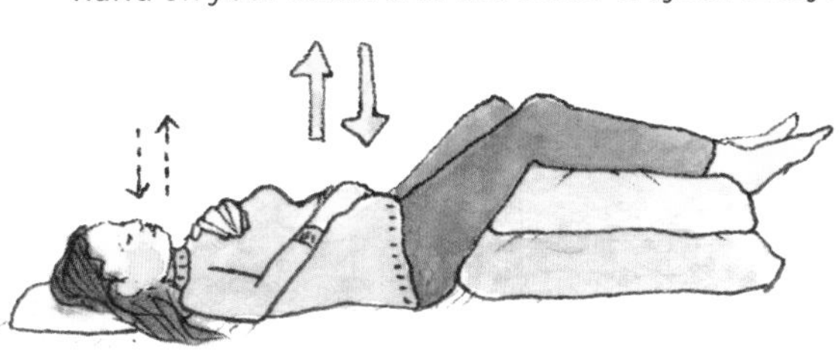

**GENTLE MOVEMENT:** When getting up out of bed, roll to your side first and use your arms to push yourself up. Do not lift loads heavier than your baby for a few weeks, and get up and down without straining your core or pelvic floor. Avoid high-intensity exercise and running until around 6 months postpartum and focus on movements that rebuild strength and balance, like walking, squatting, and natural sitting. Do not feel pressured by the 6-week mark to exercise, have sex, or do anything that feels uncomfortable. Trust that you will heal, and listen to your body.

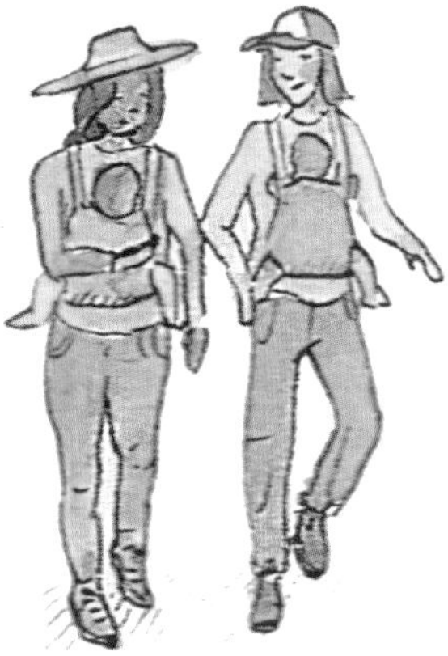

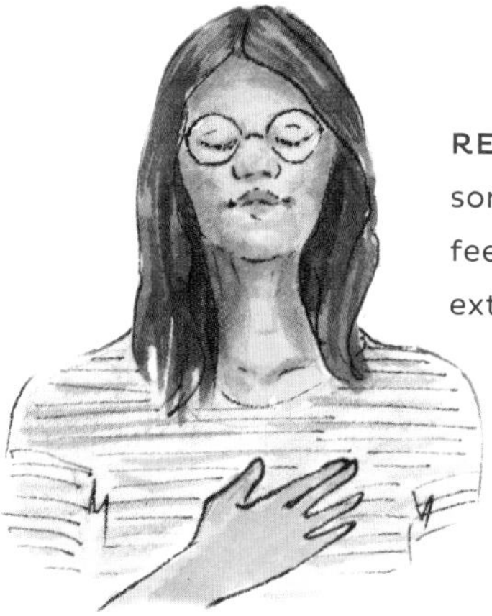

**RECONNECT TO YOUR BODY:** You may feel sore and uncomfortable. Your vagina might not feel normal for a while. Treat your body with extra care and tenderness.

**PELVIC FLOOR PHYSICAL THERAPY:** At around 6 weeks postpartum, every birthing parent should get a thorough pelvic floor assessment. Pelvic floor PTs check your abdomen for diastasis recti; address issues with pelvic pain, prolapse, and continence; and help you heal scar tissue. They are essential postpartum care providers.

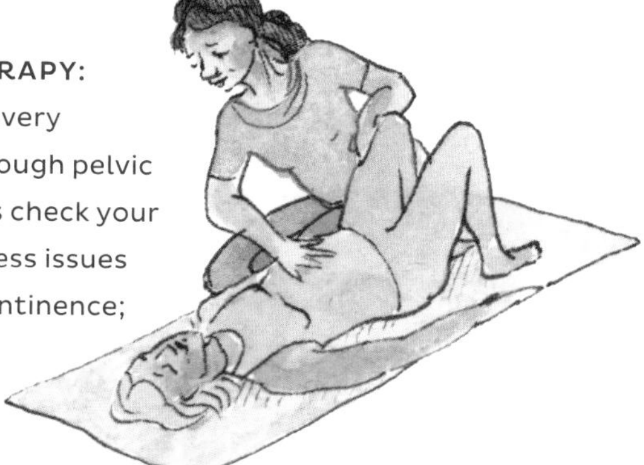

Instead of sitting all day in one position, which is uncomfortable and doesn't support balanced healing, I moved around the house, finding different areas to nest into with Holden. We spent a lot of time on the floor and outside. I'd shift him from arm to arm and sit in different positions, focusing on my breath, trying not to slump. When I was breastfeeding, I noticed I held my neck in odd positions to check his latch or watch him feed. My neck ached every day from straining, and I still have to remind myself to take extra care of my neck and keep it lined up with the rest of my body.

As I deeply considered my own recovery and gentle movement, I started to think about how Holden was learning to move in the world. On our walks, I'd carry him in my arms, shifting him from side to side, trading with Max when I needed a break. For many months, we either carried him in our arms on walks or used a carrier. Holden wasn't a big newborn, but he was a big baby. The more I carried him, the stronger I felt and the farther we could go.

When infants are carried on a walk, versus being held in one position while we sit or stand, their physiology responds. Studies have shown that when babies are transported in arms, their heart rate slows and crying decreases. This is how our babies communicate with us—through their bodies and crying. Holden didn't cry on our long walks. His body was close enough to mine that he could easily communicate if he wanted to shift positions, sleep, or nurse.

Babies move to learn. When infants are picked up and carried, they are able to feel their bodies in space. Our evolution has been molded by our relationship to gravity. The vestibular system, which is a sensory system in the inner ear, gives our brain information about the position of our bodies in space. From this information, we learn how to stabilize our head while moving, our bodies find balance, and we maintain equilibrium. Our brains need sensory information provided by gravity to change and develop normally, and our muscles develop in response to resistance.

Early on, I learned that Holden was serious about his freedom. He did not want me to roll him over, sit him up, help him crawl, or walk him by holding his hands. If he wanted my help, it was on his terms. When he was learning how to crawl, he would perform acrobatic movements like an intuitive yoga flow that was preparing his body perfectly for the next big adventure

# Respecting Your Baby's Natural Movement

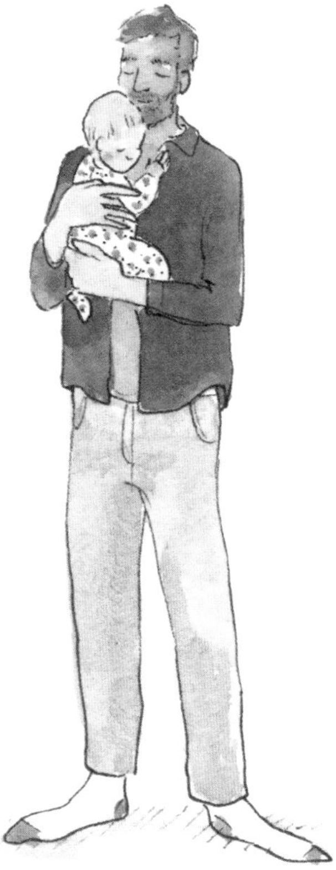

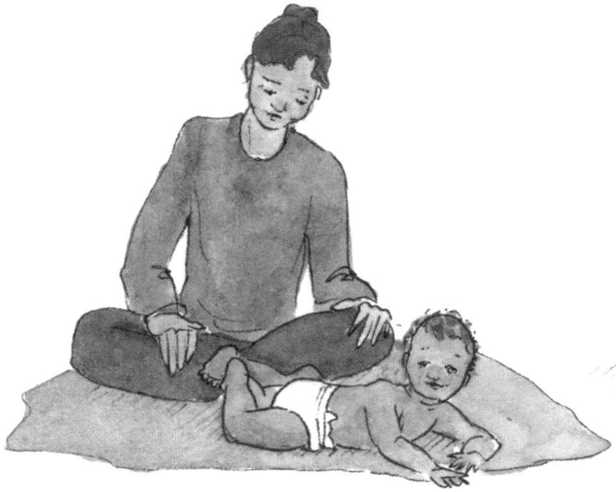

**MOVING:** Spend time carrying your baby in your arms, not always in a stroller or carrier.

**TRACTION:** Keep shoes, socks, and footy pajamas off your baby's feet when indoors.

**ENVIRONMENT:** Avoid overusing baby containers like swings, bouncy seats, and other contraptions that babies can't get out of or move freely in. Create a safe space for babies to explore.

**RESPECT:** Allow babies to develop the ability to move on their own, in their own time. Don't rush them. They are doing what they need to do.

on hands and knees. I learned to trust and respect his process. I kept socks and shoes off his feet so he had traction on our tile floor, and I didn't put him in swings, bouncy chairs, or other containment devices. As long as Holden was safe, I didn't interfere while he was learning how to move. I let him take the lead, rolling, crawling, and walking when he was ready. He didn't need me to show him or teach him; he needed to experiment, to try and keep trying until he figured it out. When we can step back and allow our babies to move freely in safe spaces, they learn how to navigate their environment and trust their bodies.

The movements I was most eager to return to after birth were the ones I performed the most while I was pregnant: walking, climbing, and working in the garden. All these movements are scalable. Walking, in particular, can start with a few steps and build into thousands of steps over time. These movements help the pelvic floor recover and find balance.

Since I carried Holden most of the time, running was gratefully out of the question. Running and other high-impact exercises performed too soon after birth can hinder the healing efforts of our pelvic floor and contribute to long-term imbalance and dysfunction. When our pelvic floor experiences stress and trauma, it tightens as a protective mechanism. Stress comes in varying degrees. The repetitive motion of running is one kind of stress; vaginal birth is another. A tense pelvic floor needs movement that allows it to lengthen. Running increases intra-abdominal pressure, which increases the load and forces placed on the organs in our pelvic container. These forces ask our pelvic ligaments, muscles, and connective tissues to take on more strain and stress. Chronic tension shows up as pain, prolapse, and the feeling that you have to pee right now and can't wait another second. Our too-tight pelvic floor muscles can cause referred pain in the abdomen, GI distress, and hip, butt, and thigh pain. Since our pelvic floor functions with our core, tension in the pelvic floor translates into tension in the core. Overtraining the core can increase the tension in the psoas muscles and thoracic diaphragm. When all these parts aren't working together, their ability to withstand forces is compromised and their instability can cause us pain and injuries.

As an athlete, I was taught that the solution to most problems in my body was to train more. Ten years ago I would have focused on running, jumping, and other high-intensity workouts after birth because that was what I knew. During pregnancy and as a new mother, I've learned that walking, squatting, and playing are the keys to feeling strong and balanced. These movements lengthen the pelvic floor muscles, decrease mental stress, and promote alignment in the body. I found that my recovery paired well with my ability to carry Holden. At first, we walked around the block. After a few weeks, we walked for miles every day.

At around six weeks postpartum, I visited a pelvic floor physical therapist again to make sure I was healing well. In other countries, pelvic floor physical therapy is a normal part of the postpartum experience. Working with a PT, surrounded by models of the pelvic floor, was oddly comforting, like an acknowledgment of this body part of mine that had just gone through so much. My vagina didn't feel like its normal self for many months. Something about the shape was unrecognizable, like I'd adopted a new body part I'd never met. Slowly my shape shifted back to the body I knew. I didn't experience any pelvic floor disorders, but I also didn't feel like I was totally myself again until about a year or so after birth. The six-week mark was an arbitrary day, and I felt like I was in the thick of healing still. At one year, I noticed a shift. I could suddenly imagine giving birth again. I was more interested in sex. I had found space for myself in relation to my baby. My first year of matrescence was complete.

## EXPERIENCE DOESN'T MAKE EXPERTS

Holden doesn't nap on me anymore, and he hasn't for a long time. Some shifts happen drastically. One day your belly is full of a baby, and the next it isn't. Other shifts happen gradually, almost imperceptibly, like how babies get bigger and claim their separate identity. There are so many questions about having a baby that other people try to answer for you. We are given advice about how and where our babies should sleep and nap, how to nurse or feed them, and how to set up our living space. We are told we can start exercising again at six weeks postpartum and go back to work at three months. Books come out to help us navigate the barrage of parenting questions that arise. But what if your questions aren't the kind that you can find in a typical parenting book? What if you are curious, like me, about how your baby develops in relationship to gravity? Or what if you intended to follow one style of parenting and find yourself on a different path? We can build a strong foundation of information about pregnancy, birth, babies, and parenting, but then we have to go on the journey and figure out who we are as parents and who our babies are as little people.

In his book *Range*, David Epstein highlights the importance of open-mindedness, experimentation, and ongoing learning. "We learn who we are in practice, not in theory," he says, meaning we have to actually go through transitions and changes to understand who we are. He found that people with experience are more confident in the advice they give, but they aren't necessarily more right. His book isn't about parenting, but this idea that experience doesn't make experts resonates with me every time another person recommends their one right way of doing something related to parenting. Leaving room for my own stories and experience helped me navigate the many recommendations I read and heard during the fourth trimester. Recognizing that I needed to learn by going through the actual thing—birth and the immediate postpartum period—helped me treat myself with gentleness and acceptance when I accidentally broke most of the rules of *zuo yue zi* that I intended to follow. The rules gave me an outline, and living through the fourth trimester wrote the actual story.

# TAKE ACTION

Discover what you need to help you heal and care for your baby. Traditional cultures focus on a defined period of rest, specific healing foods, and extensive prearranged support for the new parent-baby dyad. Our environment is just as important postpartum as it is during birth and can either support or hinder our hormonal health and our relationship with our baby. Focusing on actions that quiet, settle, and calm both you and your baby help recalibrate your physiology and support your health.

Enjoy nourishing food. The same foods that build healthy babies, including eggs, pastured meats, healthy fats, wild fish and seafood, fruits, vegetables, and fermented foods, help repair and heal our body after birth, nourish a healthy microbiome, and provide the energy and nutrient replenishment we need to care for our newborns.

Respect your body. After birth, rest is essential. Walking when you're ready and not carrying anything heavier than your baby for a few weeks helps the pelvic floor heal and protects it from stress and strain. It takes a full year for your pelvic floor and pelvis to recalibrate. Give your body time. Apply the same gentle respect for movement to your baby, and remember that babies move to learn.

Remain open and remember that experience doesn't make experts. Allow traditional wisdom and stories from others to guide you, but understand that we learn who we are when we go through an event, like pregnancy, birth, and postpartum. Because we are in progress, an open mind, and understanding that our learning is ongoing, helps us treat ourselves with gentle acceptance as we learn how to be parents.

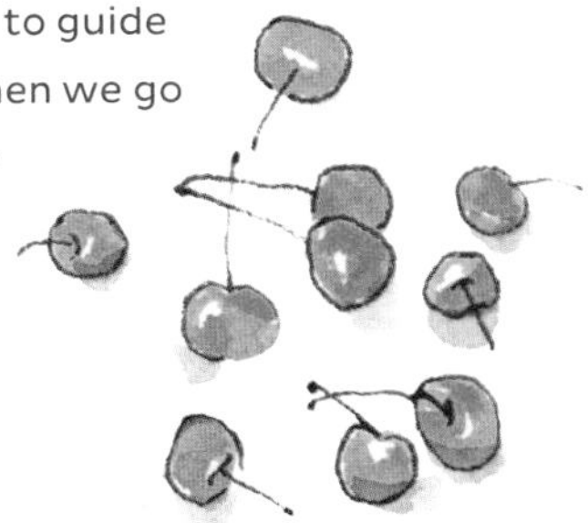

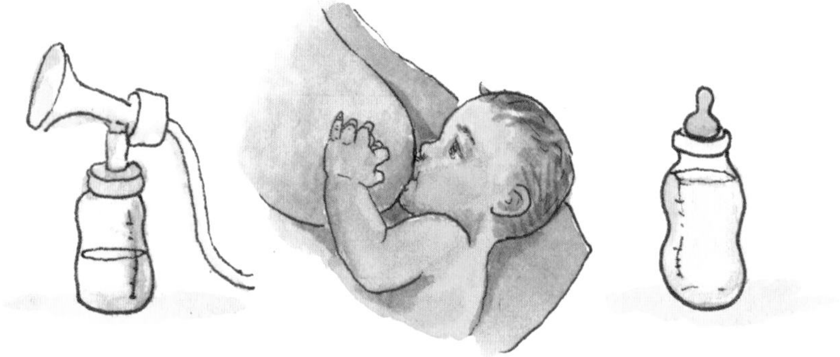

CHAPTER TEN

# Feeding Your Baby

**BREASTFEEDING OR CHESTFEEDING** is a movement much like walking. Walking may be simplified into the action of placing one foot in front of the other, but it requires complex coordination and impacts our mood, behavior, and internal physiology. Likewise, when a baby nurses, they are doing more than just suckling for food. They are also entering a relationship with their parent, and their mouth and body are performing a complex set of movements. We are not born with the immediate ability to walk, and similarly, we must learn how to breastfeed or chestfeed. For some parents, feeding their babies from their bodies is not an option, either through choice or circumstance.

What and how we feed our babies matters. But true nourishment doesn't come only from food. Nourishment comes from connecting to our babies, and connection is a product of our intentional care and attention. We connect physically when we hold our babies and emotionally when we talk and listen to them and empathize with their needs and feelings. Whether you choose to feed your baby milk from your body, donor milk, formula, or a combination of these options, the development of the parent-baby relationship is the single most important variable that impacts your baby's long-term brain development and ability to live securely in the world.

If you plan to breastfeed or chestfeed, it does not always follow that feeding your baby will feel easy or intuitive. Sometimes it's painful, frustrating, and exhausting. We are not meant to walk this path alone as new parents. Those who came before us, including our parents and grandparents, midwives and lactation consultants, and friends who have had children, may act as our guides and sources of hope and perseverance. Their diverse experiences show us that the stories of parents and babies vary greatly. There is more than one way to do this thing, and if something isn't working—for example, if breastfeeding or chestfeeding is challenging or milk supply is low—the solution is not self-hatred and shame; it is finding a different path with lots of support so that both you and your baby are nourished. This chapter dives into the fascinating science of milk from the mammary glands, but it is not meant to serve as a morality lesson on how to feed your baby.

## ORGANS THAT LISTEN

When Holden was placed on my chest after birth, he scooched and shuffled his body toward my breasts like an inchworm searching for something secure to latch onto in the breeze. I realized, watching him move across me, that he was an active participant in his survival. His body knew instinctively that safety and protection came in the shape and form of my warm breasts and soft belly.

During pregnancy, certain hormones cause mammary glands to remodel and prepare for lactation. In her book *Breasts: A Natural and Unnatural History*, Florence Williams describes how "mammary glands evolved receptors on their cells to 'listen' for and collect estrogen, progesterone, prolactin, lactogen, and many other hormones." This attentiveness allows our mammaries to respond and develop when we are pregnant so that they can accomplish their evolutionary-adapted purpose: feeding babies. They start growing their glandular network and adjust the composition of milk depending on our baby's needs. The ability of our breasts to metamorphize and feed babies shaped our evolutionary history and led to socially complex behavior. Williams describes how lactation differentiated us from reptiles by allowing our brains to grow ten times bigger, and the act of suckling shaped the structures in our mouths that we use for speech. Who we are and how we communicate started with a latch on a nipple and breasts that were primed to deliver the goods.

Breasts have been studied by evolutionary biologists as sexual objects that exist to attract mates, but the truly remarkable feat of breasts is not their ability to dumbfound or distract onlookers. When it comes to breasts, the magic is truly on the inside. Breasts are magical because they are specialized organs that produce large quantities of nutrient-rich liquid that keeps infants alive. They are filled with estrogen-sensitive cells that respond to the environment. These cells tell our breasts when to grow and expand their fat stores so that we can feed our babies. The upside of this sensitivity is a set of complex, amazing organs that evolved to perfectly nourish our babies. The downside of this sensitivity is that we've been polluting our environment with toxic compounds and putting estrogen-mimicking chemicals into our personal care products. Our breasts, which are so intricately in tune with our body and our ecosystem, respond to their environment. When the environment is polluted, our mammary glands and the milk we produce are impacted. In just a few generations, the perfection of breast milk, which was shaped by millions of years of evolution, has been degraded by our heavy-handed use of endocrine-disrupting and toxic chemicals.

I didn't test my breast milk for pesticides, PCBs, mercury, lead, or other harmful chemicals that show up in our modern milk, but this doesn't mean they weren't in there. Our breasts collect, store, and respond to the story of our lives. From conception, babies are exposed to the chemicals in our environment that live in our bodies. Our milk is a continuation of this exposure. Whether or not our babies breastfeed or chestfeed, they live in the world and their bodies adopt some of its chemical loads into their tissues.

There are many barriers to breast- and chestfeeding in our culture, and this section is not meant to add to them through fear. A few years ago I was writing a story about water. The hydrologist I interviewed told me, "Water is an expression of everything in our environment, the good and the bad." When I started writing the story, I included this quote. My editor made me take it out. She didn't want me to scare people and make them think our water was dirty and polluted. The truth is, our water has been polluted and contains some bad stuff. But we also need to keep drinking water to survive. Likewise, if we produce milk, it is an expression of our environment, the good and the bad. Whether babies drink breast milk or formula reconstituted with water, they are exposed to the realities of our ecosystem. With our responsive, intuitive bodies, we deserve to know that the milk we make is remarkable, nourishing, and likely contaminated by chemicals.

Our breasts and chests are the orchestrators of our milk. They evolved to feed our babies, and they respond and interact with the environment—which means that in addition to providing nourishment, they are also vulnerable to environmental toxins. Williams writes that "breast-feeding is an ecological act, connecting our bodies to the world in a complex web of give-and-take." This complex web of our ecology is not divided into good and bad; it is interwoven. Formula companies are trying their best to learn from breast milk and improve their products, and if breastfeeding or chestfeeding isn't an option, formula exists to keep your baby fed. Breast milk, a unique and remarkable result of our relationship to the world and to our bodies, is not perfect anymore, but if it works for you and your baby, it might feel like it is.

## THE MECHANICS OF MILK

Two days after Holden's birth, my breasts were heavy and uncomfortable. I wanted to hide them. What if they never returned to normal? I was overwhelmed by their size and shape, which felt alien and unruly. But these overflowing fountains had a purpose. They were full of milk rich in fat, carbohydrates, proteins, vitamins, minerals, and water. Within them, thousands of bioactive compounds were waiting to help build Holden's immune system and develop his organs and to cultivate healthy microbial communities in his body. Protecting him against infection and inflammation, my dynamic, burgeoning milk supply was here not to make my breasts look good, but to grow my baby.

Human milk has a significant job. It must nourish a quickly growing infant without help from any other food sources. Because of this survival pressure, milk has evolved into a highly organized, complex food. The parts of milk we think of as nourishment—the proteins, lipids, peptides, macronutrients, water, and other essential nutrients—provide the necessary tools for growth in a highly absorbable form that coincides with our baby's developmental stage. Then there are the parts we don't consider food, like the complex carbohydrates called oligosaccharides that coevolved with intestinal bacteria. Babies don't have the enzymes required to break down oligosaccharides, but specific bacteria are able to break them down and build their dominion in our babies' guts. When beneficial microbes lock down the gut as their habitat, they outcompete pathogenic microbial strains and give our infants certain advantages that help them survive. These advantages include immune function regulation, toxin binding, and certain growth factors.

Oligosaccharides feed friendly bacteria in babies' guts and act as antibiotics for pathogenic bacteria. Through their antiadhesive effects on "bad" bacteria, they directly reduce infections. They also impact the bacterial communities in our mammary glands. The milk of every individual lactating person is unique, containing different bacterial communities and structures and numbers of oligosaccharides. In the same way that oligosaccharides protect infants, they protect us from infection and diseases. Human milk contains more abundant and structurally complex oligosaccharides than any other mammalian milk source.

# What's in Breast Milk?

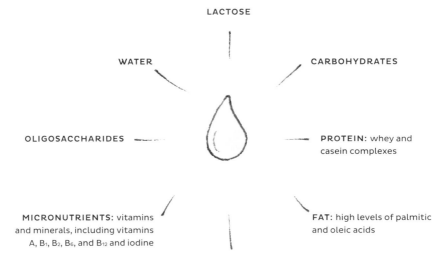

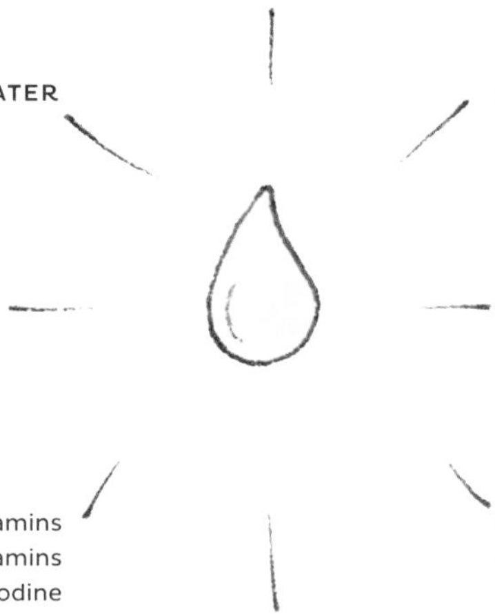
LACTOSE
WATER
CARBOHYDRATES
OLIGOSACCHARIDES
**PROTEIN:** whey and casein complexes
**MICRONUTRIENTS:** vitamins and minerals, including vitamins A, $B_1$, $B_2$, $B_6$, and $B_{12}$ and iodine
**FAT:** high levels of palmitic and oleic acids
**BIOACTIVE COMPONENTS:** immunoglobulins, growth factors, macrophages, stem cells, lymphocytes, cytokines, chemokines, hormones, antimicrobials, metabolic hormones, gangliosides, glycosaminoglycans, mucins

The first milk Holden drank after birth was colostrum. This unique breast milk provides infants with their first dose of immune protection as they are exposed to a world full of bacteria competing to inhabit their desirable ecosystems. In preparation for larger quantities of milk, colostrum urges the cells in the gut lining to arrange themselves in a way that allows for efficient absorption of nutrients. Further mammary gland remodeling allows our milk supply to ramp up. The changes in the structure of mammary glands changes the composition of breast milk. Transitional milk, which usually arrives the first few days after delivery, is the milk that engorges breasts when milk "comes in." It is higher in fat, lactose, and other nutrients than colostrum. After about two weeks, our breast milk is considered mature as its composition stabilizes.

For milk to leave the breasts and enter our baby's body, a series of coordinated movements and hormonal actions must occur. The almighty "good latch" is the ticket to creating subatmospheric pressure in the baby's mouth. This negative pressure allows the baby to suckle and their central nervous system to coordinate suckling with swallowing and breathing. Babies' jaws move in specific motions and their tongues undulate, and they must coordinate these movements with the milk ejection reflex. With a good latch, the jaw, gums, and front part of the tongue work together to compress the areola and milk ducts so that milk flows into babies' mouths. Part of the tongue directs milk into the throat, which triggers the swallowing reflex, while the back part of the tongue undulates in a gentle pattern that facilitates swallowing.

Movements performed by babies to obtain milk build strong muscles in their jaw, mouth, and surrounding structures and shape their palate and craniofacial structure. When the baby pulls the areola and nipple into his or her mouth and latches, the nipple lengthens and moves back and forth with the rhythm of nursing. The ability of the nipple to become elongated and compressible helps construct the soft palate. The shape of the soft palate and the pressure on the gums impact the position of the teeth. Objects in babies' mouths other than nipples, like pacifiers, thumbs, and bottles, require babies to adjust their mouth position. This adjustment causes an elevation in the soft palate and alters the action of the tongue, which impacts the morphology of the developing face and the position of future teeth.

# The Physiology of Lactation

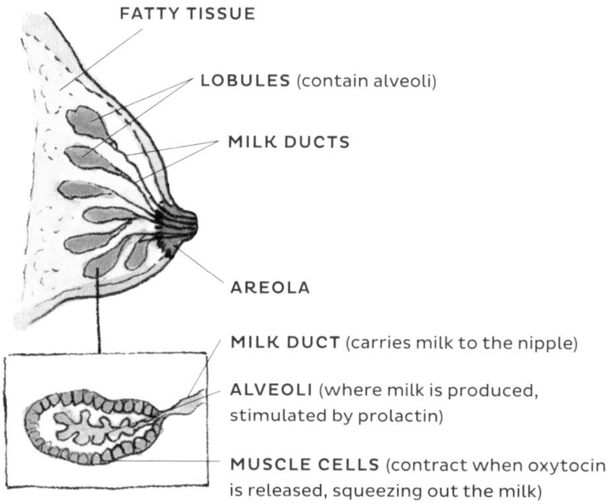


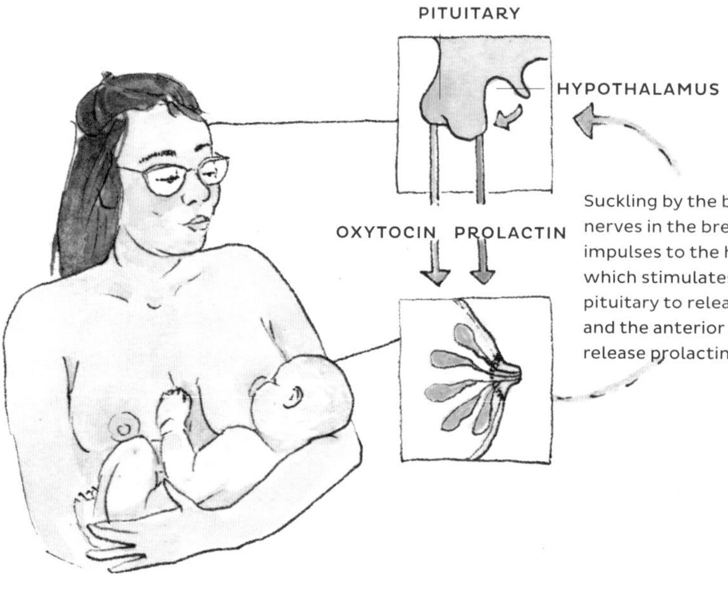


Suckling by the baby stimulates nerves in the breast that send impulses to the hypothalamus, which stimulates the posterior pituitary to release oxytocin and the anterior pituitary to release prolactin.

Breasts are composed mostly of fat and collagen, with just a small portion dedicated to mammary glands. These glands, which are modified sweat glands, have lactiferous ducts that allow milk to flow through them like a river. High levels of cortisol, prolactin, growth hormone, and estrogen expand the branches of the river during pregnancy. Increased progesterone encourages breast alveoli to enlarge and reach toward the chest wall. Milk-secreting lactocytes fill up the alveoli, which then pour milk into the ducts. At the head of the river there are clusters of alveoli, called lobules, that are organized around the nipple like a mosaic wheel.

When Holden nursed, a tingling sensation started in my breasts and then spread throughout my whole body. Initially it wasn't necessarily painful, but it also wasn't comfortable. I was feeling this sensation because his suckling caused sensory nerve fibers in my areola to tell my brain to release oxytocin. Oxytocin told my lactocytes to send their milk into my alveoli and through my lactiferous ducts, all the way down to my nipple pores, where milk shot into his mouth. Oxytocin is the hormone of the present, while prolactin prepares for the future.

High levels of estrogen and progesterone during pregnancy block prolactin from secreting milk from breast alveoli, but prolactin helps our mammary tissue develop in preparation for breastfeeding and is necessary for milk secretion after birth, when estrogen and progesterone levels drop. Suckling increases prolactin levels, which peak about thirty minutes after we start feeding our baby. One of prolactin's most important jobs is to tell the body to make milk for our baby's next feed. It does this through communication with our pituitary. The more our baby suckles, the higher our prolactin levels and the more milk we produce. Our prolactin levels are highest at night and in the morning, the times babies generally like to nurse the most, and this hormone helps us feel sleepy and relaxed so that we may still feel somewhat rested even when we nurse at night frequently.

Perhaps it was the effect of relaxation and sleepiness, but prolactin also had an amnesic effect on me. After a night of nursing and caregiving, I could not recall how frequently Holden nursed in the morning. While I faced occasional exhaustion, I was more often surprised that I somehow felt rested in the morning. The story didn't track with logic. I knew my sleep was disrupted at night, my culture told me I should feel depleted and exhausted, and yet, more often than not, I was OK.

The hormones of breastfeeding have a physical and psychological effect in the body that encourages nursing parents and babies to stay close to each other. Oxytocin keeps us calm and promotes bonding and affection. Both prolactin and oxytocin are stimulated by skin-to-skin contact and pleasurable forms of touch. Babies get a small dose of oxytocin from our milk and a significant release from suckling. The sensory nerves in babies' mouths are activated while they nurse, and once milk reaches their GI tract, even more oxytocin is released.

Oxytocin is a form of communication, mediated by the breasts, between nursing parents and babies that allows us to integrate and synchronize our interaction. One of the ways it best supports our relationship with a new baby is through its antistress effects. Stress can disrupt the physiological harmony between nursing parents and babies. Oxytocin is there to take sensory information from suckling and skin-to-skin contact and bathe your brain in messages that tell you to stay calm and keep caring for this baby.

Other compounds in our milk communicate time of day to our babies and help them develop their circadian rhythms. For this reason, our milk is considered chrononutrition. In the morning our milk contains three times more cortisol, a hormone that helps us stay alert, than our nighttime milk, which contains much higher melatonin. Nighttime milk has higher levels of specific types of DNA building blocks that promote sleep, while daytime milk is higher in amino acids that support higher activity. Magnesium, potassium, zinc, and sodium levels are highest in the morning. Iron levels peak at noon, and vitamin E peaks in the evening.

If babies continue nursing into toddlerhood, our milk supply goes down but the amount of fat and cholesterol in our milk goes up, and it continues to offer immunological support. When babies hit a growth spurt, our milk increases in fat content. When babies are sick, our breasts respond with increased infection-specific antibodies and lactoferrin, a glycoprotein with anti-infective, antioxidant, and anti-inflammatory properties. The beginning of a feeding is made up of watery foremilk, while the milk at the end of the feeding, hindmilk, is richer in fat.

# Chrononutrition

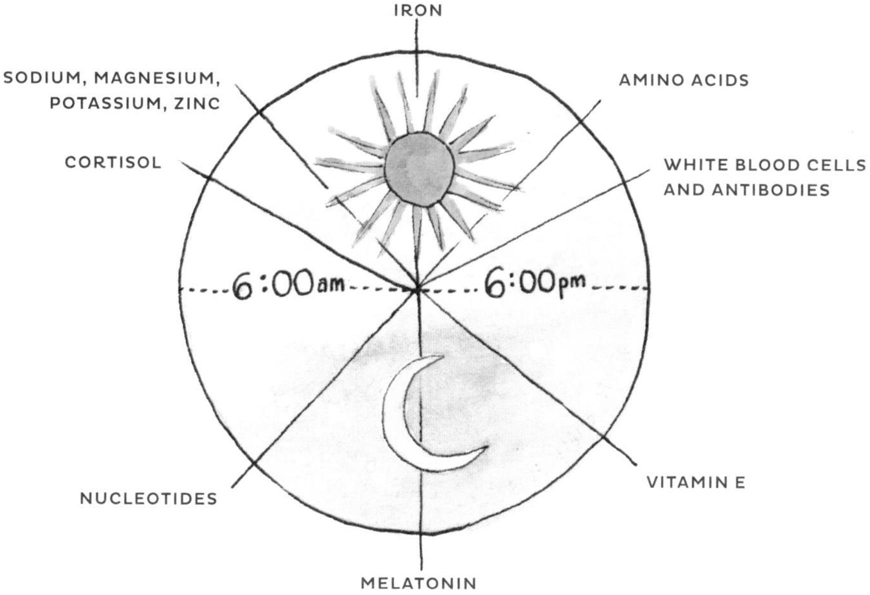


Milk communicates the time of day to infants, helping them feel alert during the day and sleepy at night.

**DAYTIME MILK:** Cortisol levels are three times higher in morning milk than in evening milk. Sodium, magnesium, and zinc are highest in the morning; iron levels peak midday; and immune components, like white blood cells and antibodies, are higher during the daytime.

**EVENING/NIGHTTIME MILK:** Melatonin, the sleepy hormone, rises in the evening and peaks around midnight. Vitamin E levels peak in the evening. Nighttime milk contains nucleotides, which are the building blocks of DNA and promote healthy sleep.

***For parents who pump:** If possible, continue nursing directly from the breast at night. Label the pumped milk by the time of day and feed daytime milk during the day and nighttime milk at night.

# Benefits of Ogliosaccharides in Breast Milk

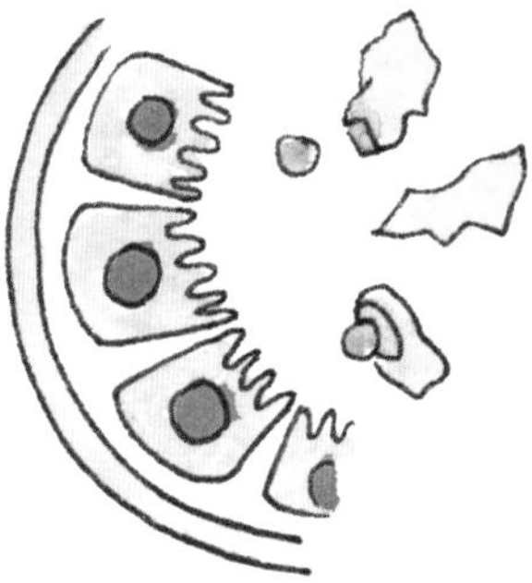

**GUT:** The combination of oligosaccharides and short-chain fatty acids helps mature the epithelial cells of the intestines by promoting the barrier function in the cells in the wall of the gut. Oligosaccharides act as prebiotics for commensal bacteria, like *Bifidobacteria*, which metabolize oligosaccharides and grow while pathogenic bacteria growth is suppressed. This allows commensal bacteria to colonize the gut, which contributes to an anti-inflammatory state.

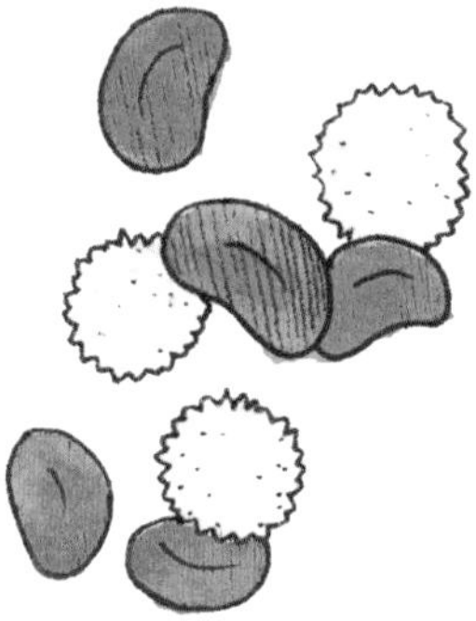

**IMMUNE SYSTEM:** Oligosaccharides have antiviral and antimicrobial effects. By binding to viruses, bacteria, and toxins, they protect against pathogenic infections.

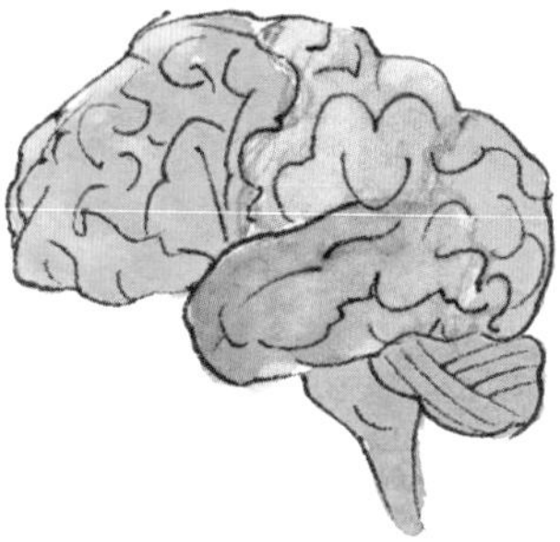

**BRAIN:** Oligosaccharides provide nutrients for neurological development, playing a role in neuronal transmission and synaptic function.

## A DELICATE BALANCE

Newborns' immune systems are often called immature, but this immaturity is a deliberate vulnerability devised by their bodies to allow beneficial microbes to colonize the lungs, mouth, skin, and gut. Thinking about newborns' immune function requires a shift in the way we think about immunity and bacteria. When we get sick as adults, our bodies fight against the pathogen responsible for the illness. Instead of this seek-and-destroy immune response, newborns have a tolerate-and-resist balance mechanism.

Tolerance refers to babies' reduced immune system response to high levels of pathogens, which allows them to establish their beneficial bacterial community. Without tolerance, their small bodies would launch a dangerous inflammatory response against the onslaught of bacteria they are exposed to at birth. This response may compromise their burgeoning microbial communities, which are crucial to their developing immune system. If babies didn't exhibit some resistance against pathogenic bacteria, their bodies and bloodstreams would be infiltrated by dangerous microbes.

Babies need to develop a healthy microbiome teeming with diverse bacteria for their immune system to function properly. Cultivating an environment that allows for safe colonization helps their bodies navigate the new world of microbial pressures. This brings us back to breast milk. The microbes found in breast milk, and the oligosaccharides that nourish beneficial microbes, help infants resist invasion by dangerous pathogens.

One of the built-in ways newborns are protected from diseases is by avoiding other foods and taking in only breast milk, which helps educate the immune system by populating the gut with specific populations of microbes. (Formula also shapes infants' gut bacteria, but it shapes it differently than breast milk. For now, breast milk and formula are not equivalent, but researchers are continually working to improve the composition of formula so that it more closely mimics breast milk.) Babies' guts are going through continual architectural changes as they develop, and microbes need ongoing nourishment from our milk so that they can boost babies' disease tolerance. The idea is that these beneficial colonizers help us build up a thick mucus layer filled with molecules that protect us from pathogens we're introduced to in various foods. This is why we wait on solid foods for babies. They need to build up their intestinal scaffolding, in coordination with their beneficial bugs, to resist and fight diseases later. Babies also receive the benefit of the anti-inflammatory environment these microbes promote. Their tolerance to and resistance of pathogenic bacteria improves, and they recover faster from infections and diseases.

Breast milk coevolved over millions of years with our unique needs for both nutrition and a healthy population of microbes. Each day, a breastfed baby takes in around 800,000 bacteria. Over time, the populations of bugs in our baby's body starts to mirror our own. Our health and microbial communities as nursing parents directly impact the diversity and type of microbes we pass to our babies. The foods highlighted again and again in this text tend our garden of beneficial commensals, which then flow like a river to our babies.

Just as in pregnancy, there are certain foods we need in greater abundance while we breastfeed or chestfeed. The food we eat impacts the microbes we pass on and the nutritional quality of our milk. The superstars of breast milk quality include plentiful healthy fats, like butter from grass-fed cows, extra virgin olive oil, lard or tallow, coconuts, avocados, and nuts and seeds. When fat is plentiful in our diet, the fat content of our milk is higher. Healthy fat builds healthy babies and impacts their gut microbiota by directly feeding bacteria and by triggering the baby to release bile acids and hormones that both regulate bacteria populations and promote beneficial bacteria.

Nursing a baby is a full-time, energy-intensive job, and fat happens to be rich in energy and uniquely delicious. It goes well with foods that contain the types of nutrients our babies require in abundance to develop optimally. Take choline, a nutrient we need in greater quantities while nursing than at any other time in our life, as our babies use it to grow their brains. The best food sources of choline are pastured eggs and liver. Eggs taste delicious fried in olive oil or butter, and liver loves to be quickly seared in bacon fat. Foods rich in B vitamins include vegetables and leafy greens (like chard, spinach, and kale) and grass-fed and pastured meats. Seafood like mackerel, salmon, sardines, anchovies, oysters, and caviar are full of omega-3 fatty acids and DHA, and the more of these foods we consume, the higher the concentrations in our breast milk. Babies use these fatty acids to build their brains and vision.

When we add healthy fat to foods like vegetables, our absorption of fat-soluble vitamins is improved. Of equal importance, high-quality fats make vegetables not only tolerable but delicious and satisfying. Kale would be a disappointment without a healthy drizzle of olive oil and sea salt. Sweet potatoes are infinitely tastier when they are slathered in butter. Nutritional information and benefits become secondary to the delight we can take in eating these foods that are growing our babies and nurturing their beneficial microbes.

## CARRY MAMMALS

The work of Dr. Nils Bergman has found its way into many important books about breastfeeding and chestfeeding. He explained that there are four different types of mammals who care for their infants in very different ways and whose breast milk composition reflects these differences. There are cache mammals, like deer, who are mature at birth. The mother stashes the infant in a safe place and returns to them every few hours. Their milk is high in protein and fat, providing long-term sustenance to the baby. Cats and dogs are nest mammals, who need to stay close to their littermates for warmth and security. Their milk is higher in protein and fat than that of follow mammals, which allows them to leave the nest and return every few hours, but lower in protein and fat than that of cache mammals. Follow mammals, like cows, can walk around after their mothers and feed frequently. Cow milk is lower in protein and fat than the milk of cache mammals because the calves are able to feed more often. Finally, there's us, the apes, and the jealousy-inducing marsupials. We are all carry mammals, but one of us gets a built-in pouch to store our infants!

As carry mammals, human infants need their parent's body to stay warm, and they need to feed often because they are the most immature of all the mammals at birth. Our breast milk is low in fat and protein, lower than in the milk of any other mammals, so our babies need to eat often. We can't store them in nests, or cache them away, or expect them to follow us around asking

# *Carry Mammals*

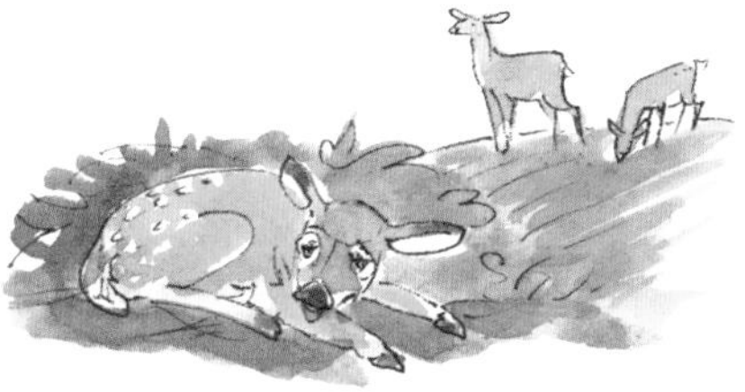

**CACHE MAMMALS** are more mature at birth than other mammals and receive milk rich in protein and fat, which keeps them full and quiet for many hours.

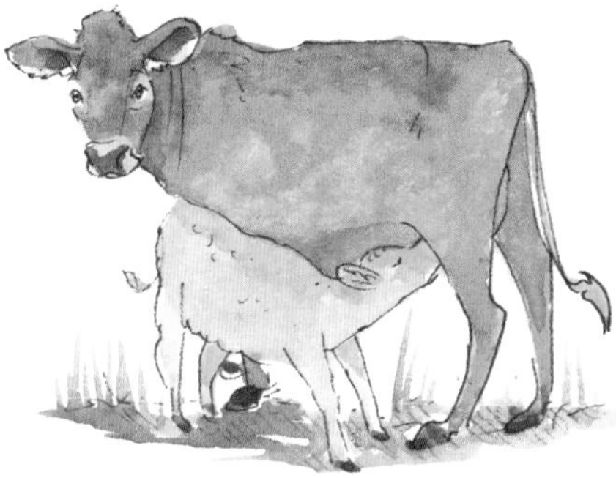

**FOLLOW MAMMALS** can walk well enough at birth to follow their mothers around and feed frequently.

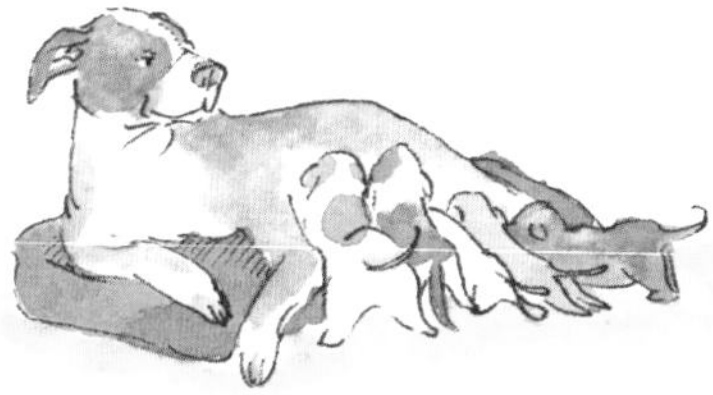

**NEST MAMMALS** need to stay close to their littermates for warmth and security, and their mother returns to feed them every 2–4 hours.

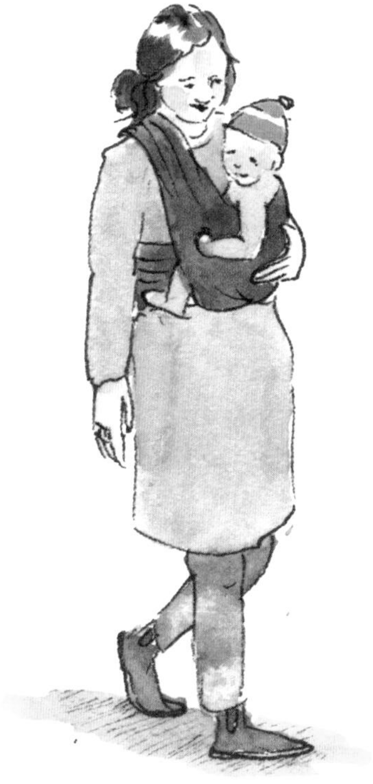

**CARRY MAMMALS** are the most immature at birth. They need to eat frequently day and night because their parent's milk is low in protein and fat, and parents hold them constantly for protection.

for milk (until they are toddlers, when they suddenly shape-shift into follow mammals).

Food, lots of water, and frequent breastfeeding or chestfeeding go hand in hand. When I was nursing Holden and my hands were full, I taught Max how to make dashi broth from kombu seaweed and bonito (dried, smoked fish) and serve it with wild salmon, tons of roasted vegetables, avocado, pickled radishes, and kimchi. He slow-cooked chicken until it was tender and then simmered the leftover bones into a stock. We ate sweet potato fries covered with parmesan cheese, bone broth with eggs and seaweed stirred into it, and big roasted cuts of grass-fed beef. Our meals were rich and simple. We'd curl up together and I'd luxuriate in the food he made while Holden continued on his mission to fill his body all the way up with my milk.

## ARE BABIES PARASITES?

Breastfeeding and chestfeeding are transfers of the nursing parent and their ecosystem to their baby. Evolutionary biologists consider breastfeeding an act of eating one's mother, or matrotropy. I didn't like this idea at first. Babies are sometimes described as life-sucking parasites, but it doesn't help me to think of my son this way (even when he feels like a life-sucking parasite). But, learning more about parasites and how breastfeeding benefits my body did help me navigate this odd relationship.

We think of parasites as creatures that take advantage of their hosts' bodies and exploit and deplete them from the inside out. The technical definition of a parasite is an organism that benefits at the expense of its host. And while we've historically considered this relationship good for the parasite and detrimental to the host, we're finding out that some parasites may form mutually beneficial, or symbiotic, relationships with their host. When it comes to babies, the act of nursing does deplete us of our vitamin and mineral stores, but, according to Florence Williams, breastfeeding also protects our cardiovascular health and shifts our metabolism so that we can recover quickly from

# Optimizing the Breastfeeding Relationship

- Find an IBCLC-certified lactation consultant (some will conduct home visits).
- Attend lactation consultant–led parent-baby classes and find a supportive community of parents.
- Prioritize rest and sleep. Create a calm and supportive environment to reduce stress. Ensuring physical and psychological comfort is essential for both you and your baby.
- Increase nourishing food and liquid intake. Energy needs are high while breastfeeding or chestfeeding, so make sure your food contains iron, protein, and healthy fats. Drink plenty of water.
- Feed your baby on demand and go skin-to-skin when you can. Frequent skin-to-skin contact encourages the baby to instinctively search and attach to the breast and can relieve stress.
- Take care of your breasts: avoid underwire bras and rotate sides and positions.
- Be flexible and avoid attempts to schedule your baby.
- Experience soothing touch from your partner or a bodyworker, or practice self-massage.

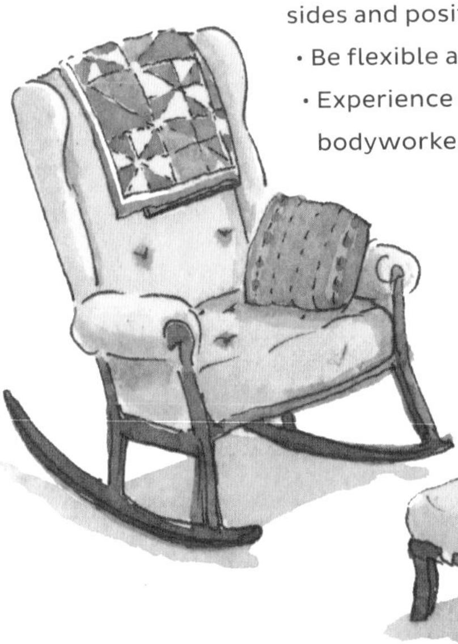

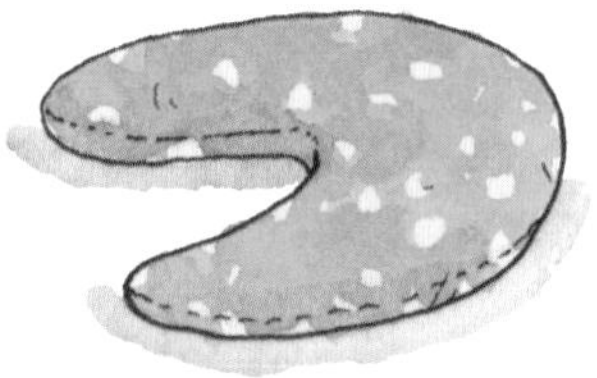

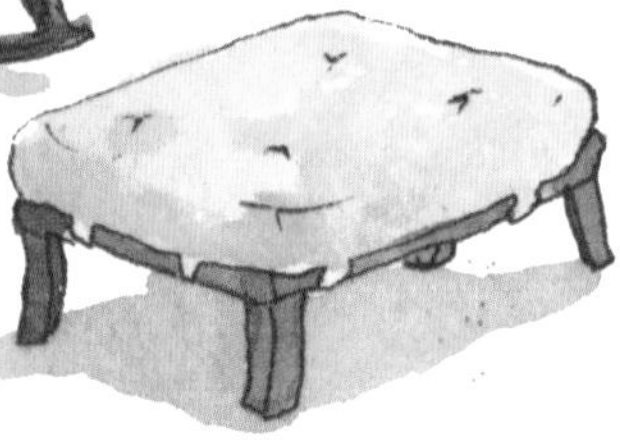

the toll pregnancy, labor, and birth take on our bodies. The mutual benefit of lactation, Williams writes, is a "critical part of how the enterprise was designed for our benefit as well as our baby's."

Babies aren't actually, technically, parasites. They are probably closer to symbiotic mycorrhizal fungi, which form mutually beneficial relationships with plants. Really, though, they are mammals through and through. The words used to describe how babies' immune systems form—"resistance" and "tolerance"—are good metaphors to describe the psychological and physiological tension we face each day we decide to continue nursing. Part of us resists. As I write about breast milk as a magnificent, evolutionary food source, I find it challenging when I have to stop working and actually nurse. Then as I settle in and he latches on like he's never eaten in his entire life, I find tolerance and am grateful to have this handy organ to soothe and nourish him.

Breastfeeding and chestfeeding is a loaded topic in our culture. As much as I like to navigate around the various axioms people use in relation to infant feeding (like "Breast is best!," "Fed is best!," and "Normalize breastfeeding!") by focusing on evolutionary biology and the nuts and bolts of milk, I worry that my discussion of breast milk and nursing might be misinterpreted as a judgment of value or worth. While new birthing parents are consistently encouraged to breastfeed, our social structures—like our lack of adequate parental leave and inadequate parental support—do little to actually support nursing parents. Breastfeeding rates and duration are impacted by systemic racism and social injustice such that before nursing parents even make a choice about whether or not breastfeeding is right for them, cultural systems of oppression choose for them and limit their ability to feel empowered and supported as parents who have the huge, daunting task of keeping a baby fed, healthy, and alive.

The words "breastfeeding" and "chestfeeding" are used to encompass a range of human behaviors, variables, and relationships. Clearly, breastfeeding happens between a nursing parent and baby, but this relationship is impacted by our habits and our ecology. Some babies are fed only formula or only breast milk from bottles, others only from the breast, others get a mix of bottle and breast, and still others get a mix of formula and breast milk. Not all breast milk is the same, and not all formula is the same. Babies also occupy different habitats in our homes, either in their cribs, in cosleepers next to our beds, or with us in bed. Parent and family structures don't all look the same. Some parents receive more support than others, and the stories from our cultures and our parents impact how we think about what is normal and what isn't when it comes to our baby's behaviors and feeding habits.

This explains why breastfeeding and chestfeeding—how we do it and for how long—varies so much from parent to parent. Each of us must form a relationship with our new baby in different contexts, and we have access to varying levels of support and information. For me, understanding the mechanics of breastfeeding and the evolutionary history of my milk encouraged me to think of breastfeeding as a dynamic relationship between me and my baby. I wondered, How do I make this work for us in the context of our life? I found that, after the initial learning phase of breastfeeding, I didn't want to sit at home all the time and breastfeed. We figured out how to breastfeed while hiking, outside in the garden, and in a side-lying position. I needed to clearly define what feeding my baby meant to me and how I was going to make it work in the context of my life and habits.

Our milk has been politicized, moralized, feminized, and economized, and the result is that we feel stress and shame when we struggle. Nursing has become a symbol of our parenting and lifestyle philosophy instead of a way to feed babies. It is possible to choose to breastfeed or chestfeed and not think all others must make the same choice as you. If you cannot, or choose not, to nurse, you are not failing. And whether you chose to nurse or not, you may still end up facing criticism and obnoxious comments daily. Parents who can't breastfeed are often told to "keep trying!," as if their stubbornness and will are the only determining factors. And when I nurse my twenty-month-old, other moms say with shock, "You're still breastfeeding! How long are you going to nurse him?" Florence Williams writes that what breasts need is "a safer world more attuned to their vulnerabilities, and they need good listeners, not just good oglers." In our complex world, we need less judgment and more understanding and support. We need what our breasts need.

# TAKE ACTION

Recognize that nursing a baby is a movement much like walking. It can seem simple, but it is a learned, complex movement and can be challenging and frustrating. If you choose to breastfeed or chestfeed, there are steps you can take—such as working with a lactation consultant, choosing nutrient-dense food, keeping well hydrated, and managing stress levels—that help optimize the nursing relationship.

Carry your mammal. Humans are carry mammals, meaning that babies need to stay close to their parent's body to stay warm and need to eat often because the composition of human milk is low in fat and protein, requiring consistent, on-demand feedings.

Understand that how you feed your baby varies based on the context of your life. Our habits and ecology, the amount of support we receive, the requirements of our jobs, where our babies sleep, and our parent and family structures are diverse, so the way we nourish our babies varies and won't look the same from family to family. Define what feeding your baby looks like for you in the context of your life and habits.

Treat yourself and others with less judgment and more understanding when it comes to feeding babies. It is possible to choose to breastfeed or chestfeed and not think all others must do the same. If you cannot, or choose not, to nurse, you are not failing. Offer yourself the same empathy, respect, and love you offer your baby, and remember that our number one job as parents is building meaningful connections and relationships with our babies.

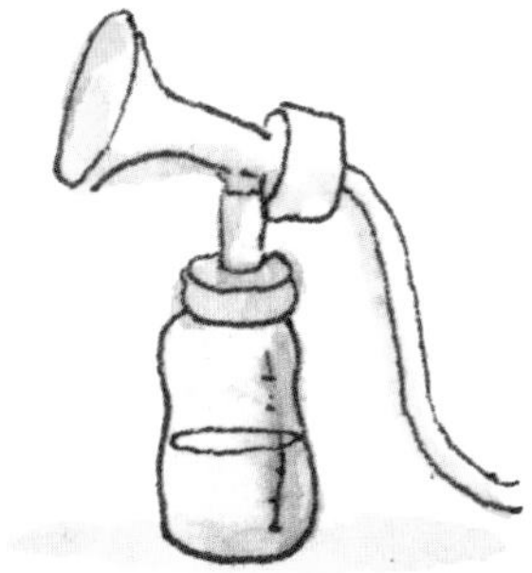

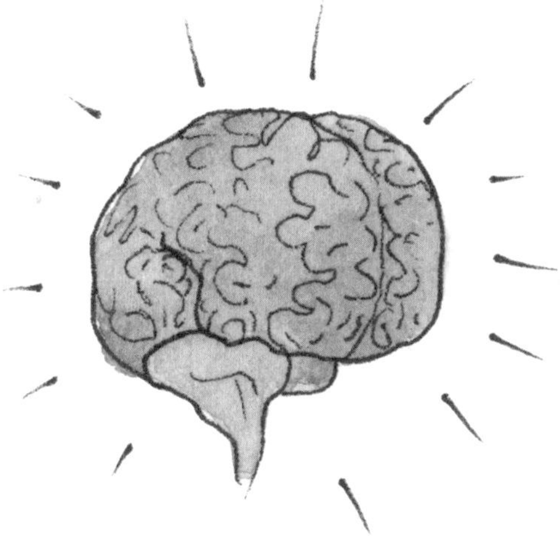

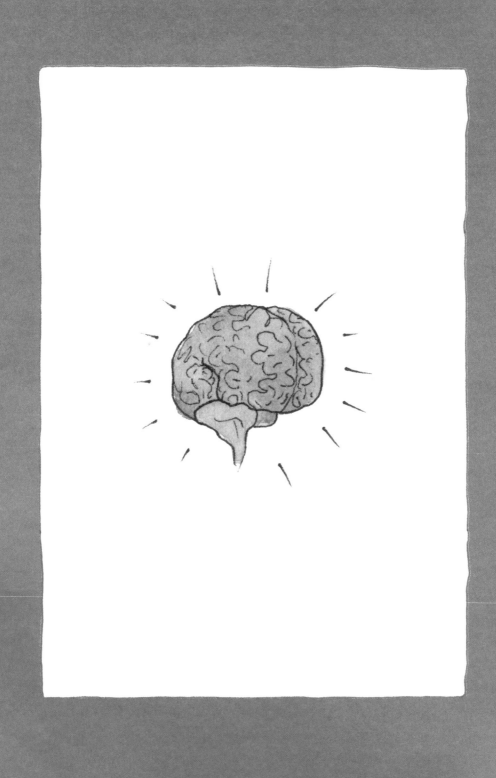

CHAPTER ELEVEN

# Your Brain on Baby

**IT WAS AROUND THREE** or four in the morning, and Holden was three days old and asleep next to me. He was so fresh and new, I struggled to physically separate myself from him. But I had to pee and I couldn't hold it. "Max," I said in a whisper to the soundly sleeping lump on the far side of the bed. Then "MAX" in a louder whisper. Finally, with a strong nudge and a full-volume utterance of his name, he roused and squinted his eyes open in the dark and looked at me with a sleepy yet kind "what do you need" expression on his face. "I have to pee," I said. "Watch Holden." I didn't know exactly why I needed him to watch Holden, who was asleep and not going anywhere on his own, but he nodded and I hopped up.

I walked the five feet to our bathroom and, mid-pee, heard Holden start to stir, then cry a little, then cry a lot. His cry grew louder and I swore at myself and my body for taking so long to empty my bladder. I didn't hear any other sounds, just the volume of his cry increasing, a crescendo that filled my body with a frantic, panicked energy. I finished peeing and jumped up: mama to the rescue! As I approached Holden and picked him up to comfort him and soothe his cries, I saw that Max was soundly, peacefully, ridiculously asleep.

Watching Max sleep filled me with an all-encompassing and surprising feeling of rage. What the hell, I thought. How is this fool asleep? How could anyone sleep when a baby is crying? Should I wake him up and yell at him? *I* was tuned in to Holden. I would wake up and feed him *before* he cried and recognize his needs through facial expressions and instinct. It was unimaginable that a person, especially *my* person, could sleep through the sharp, clear, "I need you!" cries of a newborn.

It turns out that I was primed, in a hormonal and neurological sense, to meet Holden's needs long before Max was. While my brain had been adapting in response to my dynamic hormones and altered internal physiology throughout my pregnancy, Max's brain was right at the beginning of its journey of reshaping its neural connections so that he could become a more attuned parent. Our brains are ever-changing, adaptive organs that are able to respond and adjust to our life circumstances. Pregnancy initiates structural and functional changes in the brain to help us adapt behaviorally to our infants.

The structures of the brain that are impacted early on, during the second and especially the third trimester, enhance sensitivity to environmental threats. Later in the third trimester, we tend to start feeling attached to our fetus, and we are more aware and sensitive to the cries, smells, and smiles of other infants. Our ability to perceive the perspectives and feelings of others improves. Our brain changes so that we experience greater empathy.

For a few decades, scientists have understood that stress, trauma, learning, and enriching environments can cause brain cells to reorganize, adapt, replenish, regrow, and reconnect. The ability of our brains to change how neural pathways are connected and form new connections is called neuroplasticity.

Neurogenesis is the ability of the brain to grow and potentially regenerate. Our malleable brains experience both increased neuroplasticity and neurogenesis in response to growing, birthing, and parenting babies.

Parenting, the verb, is defined by key behaviors that protect and nurture our offspring. Changes in specific regions of the brain mediate and encourage these behaviors. Gray matter, the prefrontal and temporal cortex and other parts of the brain involved in social cognition, appears to thin and reduce in size during pregnancy and postpartum. While some headlines describe this adaptation as our brains "shrinking" in a way that makes us wonder if we are getting dumber at the same time our bellies are getting bigger, the reality is that these adaptive changes improve and refine our neural circuitry so that we are more capable caregivers. It is possible that our degree of attachment, or hostility, toward our babies is impacted by the degree that our brains change both before and after the baby's birth.

In order to give the kind of all-encompassing care that a baby needs, our brains focus on a few key areas of change, also known as functional plasticity. First, we become more sensitive to environmental threats, and we experience changes in our emotional processing and regulation. When the baby arrives, it is normal to frequently worry about the baby and check if they are OK. For example, I constantly checked if Holden was breathing and was reassured by the rise and fall of his belly for a period of time before I needed to check again. Our brains, specifically regions of the brain associated with reward and motivation, become more sensitive to the cues from our infants. The dopamine-activated neural circuit that processes rewarding substances like sex, food, and drugs is sensitized by a combination of oxytocin and dopamine. The result is that our reward centers light up when we look at our baby's cute face, and we are specifically tuned in to their cries and needs.

We also experience activation of our neural circuits that increase our understanding of social information and promote empathy. This social information circuit can be thought of as the ability to understand the language of our infants. It allows us to accurately understand and appropriately respond to information that others might not even be able to see. Finally, because early postpartum is particularly stressful, our brains appear to change the way we process negative emotions. The emotional regulation circuit is activated,

# *Remodeling the Parental Brain*

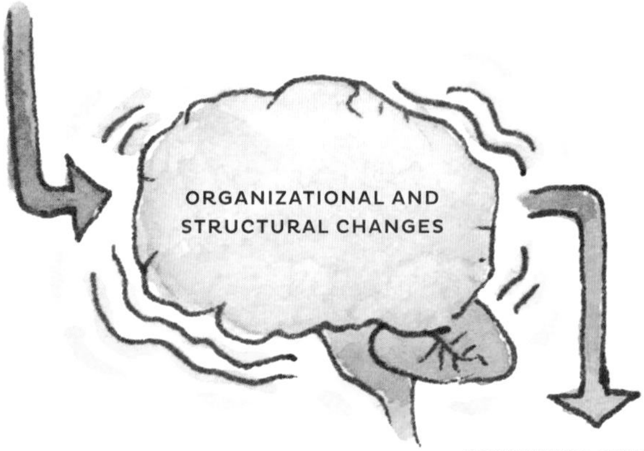


**PREGNANCY:** The huge increase in progesterone and estrogen during pregnancy causes organizational and structural changes in the brain. Part of that restructuring includes site-specific gray matter concentration, which researchers believe is an adaptive change that allows us to become more responsive to our baby's needs. As pregnancy progresses, we become more sensitive to infant cues and more aware of threats, and we experience greater emotional attachment to our baby. These changes are an evolutionary strategy that puts us in tune with our baby so we can keep them alive and healthy.

**POSTPARTUM:** After birth, activity in the amygdala increases and impacts behavior. A more active amygdala is associated with parenting behaviors like attachment and improved sensitivity and responsiveness to our baby's cues. Our dopamine-activated neural circuitry rewards us when we care for our babies. We also experience enhanced empathy and improved social processing and emotional regulation.

allowing us to cope with the high demands and stress of caring for a newborn. This circuitry allows us to keep our cool and respond sensitively when we might otherwise feel overwhelmed.

To recap, in response to a newborn, certain parts of our brains are activated that give us a hit in our reward and motivation circuits when we care for our infant. Our ability to understand our infant's cues and empathetically respond is enhanced, and we are encouraged to keep our cool in response to stressors. Throughout pregnancy, our brain size and volume decrease, reaching their shrinkage peak right at birth. At six months postpartum, our brains regain their original, prepregnancy size and volume, but the contents have been restructured. This structural and functional reshaping of our brain impacts how we adapt to parenthood and care for our infants. With our brain in a highly plastic state during pregnancy and postpartum, we are more vulnerable to both positive and negative experiences.

## NEURAL VULNERABILITY

Worrying about our infant's well-being and frequently checking to make sure they're OK are considered normal and healthy behaviors for new parents. Our anxiety is designed to draw us close to our infants, where we can meet their needs in the form of a secure embrace or, more often, a nipple in their mouth. Anxiousness and preoccupation peak right after birth and start to subside at around three or four months postpartum, like a gentle exhale that coincides with smiles and giggles from our baby. However, the increased sensitivity to threat we experience can increase our vulnerability to extreme anxiety and lead to mood disorders like depression.

Like birthing and breast milk, our brains respond to our environment, and plasticity is an evolutionary adaptation that helps us meet our baby's needs. When the environment is peaceful, supportive, and safe, the neural activation we experience in response to our baby's stimuli (i.e., cries, expressions, sounds) is positively linked to our caregiving behaviors. But our heightened plasticity makes us especially vulnerable to stress and psychopathology. Depression, trauma, chronic stress, and substance abuse can dampen neural responsiveness to infants and decrease empathy and emotional regulation. People whose own parents were dismissive or didn't treat them with care and warmth, or who were separated from their parents or raised with inadequate parenting, may experience disturbance and disruption of the normal changes in the brain during pregnancy and postpartum. This disturbance impacts the big three activated neural circuits that help us care for our baby: empathy, reward for caretaking behaviors, and emotional regulation. This means that a disturbance in brain rewiring, or dampened activation, makes it harder to understand babies and respond empathetically. Further, the brain is not rewarded while caring for the baby, which increases vulnerability to emotional dysregulation and stress.

The downside of our neural plasticity is our vulnerability to mood disorders throughout our life span and especially postpartum. The upside is our brain's openness to interventions. Our brains and behaviors are not set; they are able to change, heal, and repair.

There are ways to nurture neurogenesis and neuroplasticity. The first one I want to talk about is called environmental enrichment. Picture a laboratory mouse in its cage with just a bowl of dry food and water and a place to sleep. This mouse is all alone in this dark, monotonous, sensory-poor environment. Now imagine that same mouse placed back into its natural habitat. It is surrounded by other mice and by free open spaces where it can explore and run and eat diverse foods. In the lab, scientists simulate environmental enrichment by placing animals together with enhanced multisensory stimulation in the form of games and toys, increased physical activity, and social interactions.

When the mouse's environment is enriched, the central nervous system responds and cognitive functions, especially memory and learning, improve, as does the mouse's reactivity to emotional and stressful situations. Compared to mice in sensory poor environments, mice in enriched environments give their young more physical care and contact and spend more time with their pups in the nest, licking and grooming them. A seemingly simple shift in the environment causes animals to produce new neurons, mainly in their hippocampus, which is largely involved in memory and spatial learning. The longer animals stay in an enriched environment, the more these new neurons proliferate, differentiate, and survive.

OK, so what about us human animals? While most of us don't live in sensory-deprived cages, the sensory richness of our lives varies greatly. We experience wide-ranging levels of physical activity, social interaction, exploration, and types of spatial learning, and the degree of difference impacts our brains in a way that is similar to animals. Our senses—what we smell, hear, see, taste, and feel—affect the way our brains develop and function. Environmental enrichment can really be thought of as a way of nurturing all our senses. We can do this while we're pregnant and after through movement outside in nature or other beautiful places, by smelling soothing or delicious smells, by eating nourishing, vibrant food, through massage or other types of touch therapy, by listening to beautiful music or enjoying the quiet, or by spending time with people we love.

Negative environments increase the risk of maternal insensitivity toward the infant and the risk of psychopathology. The stakes are high. Postpartum blues and depression are common for parents. The brain plasticity inherent to reproduction paired with the task of caring for a newborn create a delicate period where we're more vulnerable to anxiety and mood disorders. Beyond taking steps to improve our environment, other evidence-backed interventions, like cognitive behavioral therapy (CBT), support neurogenesis and neuroplasticity. CBT focuses on cognitive restructuring, interpersonal support, and behavioral activation. In one study, depressed cisgender pregnant mothers received weekly CBT sessions that also focused on the transition into motherhood and other issues related to pregnancy, birth, and parenting. In the study, CBT during pregnancy reduced depressive symptoms and increased responsiveness to infants to the same level as the nondepressed control group. CBT, like environmental enrichment, is an intervention that focuses on supporting a positive neural and behavioral transition into parenthood. The result is improved health for both parent and baby.

People with a history of anxiety and depression, or those who experience these mood disorders during pregnancy, are perfect candidates for CBT starting early in pregnancy. Just like walking many miles outside and squatting a lot prepares our bodies to birth babies, supportive and enriching environments help us train, in a neurological sense, for taking care of our babies. All of us, regardless of our mental health status, deserve enriching and supportive environments. CBT and environmental enrichment are just two brain-centric examples of interventions that can help during the neurologically sensitive period of becoming a parent. Other evidence-based treatments for postpartum mood disorders include interpersonal therapy, psychodynamic psychotherapy, and pharmacological treatments. Peer and partner support, acupuncture, massage, omega-3 supplementation, physical activity, and bright light therapy have also been studied as interventions that may benefit you and your and baby during the postpartum period.

## Environmental Enrichment

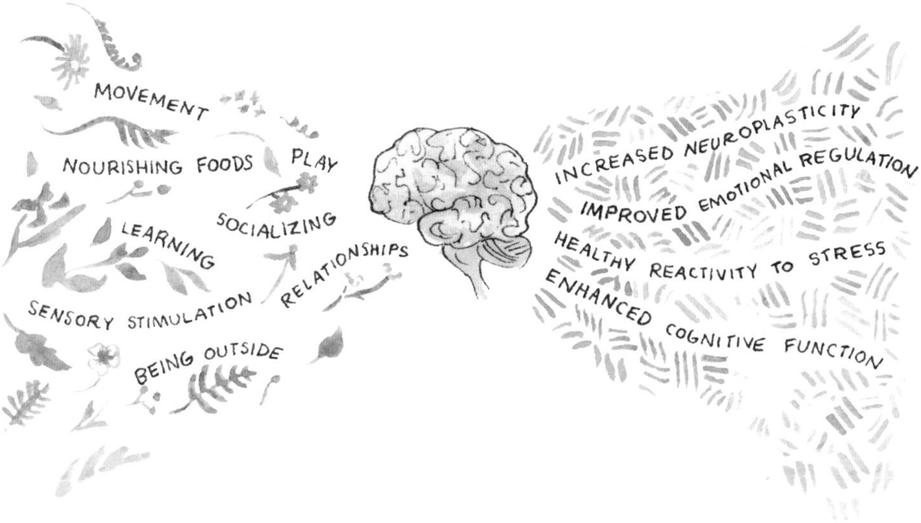
MOVEMENT
NOURISHING FOODS
PLAY
LEARNING
SOCIALIZING
RELATIONSHIPS
SENSORY STIMULATION
BEING OUTSIDE
INCREASED NEUROPLASTICITY
IMPROVED EMOTIONAL REGULATION
HEALTHY REACTIVITY TO STRESS
ENHANCED COGNITIVE FUNCTION

## EVOLUTIONARY INTELLIGENCE

Pregnancy initiates a kind of specialization of the brain, a neurohormonal-guided graduate degree that encourages us to keep our babies close, fed, and nurtured. Hormone changes and experience act as the master molders of our brains. High progesterone during pregnancy encourages us to nap and to stay away from dangerous and disgusting food, and it causes us to find unhealthy people repulsive. High estrogen helps us identify and avoid threatening people and situations. We tend to feel these effects the most during the first trimester, when our developing baby is the most vulnerable. In her book *Hormonal*, Martie Haselton writes that the most dangerous time of life, for both birthing parent and baby, are the minutes, days, and hours following birth. To get ready for this period of heightened danger, we start preparing our environment during the third trimester. Nesting is an adaptive behavior aimed at reducing pathogens, and it helps create a safe, secure, and hygienic environment for our baby.

The hormones involved in lactation further support our parenting. Lactating parents tend to report lower levels of stress overall but higher levels of aggression when needed. As a lactating mother, I can report that most of the time I feel pretty unperturbed and calm, but if I perceive a threat to my baby, I transform into a fierce, wild animal ready to fight and protect my baby. Our hormones help us remain calm while caring for our young but also keep us ready and primed to bite the head off a dangerous intruder.

Hormones, and the impact hormones have on the body and brain, are a form of evolutionary intelligence. There is remarkable, dynamic intelligence involved in caring for babies. The behaviors of parenting come from our ancient mammalian brain structures that are involved in motivation and reward, vigilance, and emotional processing. This ancient parenting network developed as a survival mechanism. If parents are able to respond to their infant's needs, they are better able to keep them alive.

Intimately caring for an infant triggers global changes in our neural networks that are involved in emotional processing and social understanding. Our parenting networks bring us into a rhythm with our baby so that we can

# Your Partner's Brain Changes Too

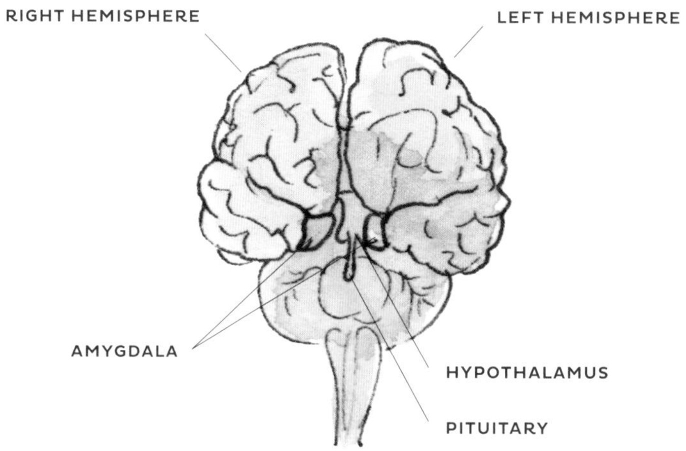


Parents who are more involved in taking care of their babies experience increased amygdala activity. This region of the brain is responsible for emotional processing and social understanding. New cisgender male fathers experience increased oxytocin and decreased testosterone, which is thought to promote bonding and decrease aggression. The day-to-day experience of parenting is an act of learning and adapting, which consequently changes the brain and allows us to focus our emotional and mental energy on our babies.

stay in tune with their emotional and physical state, make parent-like decisions, and keep providing high-level care. The more time fathers and other nonbirthing parents spend affectionately caring for their baby, the higher their oxytocin production and the more their brain shifts to connect them to their offspring.

Throughout human evolution, we humans were involved in an alloparenting caregiving system wherein both parents and nonparents provided care for babies and children. Because of our dynamic and flexible history, caregivers who are responsive and committed to a child's well-being experience activation of their parenting brains. Through practice, paying attention, and day-to-day caregiving, we get better at our job of taking care of little people.

## BABY BRAIN

Different types of movements and sensory input establish babies' neural networks. When we sing to our babies or they reach for a ball, their neural circuits, which depend on repeated activation, are strengthened. Their brains respond to patterns and sequences in our language, homing in on our phonetics so that they may one day use this language to understand us and their experience of being in the world.

Some of the most profound experiences that shape our babies' brains are their relationships and exposure and response to stressors. Attachment is a reciprocal, complex dance that most often occurs between the birth parent and baby. Each contributes to the relationship. In utero, olfactory and auditory systems develop that prime babies to recognize your smell and voice. This sensory experience and learning in the womb allows infants to orient to us when they are out in the world. We give food, warmth, safety, and comfort, and our babies cry and reach out for us. Our babies learn to smile and coo, and our neural systems and hormones tell us that their round squishy faces are highly likable, very cute, and worth protecting.

The quality of care provided by parents programs and regulates the infant's behavioral expression and brain function. Long-term emotional and cognitive development in our children is shaped by the way we care for them as infants. Part of this development includes developing a healthy response to stress. When babies and children experience stressors within a supportive environment, their stress response system activates and they experience an increase in their heart rate and stress hormone levels. Because they are supported, their physiological response is brief and quickly brought back down to their baseline. This is known as a positive stress response, and it is essential for normal development. The next level is the tolerable stress response. The baby's physiological response is more profound and lasts longer. The stress may come from something like an injury or natural disaster, and supportive relationships are essential to prevent long-term brain and organ damage. The toxic stress response is the most damaging and dangerous. Frequent, prolonged, or strong stressors in the form of neglect, abuse, exposure to violence, mental illness, or substance abuse without supportive relationships disrupt the development of the brain and predispose infants and children to cognitive impairments and stress-related diseases.

Through our body and behaviors, we create the primary environment our baby experiences, which in turn shapes their very plastic brains. The warmth and smells of your body, the sound of your voice, the way you hold your baby while you feed them, and your face and expressions create the rich, multisensorial experience that builds and shapes your newborn's brain. Just as we are attuned to our newborns, they are sensitive and susceptible to our well-being or distress. When babies and young children receive attentive and nurturing care in emotionally supportive environments, the structure and function of their brains reflect these environmental inputs. Their thinking and memory, emotional regulation, language, reasoning, and planning develop rapidly as new neural circuits form and neurons get wired together. By the time your baby turns three, he or she has developed around a hundred trillion connections.

# Nurturing Your Baby's Emotional Development

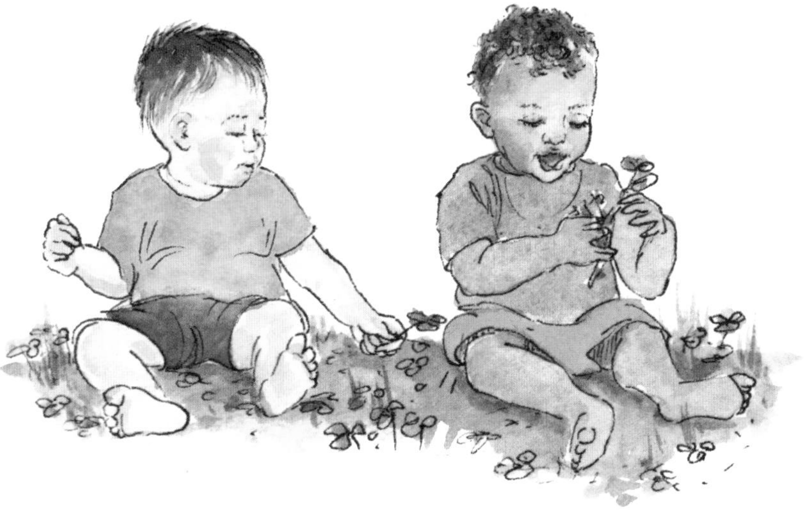

**GIVE CONSISTENT LOVING CARE:** Responsive and emotionally supportive care impacts thinking, memory, emotional regulation, language, reasoning, and planning and allows the brain to fully develop.

**CUDDLE, HUG, HOLD, MASSAGE:** Gentle physical touch allows babies and children to feel secure.

**NOURISH:** Brain-building foods (introduced at 6 months) include healthy fats, eggs, organ meats, wild fish, pastured and grass-fed meats, yogurt, kefir, sweet potatoes, fruits, and vegetables.

**TALK TO YOUR BABY:** Name what you see and ask them questions. Repetition forms neural connections.

**ALLOW YOUR BABY TO TOUCH, FEEL, SMELL, HEAR, TASTE, AND SEE:** Explore the environment safely. Spend lots of time playing outside in natural environments. Limit or eliminate screens and electronic toys.

## THE REDEMPTION OF PAPA

When Holden was a few months old, I had a nightmare that I couldn't find him. Half-asleep, I sat up in bed, utterly panicked, searching for my baby. Out of nowhere, Max leapt out of bed, turned on the light, and assumed what I'm quite sure was a Taekwondo-ready stance, with his feet slightly staggered and his arms flexed out in front of him, prepared to fight. The fog that had settled on my sleep-dazed brain cleared, and I saw that Holden was right next to me, soundly asleep. Then I had a moment to ponder the fighter my partner had morphed into at the foot of the bed. It was as if I could see his parenting brain firing, his neural circuitry primed over the last few months to fiercely protect our creature. Babies are often described as defenseless, but they mold and shape us to be their soldiers, willing to stand on the front line and guard their bodies with our own.

Our brains continue to support us and to adapt our biology to our current roles. Like the brains of our children, our brains grow and develop when they are engaged, active, playful, and flexible and when they get adequate sleep. They thrive in supportive environments and are designed by evolution to help us care for our young. The architecture of the human brain is gratefully able to reshape and regenerate, which allows us to transition from sleeping lumps who can't hear our babies cry into fiercely protective parents who are ready for battle at the slightest hint of a threat.

# TAKE ACTION

Embrace change. The regions of the brain involved in reward and maternal motivation, social information, empathy, and emotional regulation are activated during pregnancy and parenting. These changes structurally and functionally transform our brains and help us adapt, through our behavior, to our infants, who require a high level of our attention and care.

Enrich your environment to foster your brain's neurogenesis and neuroplasticity. Our brains adapt and respond to our environment, and environmental enrichment can be thought of as nurturing all our senses. Moving outside in beautiful places, spending time with people we love, eating delicious foods, smelling delightful smells, hearing soothing sounds, and experiencing healing touch affect the way our brains develop and function and cultivate our parenting brains. The degree that our brains change during pregnancy and parenting impacts our ability to provide high-quality care to our babies and requires support.

Connect with your baby and nurture your relationship. When children receive attentive and emotionally supportive care, their brains reflect these environmental inputs. Their thinking and memory, emotional regulation, language, reasoning, and planning are shaped by the care they receive and their relationships with their caretakers.

Give yourself and your partner time to adapt to parenting. Our partners also experience dynamic hormonal and brain alterations that cultivate their ability to accurately understand and appropriately respond to our babies, but they might not experience these changes at the same time as you. Through the practice of deeply paying attention and day-to-day caregiving, our rhythms become more in sync with our baby's and we get better at taking care of them.

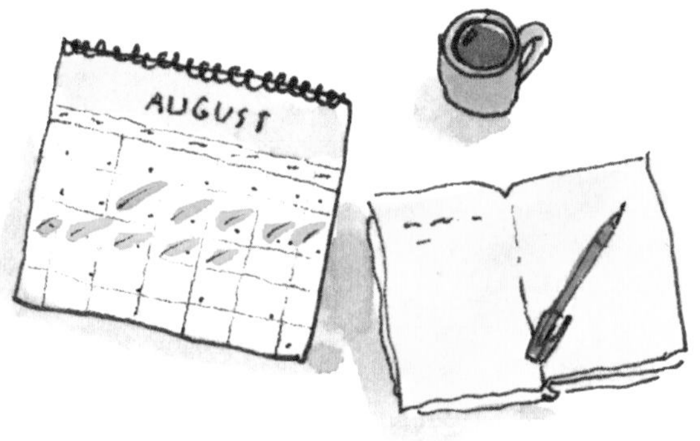
AUGUST

CHAPTER TWELVE

# Family Planning

WHEN HOLDEN WAS a little over one, my friends who had babies a few months older than him started getting pregnant with their second child. I felt a little jealous of their readiness. My cycle had just returned on Holden's first birthday, and I was feeling a shift in my body and identity as a mother. I was going on long hikes by myself again while Holden played at home with Max, and I enjoyed moving in my own body without carrying him for miles. I also wasn't sure if I was fertile yet. Holden was still nursing frequently—not like a newborn, but enough that we still couldn't see his ankle bones under the layer of chub on his legs.

The milk-producing hormone prolactin suppresses estrogen and other hormones that contribute to fertility. Specifically, prolactin inhibits follicle-stimulating hormone (FSH) and gonadotropin-releasing hormone (GnRH), two hormones that encourage follicles to develop and trigger ovulation. When estrogen and progesterone are still low, the uterine lining cannot support and nourish an egg for implantation even when FSH and luteinizing hormone (LH) resume their normal levels, allowing for ovulation. However, some people can ovulate and get pregnant before their cycles return. The length of postpartum amenorrhea, or the amount of time we don't have a menstrual cycle after birth, varies depending on age, frequency of breastfeeding or chestfeeding, and whether we exclusively nurse versus supplement with food or formula. When babies are six months and under and are exclusively breastfed on demand (day and night directly from the breast), high prolactin levels act as a pretty reliable form of birth control known as the lactational amenorrhea method (LAM), or ecological breastfeeding.

LAM requires three conditions to be effective at preventing pregnancy: the birth parent's menstrual cycle has not returned; baby is exclusively breast- or chestfed day and night on demand; and baby is less than six months old. This method is 98 percent effective. Ecological breastfeeding is based on seven standards: exclusive breastfeeding or chestfeeding for the first six months, comforting and pacifying baby at the breast, not using pacifiers or bottles, sleeping with baby for night feedings, sleeping with baby for daily nap feedings, nursing frequently day and night without a schedule, and avoiding any practice that separates you from baby. Ecological breastfeeding and LAM, while effective at preventing pregnancy, especially when babies are under three months old, are not methods that are accessible, desirable, or realistic for all parents.

When Holden was under six months, I was pretty confident in my infertility based on his habits. This isn't to say I was sure I wasn't fertile, because, even with perfect use of LAM, one to two people out of one hundred may get pregnant during the first six months following childbirth. After six months, I entered an unknown and undefined time where my cycle hadn't returned yet and Holden was eating solid food and nursing frequently. While nursing delays the return of menses, it is relatively common to ovulate before menses resumes. In nonlactating people, ovulation can occur as early as twenty-five days postpartum, but the average return is forty-five to ninety-four days after birth. In lactating people, 20 percent ovulate by six months and 64 percent ovulate by twelve months.

While I had used fertility awareness–based methods prior to my pregnancy, I wasn't sure how my signs of fertility would look now in my hormonally altered postpartum landscape. For example, basal body temperature becomes less accurate at determining the return of fertility because temperature changes happen after ovulation, so if you're not ovulating, your temperature is rather meaningless. Cervical mucus, which has always been my favorite and most accurate sign of fertility, becomes a less reliable indicator while nursing since the changes in our cervical mucus don't always coincide with our hormonal variations. That said, cervical mucus can still provide valuable information about fertility, and it quickly regained its status as my favorite sign of fertility once my cycle returned.

Because of the challenges of fertility tracking postpartum, especially identifying fertile versus nonfertile mucus, it's a good time to work with a professional fertility awareness educator. In this time of physiological flux and person-to-person variability, support and guidance from someone trained to help you read the signs of your cervical mucus can be indispensable. There are different options for preventing pregnancy postpartum, like the Marquette postpartum protocol, which combines charting, education, support from a professional, and an electronic hormonal fertility monitor. This high-tech method helps those in the postpartum phase identify their fertile window and avoid unintended pregnancies. A trained fertility awareness educator can help guide you through this or other methods while you learn to navigate the cycles of your body after baby.

Natural forms of birth control like LAM and ecological breastfeeding require flexibility, commitment, and a parent who isn't required to go back to work after three months of leave. For our ancestors, whose children probably weren't totally weaned until they were closer to three years old, breastfeeding put the brakes on their fertility until their babies were less dependent and their bodies were ready. For most of us, these forms of birth control may be impractical or impossible, and they expire at six months postpartum, aka

# Family Planning Methods

Has your period returned? NO YES

Are you pumping or supplementing with formula? NO YES

Is your baby older than 6 months? NO YES

You might try the lactational amenorrhea method (LAM), which is 98%–99% effective.

Male condoms: 98% effective
Fertility awareness method: 98%–99% effective
Withdrawal/pullout: 80%–96% effective
Nonhormonal IUD: 99% effective
Hormonal IUD: 99% effective
Hormonal contraceptives: 99% effective
Vasectomy: almost 100% effective

Note: These rates of effectiveness are based on perfect use.

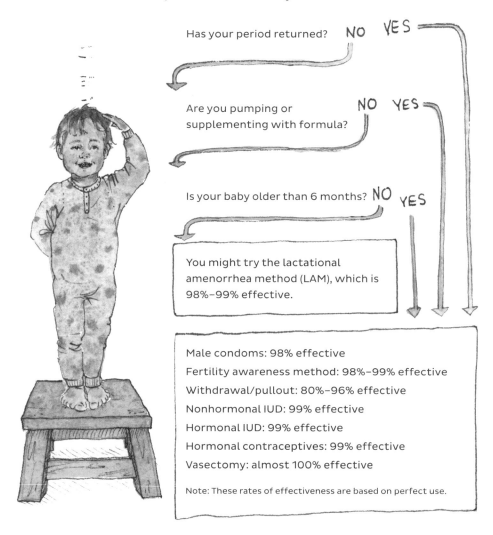

when you might want to have more sex again. I took the careful curiosity approach, which meant paying close attention to my cervical mucus and following the recommendations from *The Fifth Vital Sign*, where Lisa Hendrickson-Jack advises that we prepare for pregnancy for six to twelve months, allowing our menstrual cycle to normalize for three full cycles and focusing on replenishing nutrient stores before considering conception.

Fertility returns in stages as our hormones come back into balance. After getting to know my cycle and feeling like I understood the rhythm of my body for the years before I was pregnant, I entered a new, unknown landscape postpartum. My regular, predictable cycle was gone. The length of my cycle was variable, my skin changed, and my brain was shifting again too. As I adjusted to my returning fertility, I also felt a shift in my sexuality. My parenting brain started to overlap with my autonomous, mating brain, and navigating these roles required some practice.

## BABY SPACING AND THE MATING BRAIN

My mating brain started whispering to me when Holden was around eighteen months old. My parenting brain would say, "Look, it's 8:30, time for us to sleep," and mating brain would respond, "It's still before 9, there's plenty of time to have sex!" Max payed close attention to my internal dialogue, always at the ready when mating brain won the argument, but gratefully, never showing disappointment when parenting brain enforced bedtime. This time frame lined up with research that encourages waiting a minimum of eighteen months before conceiving another baby. The World Health Organization (WHO) recommends waiting at least twenty-four months. This specific recommendation came about when one group of people at the WHO birth-spacing meeting recommended waiting a minimum of eighteen months, while another group recommended twenty-seven months. The WHO also recommends breastfeeding for at least two years. Twenty-four months lined up well with both recommendations and was the happy compromise.

The length of time between delivery and conception, known as an interpregnancy interval, is associated with pregnancy outcomes. Adverse outcomes such as preterm delivery, low birth weight, and infant mortality are associated with interpregnancy intervals shorter than twelve months. An interpregnancy interval shorter than twelve months increases the risk of health problems for babies and birthing parents. For birthing parents under age thirty-four, shorter interpregnancy intervals increase health risks for babies, while those over thirty-five experience similar risks to their infant's health, but also increased risk to their own health.

One of the leading theories as to why interpregnancy spacing matters and impacts fetal health is that after building a baby, the birthing parent's body is depleted of key nutrients like folate and iron. The folate depletion hypothesis claims that since folate levels start to drop midpregnancy and stay low from four to twelve months postpartum, conception during this time isn't supported by enough folate, which can alter fetal neurodevelopment. Other theories include increased prenatal stress and inflammation.

In traditional hunter-gatherer societies, where mothers typically carried their children under the age of four, interpregnancy intervals jump up to thirty to forty months or more. Waiting until the first baby can walk long distances on his or her own makes sense; it is a lot of work to walk around with two small children on your back. As humans became more sedentary and our access to high-calorie foods became steady and limitless, birth spacing intervals shortened. Now our decision about when to make another baby is limited not by our environment but by our choices. For me this freedom of choice in all parts of life—What should I be when I grow up? When should we make another baby?—can travel hand in hand with stress. When I feel the anxiety of freedom, I have to remember that I'm getting a cue to pause and listen before I make a decision. When freedom feels threatening, a long walk gives me a break from the deciding and allows me to come back to my body. Moving through the world on my feet gives me answers. Perhaps the feeling of deep knowing can happen only when I'm moving.

If you decide you want another baby, the most important signs of readiness aren't necessarily the dates on a calendar. I needed to feel like my body was recovered fully and replenished with essential nutrients before my mind could start shifting toward the idea of growing another baby. Regardless of when or if we choose to conceive again, we can eat restorative food and move and care for our bodies during the interim so that we're well nourished no matter what we choose. Continuing to take a high-quality prenatal vitamin, eating the foods that support hormonal and fetal health, and moving in a way that allows your body to heal and become strong and balanced are crucial for living well in your body after having a baby.

## INTEGRATING THE PARENTAL AND THE EROTIC SELVES

Some mammals can have sex only when they are able to reproduce, but we humans aren't those mammals. Sex, after a baby, is an act that must be reclaimed by the partnership as an expression of connection and mutual desire. I wanted to reclaim the laissez-faire attitude of not *not* trying and linger in the space of present pleasure and an unknown future.

Of course, the environment around us had changed now that it wasn't just Max and me. We were in new territory with an old map, and finding our way took patience and an intact sense of direction. In her book *Mating in Captivity*, Esther Perel describes how for women especially, there is a kind of sensuality involved in parenting that can replace and displace sensuality with a partner. The sensory experience of caring for our children is the same feeling as falling in love, and it exists, from an evolutionary standpoint, to allow us to deeply bond to our babies and keep them alive.

When caring for our children shifts from this initial falling in love to a feeling of constant scheduling and organizational stress, intimacy between partners suffers. The modern style of parenting lacks the kind of support networks humans historically enjoyed while raising their babies. Imagine a baby in a village with dots connecting them to parents, aunts, uncles, grandmas, grandpas, older women, other children, and community members. The baby is part of a constellation, one of the stars in the sky of the village. In our modern, isolated homes, there are far fewer connection points, and the baby is usually at the center of the universe. "This unprecedented child-centrality," Perel says, "is unfolding against the backdrop of romanticism that underscores modern marriage." With the child in the middle of the universe and our expectations of our partnerships to fill our need for emotional closeness, intimacy, and sex, we risk feeling overwhelmed and like we're failing either our children or our partners.

Sexuality is wrapped up in our identity and sense of self. Our culture doesn't teach us that the parental and the erotic can live together and thrive in our bodies. Being a parent doesn't negate our independence, freedom, and desire for pleasure. Women, in particular, have experienced greater sexual freedom over the last few decades, but mothers have not broken free from expectations of sanctity. Perel ponders the perpetuation of the virtuous mother:

> Desexualization of the mother is a mainstay of traditionally patriarchal cultures, which makes the sexual invisibility of modern western mothers seem particularly acute. Perhaps it's our Puritan legacy that strips motherhood of its sexual components; perhaps we are convinced that lustfulness conflicts with maternal duty.

Upon reading this, I realized that resexualization of the mother has the potential to empower us and subtly undermine the cultural identity we're assigned when we have children. After giving myself plenty of time to fully heal and reconnect with my body after birth, I noticed the moments in the day when sex became an exhilarating and possible thing to do.

This doesn't mean each waking hour must be dedicated to stoking the erotic flame with your partner. Our desire for intimacy ebbs and flows. It is deeply personal and is not based on quantity. When our babies are still very young, they need us, and we must surrender part of ourselves to the cause of their survival. The postpartum period, which lasts our entire life after children, feels like a new puzzle we need to put together. There are the pieces of us that make us feel alive and individual, like our relationships, interests, and desires. And there are the parental pieces that may also make us feel vital, alive, and important. The parental pieces don't replace the other pieces; they integrate and form a new version of you.

# Integrating the Parental and the Erotic Selves

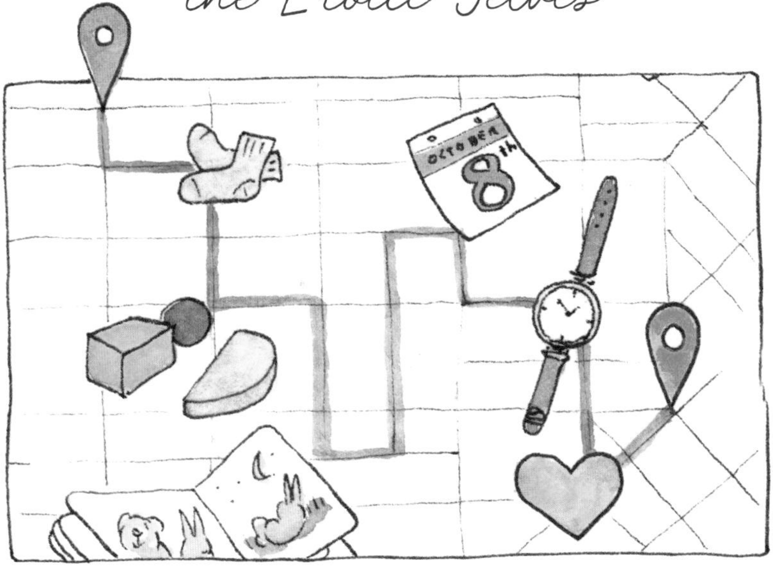


**PARENTAL**
Nurturing, selfless, safe, routined, stable, attentive, responsible

**EROTIC**
Sexually desirous, free, adventurous, pursuant of one's own interests, spontaneous, surprising, sensual

## CONTROL VERSUS COLLABORATION

In 2018, Michaeleen Doucleff wrote the article "Secrets of a Maya Supermom: What Parenting Books Don't Tell You," which highlights the mothering style of Maria de los Angeles Tun Burgos. This mother to five children was described as calm, collected, and unfazed, and Doucleff discovered through her interview with Burgos that in the Mayan language, the word "stressful" is not used to describe parenting. In one of my favorite quotes from the article, Burgos said, "I know that raising kids is slow. Little by little they will learn."

We must also learn how to parent little by little. Most of us in the US learn how to take care of young children when we have our own babies, whereas Burgos learned through firsthand experience by helping and watching other women in her community mother their children. The world of parenting in the US is often mediated by the advice of "experts" who give parenting advice that is based on their opinions and past parenting theories and is generally centered on the experience of Westerners. In the 2010 paper "The Weirdest People in the World?," three scientists from the University of British Columbia describe how behavioral scientists make broad claims about psychology and behavior based on a small representation of Western, educated, industrialized, rich, democratic (WEIRD) societies. The authors provide several examples that demonstrate how researchers, who focus on 12 percent of the world population, universally apply their findings to all of humanity. One example is parent-child play. In Western societies, parent-child play signals strong attachment, while in some indigenous cultures, parent-child play tends to be rare and play is valuable because children do it on their own and it doesn't require parent involvement. The point of this example isn't to say that playing with your children is right or wrong; it's to show that what we tend to hold as the truth is highly variable, and there are many ways to parent our children.

Understanding that parenting differs based on culture is valuable because we discover that we have choices about how we interact with our children. We also have a choice about the language we connect to parenting. The word "stress" is intertwined with child-rearing in the US, but in Mayan culture, it isn't associated with the act of raising children. There is immense power in realizing that we have the ability to choose the descriptive language that colors the narrative of our life. Doucleff writes that in our society, the parent-child relationship is centered on control, while in Mayan culture, the parent-child relationship is one of collaboration. From the time they're born, Mayan children are treated with respect. Parenting is spread throughout the community. Children are included in family goals and integrated into, rather than separated from, society.

I like to think about Burgos when I'm in a hurry or when I feel isolated and like the burden of parenting is solely upon me. How can I make my

# Many Right Ways

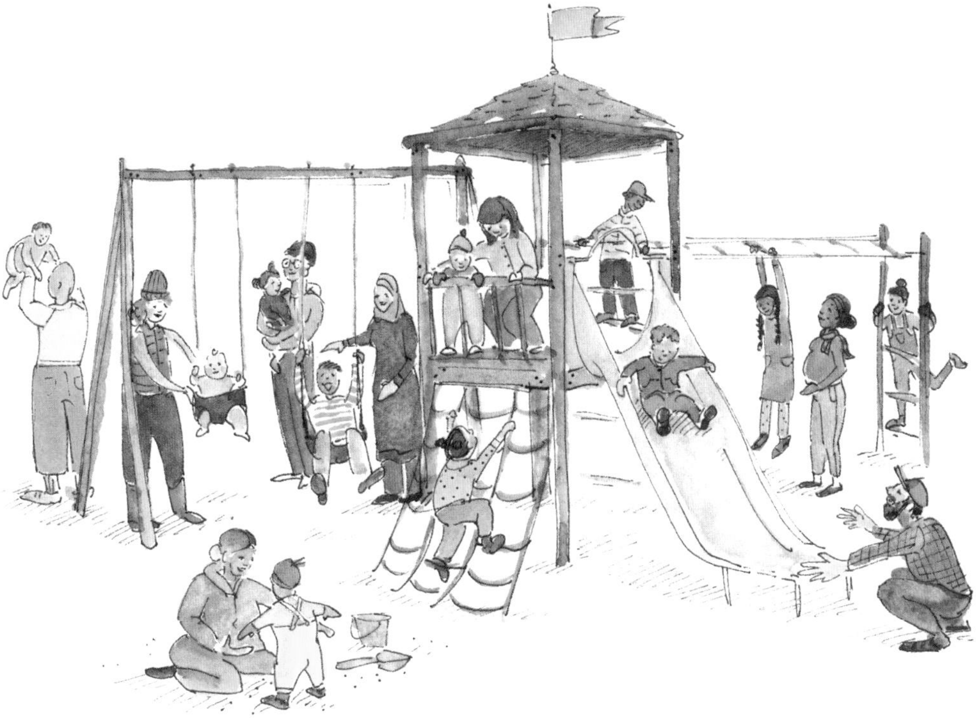

There is no one right way to parent, nor is there one right culture. We are guided by our past and by what we learn along the way, and we have a choice as we move forward.

In *individualist cultures*, emphasis is placed on stimulation, early cognitive development, and self-sufficiency. The focus is on the individual over the collective, and parenting is based less on tradition and more on upward economic mobility.

In *collectivist cultures*, emphasis is placed on self-regulation, respect, a sense of duty, living well with others, and shared dependence in a group. Tradition guides parenting.

world feel bigger and my relationship with Holden more collaborative? This question has the power to shift my perspective. It takes me out of a reactive and stressful space and into the position of observer and collaborator.

Pregnancy, birth, raising a baby, maintaining a romantic relationship with a partner, working, cooking, cleaning, and nurturing your own identity—the list of tasks can feel long and overwhelming. We feel pressured by the vision of perfection and the relentlessness of to-dos. I've found that the foundations of this book—movement, good food, and supportive communities—help me integrate and overlap the requirements of life in a way that feels meaningful and pleasurable. When I move my body often, whether I'm walking outside or cleaning the house with Holden, who does his best to help, my world expands, and I feel that Holden shares a common goal with the rest of the family. When we plant, pick, prepare, and eat nourishing food together, the act of eating feels less like one of checklist necessity and more like a valuable representation of our cultural values.

I relate, perhaps more than I should sometimes, to my willful and determined toddler. I am determined to see my partnership with Max as alive and evolving, and I'm willful when it comes to moving often, eating well, and taking care of our world and each other even when time, money, and resources feel scarce. The most important tool I have in my parenting tool kit is the ability to choose which stories shape me and inform my experience. This superpower, which we all share, allows me to remain open-minded, fascinated, and playful even when some of the cultural messages coming in are of seriousness, stress, rules, and burden. The transcendence I feel while growing my baby is not a profound feeling of becoming an adult, but rather the defiant act of reclaiming the part of me that is childlike and able to experience the world with wonder and pleasure.

# TAKE ACTION

Note the changes in your body, including signs of fertility, after childbirth. Fertility returns in stages and requires that we pay careful attention and relearn the cycles of our bodies. If you wish to avoid hormonal contraceptives, working with a fertility awareness educator can help you navigate your altered hormonal landscape and avoid pregnancy for the recommended eighteen months before conceiving another baby if you choose to do so.

Find the balance between your parental and erotic identities. Postpartum encourages us to integrate, not separate, the parts of us that are involved in caring for our children and the part of us that is sexual, that pursues our own interests and has our own desires.

Learn from other cultures and understand that the way parents care for their children varies greatly depending on where people are in the world. In Mayan culture, there isn't a word for stress in relation to parenting, collaboration is valued more than control, and children are respected and integrated into their society from the moment of their birth.

Choose the stories and language that color the narrative of your life and how you parent. Choice is a superpower that allows us to move away from stress and a task-oriented life and toward pleasure, open-mindedness, and playfulness. Little by little our babies learn, and little by little, we may also learn from them.

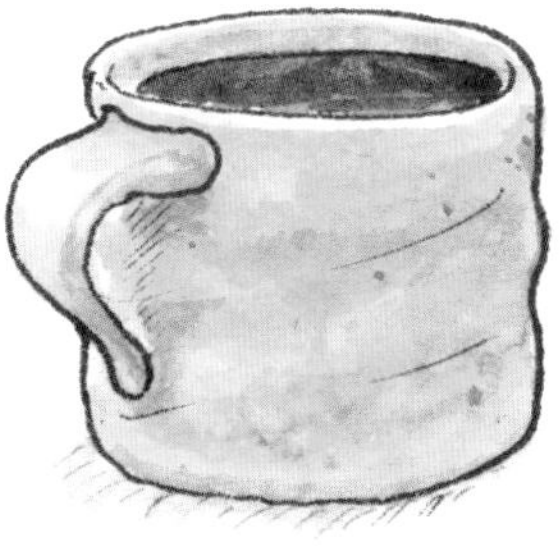

# Epilogue

**IN THE EARLY DAYS** of writing, when I was still figuring out the shape, form, and feeling of this book, I called a friend for some help. I told her I wanted this book to be full of relatable stories, fascinating and approachable science, and beautiful illustrations. More than anything, I wanted to create something that made parents feel empowered and like they could immediately put the information in this book to use while they grew their babies. The goal was to create something with foundational principles that was a delight to read.

My wise friend responded, "It sounds like you want to create the *Salt, Fat, Acid, Heat* of pregnancy books." I ran downstairs to my kitchen and grabbed this beautiful cookbook, written by Samin Nosrat and illustrated by Wendy MacNaughton. The book provides cooks with four essential elements that allow them to make inspired and delicious meals, explaining the science of each element and how they come together to create something greater than the sum of each part. No matter your question in the kitchen, the answer is probably salt, fat, acid, or heat.

I feel this way about nourishing food, movement, support, and taking care of our shared ecosystem. These four themes of this book are the ingredients that come together to allow us to grow, birth, and raise healthy babies. No matter my question during pregnancy, birth, or after, I could come back to these principles and find an answer.

The next call I made was to one of my closest friends, the illustrator of this book, Michelle Lassaline. We had talked about the project loosely, but this conversation was different. "Michelle," I said, "do you want to go all in on this project with me and create this book together?" When Michelle said yes, I could suddenly see this book, and I'd find myself flipping through the pages in my head in the middle of the night. I remember reading an article about how MacNaughton didn't like to cook when she started working on *Salt, Fat, Acid, Heat*, but by the end she was cooking everything she drew for the book and gained her own cooking education through the process. Likewise,

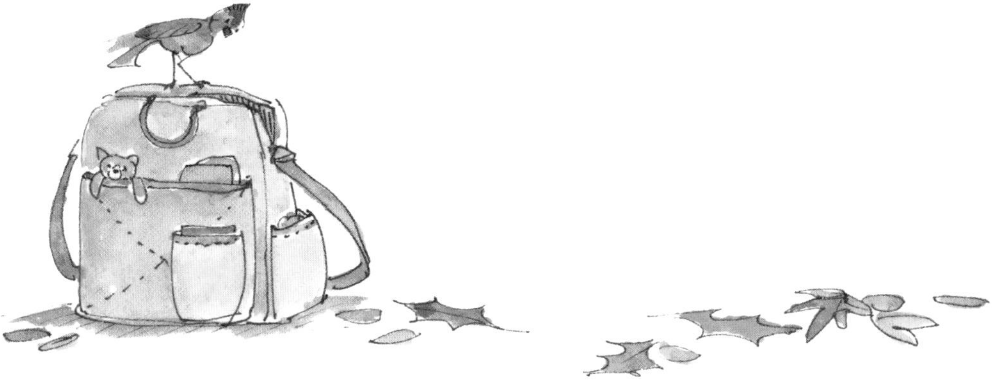

Michelle had not grown a baby. During one of our many conversations about illustrations, she told me that after reading chapter 5, she spent an hour looking at and learning about placentas. "You should see my Google search history and the tabs I have open," she said, laughing. Then she said, "I'm not going to grow a baby right now, but I feel like when I do, I'll be so ready."

For me, writing this book has been a lot like growing a baby and required the same ingredients. Long walks in the high desert allowed me to find stories and answers to hard questions. On almost every walk, ideas would stop me in my tracks, almost like I had to walk to that specific spot of earth so the idea could come up from the ground and through me. Then I'd repeat the paragraphs in my head and write them down once I got home and my baby was napping. Food, of course, was also essential. The food I write about in this book and that Michelle illustrated is the food I ate while I was pregnant and breastfeeding. When I felt deeply nourished, I could write about nourishment. This book came to life because I had consistent, indispensable support from Max.

Together, all these pieces became this book, which at its heart encourages parents to make choices that allow them to grow optimally healthy babies but also take care of our shared ecosystem. Growing a baby gives us the opportunity to reconsider how we live in the world. It is a moment of reckoning in which we realize that the life we build depends on our internal and external ecology. By understanding how the home we create in our bodies for our babies connects us to our place and to the world, it becomes easier to make choices that sustain the health of the whole.

# Acknowledgments

**BOOK WRITING IS** a happy place for a mind that constantly wanders and wonders. I wouldn't have had the space to do either without support from my family, specifically my partner, Max. The acknowledgments section isn't generally a love letter, but in this moment when I'm meditating on gratitude, all I can think about is how love facilitated this book and how truly lucky I am that I was able to work on this book with Max by my side as a partner and as a fellow creative person and storyteller. Thanks for reading every page, more than twice, and for being the best, most patient and loving partner and papa. I cannot imagine growing and raising babies without you.

Thanks to my parents and their encouragement. My mom's guidance taught me to trust my instincts and to feel powerful and capable in my body. Her example, more than anything, has shaped how I mother and how I view parenting—that is, with an open mind and a sense of adventure. My dad, ever the hard worker, gave me the gift of his stubbornness and determination, two ingredients that take a book from an idea to an actual object you can hold in your hands. To my brother Nick, thank you for reading my work and giving me honest and straightforward feedback. And to my brother Bob, thanks for being so kind and gentle.

Of any artist I've ever met, Michelle is the most academic, and yet she retains the sincerity, humor, and curiosity of a child who has just met a spiderweb glistening in the sun after a rainstorm. She stops, sees, examines, pays attention, and doesn't miss a single detail. Her talent and thoughtfulness shine through in each piece of art she created for this book. Thank you for one of the most meaningful friendships in my life and for bringing so much beauty into the world.

My deepest gratitude to the best teacher I've ever had and my favorite writer, Michael Branch. Thank you for reading my initial proposal for this book and for your guidance and encouragement. Your work and example are a guiding light and constant source of inspiration.

I'm incredibly grateful to my editor, Juree Sondker, and the whole team at Roost Books who decided to take a chance on an emerging writer and a book about growing babies. Thank you to the sensitivity reader who helped me make this book more inclusive. Thank you to the associate editor, copyeditor, and proofreader for your incredible attention to detail. And thank you to the design and marketing team for bringing the vision for this book to life. Working with such a talented team is a true honor.

Thank you to the friends who listened to me talk about this book on walks or while we shared a meal, and to the parents who shared their stories with me. Thank you to the writers and researchers I admire and reference throughout this book, and to the practitioners who read and checked my work. Thank you to all the people who supported me during my pregnancy, birth, and beyond and to the wider community of remarkable people who work in the world of babies and birth.

This book is dedicated to my son Holden. I started writing the first chapter when he was seven months old, and by the time I finished the book he was deep into his toddlerhood and a second baby was growing in my belly. I'd be remiss to leave out this second baby I grew who shared a due date with the final version of the manuscript of this book and whose kicks and nudges reminded me daily that this work matters. There is no end to my gratitude for the babies I've grown and to the land, air, water, and people that have supported and nourished me along the way.

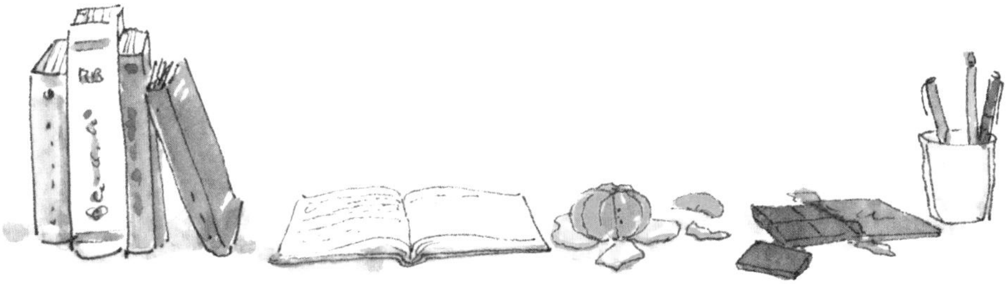

# Resources

## RECOMMENDED READING

*Braiding Sweetgrass: Indigenous Wisdom, Scientific Knowledge, and the Teachings of Plants* by Robin Wall Kimmerer

*The Bold World: A Memoir of Family and Transformation* by Jodie Patterson

*Breasts: A Natural and Unnatural History* by Florence Williams

*Family Business: Thirty Years of Innovative On-Site Child Care* by Malinda Pennoyer Chouinard and Jennifer Ridgeway

*The Fifth Vital Sign: Master Your Cycles and Optimize Your Fertility* by Lisa Hendrickson-Jack

*The First Forty Days: The Essential Art of Nourishing the New Mothers* by Heng Ou, with Amely Greeven and Marisa Belger

*The Fourth Trimester: A Postpartum Guide to Healing Your Body, Balancing Your Emotions, and Restoring Your Vitality* by Kimberly Ann Johnson

*This Is Your Brain on Birth Control: The Surprising Science of Women, Hormones, and the Law of Unintended Consequences* by Sarah E. Hill

*Gentle Birth, Gentle Mothering: A Doctor's Guide to Natural Childbirth and Gentle Early Parenting* by Sarah Buckley

*Guidebook to Relative Strangers: Journeys in Race, Motherhood, and History* by Camille T. Dungy

*Having Faith: An Ecologist's Journey to Motherhood* by Sandra Steingraber

*Home Grown: Adventures in Parenting Off the Beaten Path* by Ben Hewitt

*Hormonal: The Hidden Intelligence of Hormones* by Martie Haselton

*How to Be an Antiracist* by Ibram X. Kendi

*It's OK Not to Share and Other Renegade Rules for Raising Competent and Compassionate Kids* by Heather Shumaker

*Mating in Captivity: Unlocking Erotic Intelligence* by Esther Perel

*Mindful Birthing: Training the Mind, Body, and Heart for Childbirth and Beyond* by Nancy Bardacke

*Motherhood So White: A Memoir of Race, Gender, and Parenting in America* by Nefertiti Austin

*Movement Matters: Essays on Movement Science, Movement Ecology, and the Nature of Movement* by Katy Bowman

*Move Your DNA: Restore Your Health through Natural Movement* by Katy Bowman

*Nurture: A Modern Guide to Pregnancy, Birth, Early Motherhood—and Trusting Yourself and Your Body* by Erica Chidi Cohen

*Pelvic Liberation: Using Yoga, Self-Inquiry, and Breath Awareness for Pelvic Health* by Leslie Howard

*Period Repair Manual: Natural Treatment for Better Hormones and Better Periods* by Lara Briden

*The Power of Showing Up: How Parental Presence Shapes Who Our Kids Become and How Their Brains Get Wired* by Daniel J. Siegel and Tina Payne Bryson

*Raising Elijah: Protecting Our Children in an Age of Environmental Crisis* by Sandra Steingraber

*Raising Wild: Dispatches from a Home in the Wilderness* by Michael P. Branch

*Real Food for Mother and Baby: The Fertility Diet, Eating for Two, and Baby's First Foods* by Nina Planck

*Real Food for Pregnancy: The Science and Wisdom of Optimal Prenatal Nutrition* by Lily Nichols

*Reproductive Injustice: Racism, Pregnancy, and Premature Birth* by Dána-Ain Davis

*Wanderlust: A History of Walking* by Rebecca Solnit

*We Live for the We: The Political Power of Black Motherhood* by Dani McClain

*The Whole-Brain Child: 12 Revolutionary Strategies to Nurture Your Child's Developing Mind* by Daniel J. Siegel and Tina Payne Bryson

## OTHER RESOURCES

*Spinning Babies* www.spinningbabies.com

*Kelly Mom* www.kellymom.com

*Evolutionary Parenting* www.evolutionaryparenting.com

*Evidence Based Birth* www.evidencebasedbirth.com

# Bibliography


## PROLOGUE

Steingraber, S. *Having Faith: An Ecologist's Journey to Motherhood*. New York: Perseus Publishing, 2001.

Wilson, E.O. *Consilience: The Unity of Knowledge*. New York: Vintage Books, 1998.

## CHAPTER 1: NEW BEGINNINGS

Achermann, Yvonne, Ellie Goldstein, Tom Coenye, and Mark Shirliff. "*Propionibacterium acnes*: From Commensal to Opportunistic Biofilm-Associated Implant Pathogen," *Clinical Microbiology Reviews* 27, no. 3 (2014): 419–40. https://doi.org/10.1128/CMR.00092-13.

American College of Obstetricians and Gynecologists. "Menstruation in Girls and Adolescents: Using the Menstrual Cycle as a Vital Sign," *ACOG*, December 2015. https://www.acog.org/Clinical-Guidance-and-Publications/Committee-Opinions/Committee-on-Adolescent-Health-Care/Menstruation-in-Girls-and-Adolescents-Using-the-Menstrual-Cycle-as-a-Vital-Sign.

Ames, Bruce N. "Low Micronutrient Intake May Accelerate the Degenerative Diseases of Aging Through Allocation of Scarce Micronutrients by Triage," *PNAS* 103, no. 47 (2006): 17589–94. https://doi.org/10.1073/pnas.0608757103.

Briden, Lara. *Period Repair Manual: Natural Treatment for Better Hormones and Better Periods*, 2nd ed. Self-published, 2017.

Degnan, Patrick, Michiko Taga, and Andrew Goodman. "Vitamin $B_{12}$ as a Modulator of Gut Microbial Ecology," *Cell Metabolism* 20, no. 5 (2014). https://doi.org/10.1016/j.cmet.2014.10.002.

Dréno, B., et al. "Microbiome in Healthy Skin, Update for Dermatologists," *Journal of the European Academy of Dermatology and Venereology* 30, no. 12 (2016): 2038–47.

Hendrickson-Jack, Lisa. *The Fifth Vital Sign: Master Your Cycles and Optimize Your Fertility*. Self-published, 2019.

Horvath, Sarah, Courtney Schreiber, and Sarita Sonalkar. "Contraception," *Endotext*, 2018. https://www.ncbi.nlm.nih.gov/books/NBK279148/.

Huang, M. J., and Y. F. Liaw. "Clinical Associations Between Thyroid and Liver Disease," *Journal of Gastroenterology and Hepatology* 10, no. 3 (1995). https://www.ncbi.nlm.nih.gov/pubmed/7548816.

Lee, Seunh Hun, Se Kyoo Jeohn, and Sung Ku Ahn. "An Update of the Defensive Barrier Function of Skin," *Yonsei Medical Journal* 47, no. 3 (2006): 293–306. https://doi.org/10.3349/ymj.2006.47.3.293.

Meethal, Sivan, and Craig Atwood. "The Role of Hypothalamic-Pituitary-Gonadal Hormones in the Normal Structure and Functioning of the Brain," *Cellular and Molecular Life Sciences* 62, no. 3 (2005): 257–70. https://doi.org/10.1007/s00018-004-4381-3.

Nichols, Lily. *Real Food for Pregnancy: The Science and Wisdom of Optimal Prenatal Nutrition*. Self-published, 2018.

Palmery, M., A. Saraceno, A. Vaiarelli, and G. Carlomagno. "Oral Contraceptives and Changes in Nutritional Requirements," *European Review for Medical and Pharmacological Sciences* 17, no. 13 (2013): 1804–13. https://www.europeanreview.org/wp/wp-content/uploads/1804-1813.pdf.

Peeters, Robin, and Theo Visser. "Metabolism of Thyroid Hormone," *Endotext*, 2017. https://www.ncbi.nlm.nih.gov/books/NBK285545/.

Pieczynska, J., and H. Grajeta. "The Role of Selenium in Human Conception and Pregnancy," *Journal of Trace Elements in Medicine and Biology* 31, no. 8 (2014). http://doi.org/10.1016/j.jtemb.2014.07.003.

Powers, Hilary. "Folic Acid Under Scrutiny," *British Journal of Nutrition* 98, no. 4 (2007). https://doi.org/10.1017/S0007114507795326.

Pullar, J. M., A. C. Carr, and M. C. Vissers. "The Roles of Vitamin C in Skin Health," *Nutrients* 9, no. 8 (2017). https://doi.org/10.3390/nu9080866.

Reed, Beverly, and Bruce Carr. "The Normal Menstrual Cycle and the Control of Ovulation," *Endotext*, 2018. https://www.ncbi.nlm.nih.gov/books/NBK279054/.

Saini, Rajiv. "Coenzyme Q10: The Essential Nutrient," *Journal of Pharmacy and Bioallied Sciences* 3, no. 3 (2011). https://doi.org/10.4103/0975-7406.84471.

Spiller, Henry. "Rethinking Mercury: The Role of Selenium in the Pathophysiology of Mercury Toxicity," *Clinical Toxicology*, 2017. https://doi.org/10.1080/15563650.2017.1400555.

University of California San Francisco Health. "The Menstrual Cycle," *UCSF Health*, 2019. https://www.ucsfhealth.org/education/the_menstrual_cycle/.

Wong, Carmen P., Nicole A. Rinaldi, and Emily Ho. "Zinc Deficiency Enhanced Inflammatory Response by Increasing Immune Cell Activation and Inducing IL6 Promoter Demethylation," *Molecular Nutrition and Food Research* 59, no. 5 (2015): 991–99. https://doi.org/10.1002/mnfr.201400761.

## CHAPTER 2: MOVEMENT AND THE MIGHTY PELVIS

Ashton-Miller, James A., and John O. L. DeLancey. "On the Biomechanics of Vaginal Birth and Common Sequelae," *Annual Review of Biomedical Engineering* 11 (2009): 163–76. https://doi.org/10.1146/annurev-bioeng-061008-124823.

Bowman, Katy. *Diastasis Recti: The Whole-Body Solution to Abdominal Weakness and Separation*. Sequim, WA: Propriometrics Press, 2016.

Bowman, Katy. "High Heels, Pelvic Floor, and Bad Science," *Nutritious Movement*, 2019. https://www.nutritiousmovement.com/high-heels-pelvic-floor-and-bad-science/.

Bowman, Katy. *Move Your DNA: Restore Your Health Through Natural Movement*. Sequim, WA: Propriometrics Press, 2014.

Branco, Marco, Rita Santos-Rocha, and Filomena Vieira. "Biomechanics of Gait during Pregnancy," *The Scientific World Journal* (2014). http://dx.doi.org/10.1155/2014/527940.

Brito, Leonardo Barbosa Barreto de, Djalma Rabelo Ricardo, and Denise Sardinha Mendes Soares de Araújo. "Ability to Sit and Rise from the Floor as a Predictor of All-Cause Mortality," *European Jounal of Preventive Cardiology* 21, no. 7 (2012): 892–98. https://doi.org/10.1177/2047487312471759.

Chen, Chia-Hsin, Mao-Hsiung Huang, Tien-Wen Chen, Ming-Cheng Weng, Chia-Ling Lee, and Gwo-Jaw Wang. "Relationship Between Ankle Position and Pelvic Floor Muscle Activity in Female Stress Urinary Incontinence," *Urology* 66, no. 2 (2005): 288–92. https://doi.org/10.1016/j.urology.2005.03.034.

Easley, Deanna, Steven Abramowitch, and Pamela Moalli. "Female Pelvic Floor Biomechanics: Bridging the Gap," *Current Opinion in Urology* 27, no. 3 (2017). https://doi.org/10.1097/MOU.0000000000000380.

Herschorn, Sender. "Female Pelvic Floor Anatomy: The Pelvic Floor, Supporting Structures, and Pelvic Organs," *Reviews in Urology* 6, Suppl. 5 (2004): S2–S10. https://www.ncbi.nlm.nih.gov/pmc/articles/PMC1472875/.

Howard, Leslie. *Pelvic Liberation: Using Yoga, Self-Inquiry, and Breath Awareness for Pelvic Health*. Self-published, 2017.

Nordin, Margareta, and Victor H. Frankel. *Basic Biomechanics of the Musculoskeletal System*. Baltimore: Lippincott Williams & Wilkins, 2001.

Solnit, Rebecca. *Wanderlust: A History of Walking*. New York: Penguin, 2001.

Vernikos, Joan. *Sitting Kills, Moving Heals: How Everyday Movement Will Prevent Pain, Illness, and Early Death—and Exercise Alone Won't*. Fresno, CA: Quill Driver, 2011.

## CHAPTER 3: CULTIVATING YOUR BABY'S MICROBIOME

Anderson, Deborah Jean, Jai Marathe, and Jeffrey Pudney. "The Structure of the Human Vaginal *Stratum Corneum* and Its Role in Immune Defense," *American Journal of Reproductive Immunology* 71 (2014): 618-23. https://doi.org/10.1111/aji.12230.

Dawes, Colin. "Salivary Flow Patterns and the Health of Hard and Soft Oral Tissues," *JADA* 139 (2009). https://jada.ada.org/article/S0002-8177(14)63878-2/pdf.

Dominguez-Bello, Maria, Filipa Godoy-Vitorino, Rob Knight, and Martin J. Blaser. "Role of the Microbiome in Human Development," *Gut* 68, no. 6 (2019): 1108–14. https://doi.org/10.1136/gutjnl-2018-317503.

Edwards, Sara, Solveig Cunningham, Anne Dunlop, and Elizabeth Corwin. "The Maternal Gut Microbiome During Pregnancy," *American Journal of Maternal Child Nursing* 42, no. 6 (2017): 310–17. http://pubmed.ncbi.nim.nih.gov/28787280.

Gilbert, Scott. "A Holobiont Birth Narrative: The Epigenetic Transmission of the Human Microbiome," *Frontiers in Genetics* 5, no. 282 (2014). https://doi.org/10.3389/fgene.2014.00282.

Gilbert, Scott, Jann Sapp, and Alfred Tauber. "A Symbiotic View of Life: We Have Never Been Individuals," *Quarterly View of Biology* 87, no. 4 (2012): 325–41. https://www.ncbi.nlm.nih.gov/pubmed/23397797.

Gosalbes, María José, Joan Compte, Silvia Moriano-Gutierrez, Yvonne Vallès, Nuria Jiménez-Hernández, Xavier Pons, Alejandro Artacho, and M. Pilar Francino. "Metabolic Adaptation in the Human Gut Microbiota During Pregnancy and the First Year of Life," *The Lancet* 39 (2019): 497–509. https://doi.org/10.1016/j.ebiom.2018.10.071.

Kilian, M., I. L. C. Chapple, M. Hannig, P. D. Marsh, A. M. L. Pedersen, M.S. Tonetti, W. G. Wade, and E. Zaura. "The Oral Microbiome—An Update for Oral Healthcare Professionals," *British Dental Journal* 221, no. 10 (2016): 657–66. https://www.nature.com/articles/sj.bdj.2016.865.pdf.

Klepzig, K. D., A. S. Adams, J. Handelsman, and K. F. Raffa. "Symbioses: A Key Driver of Insect Physiological Processes, Ecological Interactions, Evolutionary Diversifications, and Impacts on Humans," *Environmental Entomology* 38, no. 1 (2009): 67–77. https://www.ncbi.nlm.nih.gov/pubmed/19791599.

Knight, Rob. *Follow Your Gut: The Enormous Impact of Tiny Microbes*. New York: TED Books, 2015.

Kunin, A. A., A. Y. Evdokimova, and N. S. Moiseeva. "Age-Related Differences of Tooth Enamel Morphochemistry in Health and Dental Caries," *EPMA Journal* 6, no. 1 (2015). https://doi.org/10.1186/s13167-014-0025-8.

MacIntyre, David, Manju Chandiramani, Yun Lee, Lindsay Kindinger, Ann Smith, Nicos Angelopoulos, Benjamin Lehne, Shankari Arulkumarin, Richard Brown, and Tiong Ghee Teoh. "The Vaginal Microbiome During Pregnancy and the Postpartum Period in a European Population," *Scientific Reports* 5, no. 8988 (2015). https://pubmed.ncbi.nlm.nih.gov/25758319/.

Nuriel-Ohayon, M., H. Neuman, and O. Koren. "Microbial Changes during Pregnancy, Birth, and Infancy," *Frontiers in Microbiology* 7, no. 1031 (2016). https://doi.org/10.3389/fmicb.2016.01031.

Planck, Nina. *Real Food for Mother and Baby: The Fertility Diet, Eating for Two, and Baby's First Foods*. New York: Bloomsbury, 2016.

Rajesh, K. S., Zareena, S. Heged, and M. S. Kumar. "Assessment of Salivary Calcium, Phosphate, Magnesium, pH, and Flow Rate in Healthy Subjects, Periodontitis, and Dental Caries," *Contemporary Clinical Dentistry* 6, no. 4 (2015): 461–65. https://doi.org/10.4103/0976-237X.169846.

Takahashi, Nobuhiro. "Microbial Ecosystem in the Oral Cavity: Metabolic Diversity in an Ecological Niche and Its Relationship with Oral Diseases," *International Congress Series 1284* (2005): 103–12. https://doi.org/10.1016/j.ics.2005.06.071.

Tiwari, Manjul. "Science Behind Human Saliva," *Journal of Natural Science, Biology, and Medicine* 2, no. 1 (2011): 53–58. https://doi.org/10.4103/0976-9668.82322.

Tsing, Anna, Heather Swanson, Elaine Gan, and Nils Bubandt. *Arts of Living on a Damaged Planet: Ghosts and Monsters of the Anthropocene*. Minneapolis: University of Minnesota Press, 2017.

Walker, R. W., J. C. Clemente, I. Peter, and R. J. Loos. "The Prenatal Gut Microbiome: Are We Colonized with Bacteria *in utero*?" *Pediatric Obesity* 12, Suppl. 1 (2017): 3–17. https://doi.org/10.1111/ijpo.12217.

## CHAPTER 4: A SPERM'S TALE

Annunziato, Anthony. "DNA Packaging: Nucleosomes and Chromatin," *Nature Education* 1, no. 1 (2008). https://www.nature.com/scitable/topicpage/dna-packaging-nucleosomes-and-chromatin-310.

Brody, Jane. "The Risks to Babies of Older Fathers," *New York Times*, March 25, 2019. https://www.nytimes.com/2019/03/25/well/family/the-risks-to-babies-of-older-fathers.html.

Canovas, Sebastian, and Pablo Ross. "Epigenetics in Preimplantation Mammalian Development," *Theriogenology* 86, no. 1 (2017): 69–79. https://doi.org/10.1016/j.theriogenology.2016.04.020.

Chevalier, N., and P. Fenichel. "Endocrine Disruptors: New Players in the Pathophysiology of Type 2 Diabetes?," *Diabetes & Metabolism* 41, no. 2 (2015): 107–15. https://doi.org/10.1016/j.diabet.2014.09.005.

Diamanti-Kandarakis, Evanthia, Jean-Pierre Bourguignon, Linda Giudice, Russ Hauser, Gail Prins, Ana Soto, R. Thomas Zoeller, and Andrea Gore. "Endocrine-Disrupting Chemicals: An Endocrine Society Scientific Statement," *Endocrine Reviews* 30, no. 4 (2009): 293–342. https://doi.org/10.1210/er.2009-0002.

Inhorn, Marcia C. "A Male Infertility Crisis is Coming. The Middle East Can Help," *New York Times*, October 21, 2017. https://www.nytimes.com/2017/10/21/opinion/sunday/male-infertility-middle-east.html.

Jóźków, P., and M. Rossato. "The Impact of Intense Exercise on Semen Quality," *American Journal of Men's Health* 11, no. 3 (2017): 654–62. https://doi.org/10.1177/1557988316669045.

Kimmerer, Robin Wall. *Braiding Sweetgrass: Indigenous Wisdom, Scientific Knowledge, and the Teachings of Plants*. Minneapolis: Milkweed Editions, 2014.

Klass, Perri. "Good News for Older Mothers," *New York Times*, April 3, 2017. https://www.nytimes.com/2017/04/03/well/family/good-news-for-the-older-mothers.html.

Salma, Umme, Harjinder Kaur Gill, Louis J. Keith, Sandra Tilmon, Christopher A. Jones, Anjali Sobti, and Ashlesha Patel. "Male Subfertility and the Role of Micronutrient Supplementation: Clinical and Economic Issues," *Journal of Experimental and Clinical Assisted Reproduction* 8, no. 1 (2011). https://www.ncbi.nlm.nih.gov/pmc/articles/PMC3183500/.

Watkins, Adam J., Irundika Dias, Heather Tsuro, Danielle Allen, Richard D. Emes, Joanna Moreton, Ray Wilson, Richard J. M. Ingram, and Kevin D. Sinclair. "Paternal Diet Programs Offspring Health Through Sperm and Seminal Plasma–Specific Pathways in Mice," *PNAS* 115, no. 40 (2018): 10064–69. https://doi.org/10.1073/pnas.1806333115.

## CHAPTER 5: THE FIRST TRIMESTER


Abramowicz, Jacques S., Stanley B. Barnett, Francis A. Duck, Peter D. Edmonds, Kullervo H. Hynynen, and Marvin C. Ziskin. "Fetal Thermal Effects on Diagnostic Ultrasound," *Journal of Ultrasound in Medicine* 27, no. 4 (2008): 541–59. https://doi.org/10.7863/jum.2008.27.4.541.

Altmae, Signe. "Uterine Microbiota: A Role Beyond Infection," *European Medical Journal* 6, no. 1 (2018): 70–75. https://www.emjreviews.com/reproductive-health/article/uterine-microbiota-a-role-beyond-infection/.

American College of Obstetricians and Gynecologists. "Ultrasound Exams," *ACOG*, June 2017. https://www.acog.org/Patients/FAQs/Ultrasound-Exams.

Arnold, Carrie. "Choosy Eggs May Pick Sperm for Their Genes, Defying Mendel's Law," *Quanta Magazine*, November 15, 2017. https://www.quantamagazine.org/choosy-eggs-may-pick-sperm-for-their-genes-defying-mendels-law-20171115/.

Arnup, Katherine. "Adrienne Rich: Poet, Mother, Lesbian, Feminist, Visionary," *Atlantis* 8, no. 1 (1982): 97–110.

Barber, Dan. *The Third Plate: Field Notes on the Future of Food*. New York: Penguin Books, 2014.

Baskett, Thomas F., and Fritz Naegele. "Naegele's Rule: A Reappraisal," *BJOG* 107, no. 11 (2005). https://doi.org/10.1111/j.1471-0528.2000.tb11661.x.

Benner, M., G. Ferwerda, I. Joosten, and R. G. Molen. "How Uterine Microbiota Might Be Responsible for a Receptive, Fertile Endometrium," *Human Reproduction Update* 24, no. 4 (2018): 393–415. https://doi.org/10.1093/humupd/dmy012.

Campo-Engelstein, Lisa. "The Fertilization Fairytale: 'Knight in Shining Armor' Sperm and 'Damsel in Distress' Eggs," *Bioethics Today*, July 15, 2013. https://www.amc.edu/BioethicsBlog/post.cfm/the-fertilization-fairytale-knight-in-shining-armor-sperm-and-damsel-in-distress-eggs.

Food and Drug Administration (US). "Avoid Fetal 'Keepsake' Images, Heartbeat Monitors," FDA, December 16, 2014. https://www.fda.gov/consumers/consumer-updates/avoid-fetal-keepsake-images-heartbeat-monitors.

Gamble, Karen L., David Resuehr, and Carl Hirschie Johnson. "Shift Work and Circadian Dysregulation of Reproduction," *Frontiers in Endocrinology* 4, no. 92 (2013). https://doi.org/10.3389/fendo.2013.00092.

Gernand, Alison D., Kerry J. Schulze, Christine P. Stewart, Keith P. West Jr., and Parul Christian. "Micronutrient Deficiencies in Pregnancy Worldwide: Health Effects and Prevention," *Nature Reviews Endocrinology* 12, no. 5 (2016): 274–89. https://doi.org/10.1038/nrendo.2016.37.

Gervasi, Maria Gracia, and Pablo E. Visconti. "Molecular Changes and Signaling Events Occurring in Spermatozoa During Epididymal Maturation," *Andrology* 5, no. 2 (2017): 204–18. https://doi.org/10.1111/andr.12320.

Ghazal, Sanaz, Jennifer Kulp Makarov, Christopher De Jonge, and Pasquale Patrizio. "Egg Transport and Fertilization," *Global Library of Women's Medicine*, 2014. https://doi.org/10.3843/GLOWM.10317.

Griffiths, Sarah K., and Jeremy P. Campbell. "Placental Structure, Function and Drug Transfer," *Continuing Education in Anesthesia Critical Care and Pain* 15, no. 2 (2015): 84–89. https://doi.org/10.1093/bjaceaccp/mku013.

Kurosaka, Satoshi, and Anna Kashina. "Cell Biology of Embryonic Migration," *Birth Defects Research Part C: Embryo Today: Reviews* 84, no. 2 (2008): 102–22. https://doi.org/10.1002/bdrc.20125.

Lee, N. M., and S. Saha. "Nausea and Vomiting of Pregnancy," *Gastroenterology Clinics of North America* 40, no. 2 (2011). https://doi.org/10.1016/j.gtc.2011.03.009.

Lyons, R. A., E. Saridogan, and O. Djahanbakhch. "The Reproductive Significance of Human Fallopian Tube Cilia," *Human Reproduction Update* 12, no. 4 (2006): 363–72. https://doi.org/10.1093/humupd/dml012.

Martin, Emily. "The Egg and the Sperm: How Science Has Constructed a Romance Based on Stereotypical Male-Female Roles," *Signs* 16, no. 3 (1991): 485–501. https://web.stanford.edu/~eckert/PDF/Martin1991.pdf.

Mor, Gil, Ingrid Cardenas, Vikki Abrahams, and Seth Guller. "Inflammation and Pregnancy: The Role of the Immune System at the Implantation Site," *Annals of New York Academy of Sciences* 1221, no. 1 (2011): 80–87. https://doi.org/10.1111/j.1749-6632.2010.05938.x.

Nichols, Lily. *Real Food for Pregnancy: The Science and Wisdom of Optimal Prenatal Nutrition*. Self-published, 2018.

Perez-Muñoz, Maria Elisa, Marie-Claire Arrieta, Amanda E. Ramer-Tait, and Jens Walter. "A Critical Assessment of the 'Sterile Womb' and 'In Utero Colonization' Hypothesis: Implications for Research on the Pioneer Infant Microbiome," *Microbiome* 5, no. 48 (2017). https://doi.org/10.1186/s40168-017-0268-4.

Russell, Darryl L., and Rebecca L. Robker. "Molecular Mechanisms of Ovulation: Co-ordination Through the Cumulus Complex," *Human Reproduction Update* 13, no. 3 (2007): 289–312. https://doi.org/10.1093/humupd/dml062.

Schoenmakers, Sam, Regine Steegers-Theunissen, and Marijke Fass. "The Matter of the Reproductive Microbiome," *Obstetric Medicine*, May 17, 2018. https://doi.org/10.1177/1753495X18775899.

Sihi, Debjani, Biswanath Dari, Dinesh K. Sharma, Himanshu Pathak, Lata Nain, and Om Parkash Sharma. "Evaluation of Soil Health in Organic vs. Conventional Farming of Basmati Rice in North India," *Journal of Plant Nutrition and Soil Science* 180, no. 3 (2017): 389–406. https://doi.org/10.1002/jpln.201700128.

Sperotto, Raul A., Felipe K. Ricachenevsky, Lorraine E. Williams, Marta W. Vasconcelos, and Paloma K. Menguer. "From Soil to Seed: Micronutrient Movement into and within the Plant," *Frontiers in Plant Science* 5 (2014). https://doi.org/10.3389/fpls.2014.00438.

Steingraber, Sandra. *Having Faith: An Ecologist's Journey to Motherhood.* New York: Berkley Books, 2001.

Wellner, Karen. "Carnegie Stages," *Embryo Project Encyclopedia*, July 17, 2009. https://embryo.asu.edu/pages/carnegie-stages.

Wolter, Justin M. "The Process of Implantation of Embryos in Primates," *Embryo Project Encyclopedia*, March 21, 2013. https://embryo.asu.edu/pages/process-implantation-embryos-primates.

## CHAPTER 6: ENDOCRINE CHANGES AND AVOIDING TOXINS


Angueira, Anthony R., Anton E. Ludvik, Timothy E. Reddy, Barton Wicksteed, William L. Lowe Jr., and Brian T. Layden. "New Insights into Gestational Glucose Metabolism: Lessons Learned from 21st Century Approaches," *Diabetes* 64, no. 2 (2015): 327–34. https://doi.org/10.2337/db14-0877.

Bleyl, Steven B., and Gary C. Schoenwolf. "What Is the Timeline of Important Events During Pregnancy That May Be Disrupted by a Teratogenic Exposure?," *Teratology Primer*, 3rd ed., January 2017. https://www.teratology.org/primer/Teratogenic-Exposure.asp.

Campaign for Safe Cosmetics and Environmental Working Group. "Not So Sexy: The Health Risks of Secret Chemicals in Fragrance," Campaign for Safe Cosmetics and Environmental Working Group, May 2010. https://www.ewg.org/sites/default/files/report/SafeCosmetics_FragranceRpt.pdf.

Cheung, K. L., and R. A. Lafayette. "Renal Physiology of Pregnancy," *Advances in Chronic Kidney Disease* 20, no. 3 (2014): 209–14. https://doi.org/10.1053/j.ackd.2013.01.012.

Environmental Working Group. "Body Burden: The Pollution in Newborns," Environmental Working Group, July 14, 2005. https://www.ewg.org/research/body-burden-pollution-newborns.

Ernst, Sara, Cem Demirci, Shelley Valle, Silvia Velazquez-Garcia, and Adolfo Garcia-Ocaña. "Mechanisms in the Adaptation of Maternal ß-cells During Pregnancy," *Diabetes Management* 1, no. 2 (2011): 239–48. https://pubmed.ncbi.nlm.nih.gov/21845205/.

Imbard, Apolline, Jean-François Benoist, and Henk J. Blom. "Neural Tube Defects, Folic Acid and Methylation," *International Journal of Environmental Research and Public Health* 10, no. 9 (2013): 4352–89. https://doi.org/10.3390/ijerph10094352.

Miller, Richard K. "What Is the Role of the Placenta—Does It Protect Against or Is It a Target for Insult?," *Teratology Primer*, 3rd ed., January 2017. https://www.teratology.org/primer/Placenta.asp.

Potera, Carol. "Indoor Air Quality: Scented Products Emit a Bouquet of VOCs," *Environmental Health Perspectives* 119, no. 1 (2011): A16. https://doi.org/10.1289/ehp.119-a16.

Schneider, Samantha L., and Henry W. Lim. "Review of Environmental Effects of Oxybenzone and Other Sunscreen Active Ingredients," *Journal of the American Academy of Dermatology* 80, no. 1 (2019): 266–71. https://doi.org/10.1016/j.jaad.2018.06.033.

Snyder, Gary. *The Gary Snyder Reader, Volume 1: Prose, Poetry, and Translations, 1952–1998*. Washington, DC: Counterpoint, 1999.

Soma-Pillay, Priya, Catherine Nelson-Piercy, Heli Tolppanen, and Alexandre Mebazaa. "Physiological Changes in Pregnancy," *Cardiovascular Journal of Africa* 27, no. 2 (2016): 89–94. https://doi.org/10.5830/CVJA-2016-021.

Steingraber, Sandra. "Household Tips from Warrior Mom!," *Orion Magazine*. https://orionmagazine.org/article/household-tips-from-warrior-mom/.

## CHAPTER 7: THE SECOND AND THIRD TRIMESTERS

Berry, Wendell. "Faustian Economics: Hell Hath No Limits," *Harper's Magazine*, May 2008. https://harpers.org/archive/2008/05/faustian-economics/.

Bowman, Katy. "Mind Your Pelvis," *Nutritious Movement*, July 2010. https://www.nutritiousmovement.com/mind-your-pelvis/.

Bowman, Katy. "Natural Mama," *Nutritious Movement*. https://www.nutritiousmovement.com/natural-mama/.

Bowman, Katy. "Natural Pregnancy, Natural Birth." *Nutritious Movement*. https://www.nutritiousmovement.com/natural-pregnancy-natural-birth/.

Braarud, Hanne C., Maria W. Markhus, Siv Skotheim, Kjell M. Stormark, Livar Froyland, Ingvild E. Graff, and Marian Kjellevold. "Maternal DHA Status During Pregnancy Has a Positive Impact on Infant Problem Solving: A Norwegian Prospective Observation Study," *Nutrients* 10, no. 5 (2018): 529. https://doi.org/10.3390/nu10050529.

Bradford, Billie F., Robin S. Cronin, Christopher J. McKinlay, John M. Thompson, Edwin A. Mitchell, Peter R. Stone, and Lesley M. McCowan. "A Diurnal Fetal Movement Pattern: Findings from a Cross-Sectional Study of Maternally Perceived Fetal Movements in the Third Trimester of Pregnancy," *PLOS* One 14, no. 6 (2019). https://doi.org/10.1371/journal.pone.0217583.

Centers for Disease Control and Prevention. "Childhood Lead Poisoning Prevention," CDC, 2019. https://www.cdc.gov/nceh/lead/faqs/lead-faqs.htm.

Chilton, Stephanie N., Jeremy P. Burton, and Gregor Reid. "Inclusion of Fermented Foods in Food Guides Around the World," *Nutrients* 7, no. 1 (2015): 390–404. https://doi.org/10.3390/nu7010390.

Collins, N. L., C. Dunkel-Schetter, M. Lobel, and S. C. Scrimshaw. "Social Support in Pregnancy: Psychosocial Correlates of Birth Outcomes and Postpartum Depression," *Journal of Personality and Social Psychology* 65, no. 6 (1993): 1243–58. https://doi.org/10.1037//0022-3514.65.6.1243.

Elsenbruch, S., S. Benson, M. Rücke, M. Rose, J. Dudenhausen, M. K. Pincus-Knackstedt, B. F. Knapp, and P. C. Arck. "Social Support During Pregnancy: Effects on Maternal Depressive Symptoms, Smoking and Pregnancy Outcome," *Human Reproduction* 22, no. 3 (2007): 869–77. https://doi.org/10.1093/humrep/del432.

Fagard, J., R. Esseily, L. Jacquey, K. O'Regan, and E. Somogyi. "Fetal Origin of Sensorimotor Behavior," *Frontiers in Neurobiotics* 12, no. 23 (2018). https://doi.org/10.3389.fnbot.2018.00023.

Gintis, Herbert. "Gene-Culture Coevolution and the Nature of Human Sociality," *Philosophical Transactions of the Royal Society of London. Series B, Biological Sciences* 366, no. 1566 (2011): 878–88. https://doi.org/10.1098/rstb.2010.0310.

Gohir, Wajiha, Elyanne M. Ratcliffe, and Deborah M. Sloboda. "Of the Bugs That Shape Us: Maternal Obesity, the Gut Microbiome, and Long-Term Disease Risk," *Pediatric Research* 77, no. 1 (2015). https://www.nature.com/articles/pr2014169.pdf.

Gribble, Matthew O., Roxanne Karimi, Beth J. Feingold, Jennifer F. Nyland, Todd M. O'Hara, Michail I. Gladyshev, and Celia Y. Chen. "Mercury, Selenium and Fish Oils in Marine Food Webs and Implications for Human Health," *Journal of the Marine Biological Association of the United Kingdom* 96, no. 1 (2016): 43–59. https://doi.org/10.1017/S0025315415001356.

Lai, Jonathan, Niamh C. Nowlan, Ravi Vaidyanathan, Caroline J. Shaw, and Christoph C. Lees. "Fetal Movements as a Predictor of Health," *AOGS* 95, no. 9 (2016). https://doi.org/10.1111/aogs.12944.

McDonald, Braedon, and Kathy D. McCoy. "Maternal Microbiota in Pregnancy and Early Life," *Science* 365, no. 6457 (2019): 984–85. https://doi.org/10.1126/science.aay0618.

Mostafa, W. Z., and R. A. Hegazy. "Vitamin D and the Skin: Focus on a Complex Relationship: A Review," *Journal of Advanced Research* 6, no. 6 (2015): 793–804. https://doi.org/10.1016/j.jare.2014.01.011.

Murray, Sharon S., and Emily S. McKinney. *Foundations of Maternal-Newborn and Women's Health Nursing*, 6th ed. St. Louis: Elsevier Saunders, 2014.

Myers, Kristin M., and David Elad. "Biomechanics of the Human Uterus," *WIREs Systems Biology and Medicine* 9, no. 5 (2017): e1388. https://doi.org/10.1002/wsbm.1388.

Narendran, Vivek, R. Randall Wickett, William L. Pickens, and Steven B. Hoath. "Interaction Between Pulmonary Surfactant and Vernix: A Potential Mechanism for Induction of Amniotic Fluid Turbidity," *Pediatric Research* 48 (2000): 120–24. https://doi.org/10.1203/00006450-200007000-00021.

Ohayon-Nuriel, M., H. Nueman, and O. Koren. "Microbial Changes during Pregnancy, Birth, and Infancy," *Frontiers in Microbiology* 7 (2016): 1031 . https://doi.org/10.3389/fmicb.2016.01031.

Reissland, Nadja, and Barbara S. Kisilevsky. *Fetal Development: Research on Brain and Behavior, Environmental Influences, and Emerging Technologies*. New York: Springer, 2016.

Reiter, Russel J., Dun Xian Tan, Ahmet Korkmaz, and Sergio A. Rosales-Corral. "Melatonin and Stable Circadian Rhythms Optimize Maternal, Placental and Fetal Physiology," *Human Reproduction Update* 20, no. 2 (2013). https://doi.org/10.1093/humupd/dmt054.

Sekulić, Slobodan R., Damir D. Lukač, and Nada M. Naumović. "The Fetus Cannot Exercise Like an Astronaut: Gravity Loading Is Necessary for the Physiological Development During Second Half of Pregnancy," *Medical Hypothesis* 64, no. 2 (2005). https://doi.org/10.1016/j.mehy.2004.08.012.

Shea, C. A., R. A. Rolfe, and P. Murphy. "The Importance of Foetal Movement for Co-ordinated Cartilage and Bone Development *in utero*," *Bone and Joint Research* 4, no. 7 (2015): 106–16. https://doi.org/10.1302/2046-3758.47.2000387.

Singh, Gurcharan, and G. Archana. "Unraveling the Mystery of Vernix Caseosa," *Indian Journal of Dermatology* 53, no. 2 (2008): 54–60. https://doi.org/10.4103/0019-5154.41645.

Stiles, J., and T. L. Jernigan. "The Basics of Brain Development," *Neuropsychology Review* 20, no. 4 (2010): 327–48. https://doi.org/10.1007/s11065-010-9148-4.

Taddeo, Lisa. *Three Women*. New York: Avid Reader, 2019.

Toscano, M., R. D. Grandi, E. Grossi, and L. Drago. "Role of the Human Breast Milk-Associated Microbiota on the Newborns' Immune System: A Mini Review," *Frontiers in Microbiology* 8, no. 2100 (2017). https://doi.org/10.3389/fmicb.2017.02100.

Ventura, A. K., and J. Worobey. "Early Influences on the Development of Food Preferences," *Current Biology* 23, no. 9 (2013). https://doi.org/10.1016/j.cub.2013.02.037.

Verbruggen, S. W., B. Kainz, S. C. Shelmerdine, J. V. Hajnal, M. A. Rutherford, O. J. Arthurs, and N. C. Nowlan. "Stresses and Strains on the Human Fetal Skeleton During Development," *Journal of the Royal Society Interface* 15, no. 138 (2018). https://doi.org/10.1098/rsif.2017.0593.

De Vries, J., and B. F. Fong. "Normal Fetal Motility: An Overview," *Ultrasound in Obstetrics and Gynecology* 27, no. 6 (2006): 701–11. https://doi.org/10.1002/uog.2740.

Wagner, C. L., and B. W. Hollis. "The Implications of Vitamin D Status During Pregnancy on Mother and Her Developing Child," *Frontiers in Endocrinology* 9, no. 500 (2018). https://doi.org/10.3389/fendo.2018.00500.

Zheng, Tongzhang, et al. "Effects of Environmental Exposures on Fetal and Childhood Growth Trajectories," *Annals of Global Health* 82, no. 1 (2016). https://doi.org/10.1016/j.aogh.2016.01.008.

## CHAPTER 8: BIRTH!

Becher, Naja, Kristina Waldorf, Merete Hein, and Niels Uldbjerg. "The Cervical Mucus Plug: Structured Review of the Literature," *Acta Obstetricia et Genecologia Scandinavia* 88, no. 5 (2009): 502–13. https://doi.org/10.1080/00016340902852898.

Bell, A. F., E. N. Erickson, and C. S. Carter. "Beyond Labor: The Role of Natural and Synthetic Oxytocin in the Transition to Motherhood," *Journal of Midwifery and Women's Health* 59, no. 1 (2014): 35–42. https://doi.org/10.1111/jmwh.12101.

Buckley, Sarah. *Gentle Birth, Gentle Mothering: A Doctor's Guide to Natural Childbirth and Gentle Early Parenting Choices*. Berkeley, CA: Celestial Arts, 2009.

Butwick, A. J, C. A. Wong, and N. Guo. "Maternal Body Mass Index and Use of Labor Neuraxial Analgesia: A Population-Based Retrospective Cohort Study," *Anesthesiology* 129 (2018). https://doi.org/10.1097/ALN.0000000000002322.

Centers for Disease Control and Prevention. "Preterm Birth," CDC, 2019. https://www.cdc.gov/reproductivehealth/maternalinfanthealth/pretermbirth.htm.

Dekker, Rebecca. "The Evidence On: Fetal Monitoring," *Evidence Based Birth*, July 17, 2012 (updated May 21, 2018). https://evidencebasedbirth.com/fetal-monitoring/.

Fleres, Jaime. *Birth Your Story: Why Writing about Your Birth Matters*. Asheville, NC: Santosha Press, 2017.

Haines, Helen H., Christine Rubertsson, Julie F. Pallant, and Ingegerd Hidingsson. "The Influence of Women's Fear, Attitudes and Beliefs of Childbirth on Mode and Experience of Birth," *BMC Pregnancy and Childbirth* 12, no. 55 (2012). https://doi.org/10.1186/1471-2393-12-55.

Ikei, Harumi, Chorong Song, and Yoshifumi Miyazaki. "Physiological Effect of Olfactory Stimulation by Hinoki Cypress (*Chamaecyparis obtuse*) Leaf Oil," *Journal of Physiological Anthropology* 34, no. 44 (2015). https://doi.org/10.1186/s40101-015-0082-2.

Lothian, Judith A. "The Purpose and Power of Pain in Labor," *Choices in Childbirth*, 2008. https://choicesinchildbirth.org/wp-content/uploads/2014/08/2008_LOTHIAN_Purpose-of-pain-in-Labor.pdf.

Lothian, Judith A. "Safe, Healthy Birth: What Every Pregnant Woman Needs to Know," *Journal of Perinatal Education* 18, no. 3 (2009): 48–54. https://doi.org/10.1624/105812409X461225.

Markman, Art. "Trauma and the Benefits of Writing About It," *Psychology Today*, October 20, 2009. https://www.psychologytoday.com/us/blog/ulterior-motives/200910/trauma-and-the-benefits-writing-about-it.

Norwitz, Errol R., Elizabeth A. Bonney, Victoria V. Snegovskikh, Michelle A. Williams, Mark Phillippe, Joong S. Park, and Vikki M. Abrahams. "Molecular Regulation of Parturition: The Role of the Decidual Clock," *Cold Springs Harbor Perspectives in Medicine* 5, no. 11 (2015). https://doi.org/10.1101/cshperspect.a023143.

Slade, P., K. Balling, K. Sheen, and G. Houghton. "Establishing a Valid Construct of Fear of Childbirth: Findings from In-Depth Interviews with Women and Midwives," *BMC Pregnancy and Childbirth* 19, no. 96 (2019). https://doi.org/10.1186/s12884-019-2241-7.

## CHAPTER 9: REST, RECOVERY, AND GENTLE MOVEMENT

Dennis, Cindy-Lee, Kenneth Fung, Sophie Grigoriadis, Gail Erlick Robinson, Sarah Romans, and Lori Ross. "Traditional Postpartum Practices and Rituals: A Qualitative Systemic Review," *Embryo Project Encyclopedia* (2007). https://doi.org/10.2217/17455057.3.4.487.

Epstein, David. *Range: Why Generalists Triumph in a Specialized World*. New York: Riverhead Books, 2019.

Gammie, Stephen C. "Mother-Infant Communication: Carrying Understanding to a New Level," *Current Biology* 23, no. 9 (2013). https://doi.org/10.1016/j.cub.2013.03.051.

Gelb, David, dir. *Chef's Table*. Season 3, episode 1, "Jeong Kwan." Aired February 17, 2017, on Netflix.

Jamon, Marc. "The Development of Vestibular System and Related Functions in Mammals: Impact of Gravity," *Frontiers in Integrative Neuroscience* 8, no. 11 (2014). https://doi.org/10.3389/fnint.2014.00011.

Memon, Hafsa U., and Victoria L. Handa. "Vaginal Childbirth and Pelvic Floor Disorders," *Women's Health* 9, no. 3 (2013): 265–77. https://doi.org/10.2217/whe.13.17.

Mutic, Abby D., Sheila Jordan, Sara M. Edwards, Erin P. Ferranti, Taylor A. Thul, and Irene Yang. "The Postpartum Maternal and Newborn Microbiomes," *American Journal of Maternal Child Nursing* 42, no. 6 (2017): 326–31. https://doi.org/10.1097/NMC.0000000000000374.

Roberts, Sam. "Dana Raphael, Proponent of Breast-Feeding and Use of Doulas, Dies at 90," *New York Times*, February 19, 2016. https://www.nytimes.com/2016/02/21/nyregion/dana-raphael-proponent-of-breast-feeding-and-the-use-of-doulas-dies-at-90.html.

Sacks, Alexandra, and Catherine Birndorf. *What No One Tells You: A Guide to Your Emotions from Pregnancy to Motherhood*. New York: Simon & Schuster, 2019.

Uvnas-Moberg, Kerstin, and Maria Petersson. "Oxytocin, a Mediator of Anti-Stress, Well-being, Social-Interaction, Growth and Healing," *Z Psychosom Med Psychotherapy* 51, no. 1 (2005): 57–80. https://www.ncbi.nlm.nih.gov/pubmed/15834840.

Yates, Jacqueline. "Perspective: The Long-Term Effects of Light Exposure on Establishment of Newborn Circadian Rhythm," *Journal of Clinical Sleep Medicine* 14, no. 10 (2018). https://doi.org/10.5664/jcsm.7426.

## CHAPTER 10: FEEDING YOUR BABY

Ballard, Olivia, and Ardythe Morrow. "Human Milk Composition: Nutrients and Bioactive Factors," *Pediatric Clinics of North America* 60, no. 1 (2013): 49–74. https://doi.org/10.1016/j.pcl.2012.10.002.

Bode, Lars. "Human Milk Oligosaccharides: Every Baby Needs a Sugar Mama," *Glycobiology* 22, no. 9 (2012): 1147–62. https://doi.org/10.1093/glycob/cws074.

Hahn-Holbrook, Jennifer, Darby Saxbe, Christine Bixby, Caroline Steele, and Laura Glynn. "Human Milk as 'Chrononutrition': Implications for Child Health and Development," *Pediatric Research* 85 (2019): 936–42. https://doi.org/10.1038/s41390-019-0368-x.

Harbeson, Danny, Rym Ben-Othman, Nelly Amenyogbe, and Tobias R. Kollman. "Outgrowing the Immaturity Myth: The Cost of Defending from Neonatal Infectious Disease," *Frontiers in Immunology* 29 (2018). https://doi.org/10.3389/fimmu.2018.01077.

Le Doare, Kirsty, Beth Holder, Aisha Bassett, and Pia S. Pannaraj. "Mother's Milk: A Purposeful Contribution to the Development of the Infant Microbiota and Immunity," *Frontiers in Immunology* 28 (2018). https://doi.org/10.3389/fimmu.2018.00361.

Moberg, Kerstin Uvnas, and Danielle K. Prime. "Oxytocin Effects in Mother and Infants During Breastfeeding," *Infant Journal* 9, no. 6 (2013): 201–6. http://www.infantjournal.co.uk/pdf/inf_054_ers.pdf.

Reardon, Sara. "Resistance to Infections is Suppressed to Prevent Inflammation from Bacterial Colonization," *Nature*, November 6, 2013. https://www.nature.com/news/babies-weak-immune-systems-let-good-bacteria-in-1.14112.

Steingraber, Sandra. *Having Faith: An Ecologist's Journey to Motherhood.* New York: Berkley Books, 2001.

Van den Elsen, Lieke W. J., Johan Garssen, Remy Burcelin, and Valerie Verhasselt. "Shaping the Gut Microbiota by Breastfeeding: The Gateway to Allergy Prevention?," *Frontiers in Pediatrics* 7 (2019): 47. https://doi.org/10.3389/fped.2019.00047.

Williams, Florence. *Breasts: A Natural and Unnatural History.* New York: Norton, 2013.

## CHAPTER 11: YOUR BRAIN ON BABY

Abraham, Eyal, Talma Hendler, Irit Shapira-Lichter, Yaniv Kanat-Maymon, Orna Zagoory-Sharon, and Ruth Feldman. "Father's Brain is Sensitive to Childcare Experiences," *PNAS* 111, no. 27 (2014): 9792–97. https://doi.org/10.1073/pnas.1402569111.

Ball, Natalie, Eduardo Mercado III, and Itzel Orduña. "Enriched Environments as a Potential Treatment for Development Disorders: A Critical Assessment," *Frontiers in Psychology* 10 (2019): 466. https://doi.org/10.3389/fpsyg.2019.00466.

Barba-Müller, Erika, Sinead Craddock, Susanna Carmona, and Elseline Hoekzema. "Brain Plasticity in Pregnancy and the Postpartum Period: Links to Maternal Caregiving and Mental Health," *Archives of Women's Mental Health* 22, no. 2 (2019): 289–99. https://doi.org/10.1007/s00737-018-0889-z.

Baroncelli, L., C. Braschi, M. Spolidoro, T. Begenisic, A. Sale, and L. Maffei. "Nurturing Brain Plasticity: Impact of Environmental Enrichment," *Cell Death and Differentiation* 17 (2010): 1092–1103. https://doi.org/10.1038/cdd.2009.193.

Belluck, Pam. "Pregnancy Changes the Brain in Ways That May Help Mothering," *New York Times*, December 19, 2016. https://www.nytimes.com/2016/12/19/health/pregnancy-brain-change.html.

Bhattacharjee, Yudhijit. "The First Year," *National Geographic Magazine*, January 2015. https://www.nationalgeographic.com/magazine/2015/01/baby-brains-development-first-year/.

Center on the Developing Child. "Toxic Stress," Center on the Developing Child, Harvard University, 2019. https://developingchild.harvard.edu/science/key-concepts/toxic-stress/.

Clemenson, Gregory D., Fred H. Gage, and Craig E.L. Stark. "Environmental Enrichment and Neuronal Plasticity," in *The Oxford Handbook of Developmental Neural Plasticity* (Oxford Handbooks Online), ed. Moses V. Chao. Published online October 2018. https://doi.org/10.1093/oxfordhb/9780190635374.013.13.

Cusick, Sarah, and Michael Georgieff. "The Role of Nutrition in Brain Development: The Golden Opportunity of the 'First 1000 Days,'" *Journal of Pediatrics* 175 (2016): 16–21. https://doi.org/10.1016/j.jpeds.2016.05.013.

Fitelson, Elizabeth, Sarah Kim, Allison Scott Baker, and Kristin Leight. "Treatment of Postpartum Depression: Clinical, Psychological and Pharmacological Options," *International Journal of Women's Health* 3 (2011): 1–14. https://doi.org/10.2147/IJWH.S6938.

Gingnell, Malin, Simone Toffolleto, Johan Wikstrom, Jonas Engman, Elin Bannbers, Erika Comasco, and Inger Sundstrom-Poromaa. "Emotional Anticipation After Delivery: A Longitudinal Neuroimaging Study of the Postpartum Period," *Scientific Reports* 7, no. 114 (2017). https://doi.org/10.1038/s41598-017-00146-3.

Hoekzema, Elseline, et al. "Pregnancy Leads to Long-Lasting Changes in Human Brain Structure," *Nature Neuroscience* 20 (2017): 287–96. https://www.nature.com/articles/nn.4458.

Kim, Pilyoung. "Human Maternal Brain Plasticity: Adaptation to Parenting," *New Directions for Child and Adolescent Development* 153 (2016): 47–58. https://doi.org/10.1002/cad.20168.

Kim, Pilyoung, Lane Strathearn, and James E. Swain. "The Maternal Brain and Its Plasticity in Humans," *Hormones and Behavior* 77 (2016): 113–23. https://doi.org/10.1016/j.yhbeh.2015.08.001.

Leuner, Benedetta, Erica R. Glasper, and Elizabeth Gould. "Parenting and Plasticity," *Trends in Neuroscience* 33, no. 10 (2010): 465–73. https://doi.org/10.1016/j.tins.2010.07.003.

Luo, Lizhu, Xiaole Ma, Xiaoxiao Zheng, Weihua Zhao, Lei Xu, Benjamin Becker, and Keith M. Kendrick. "Neural Systems and Hormones Mediating Attraction to Infant and Child Faces," *Frontiers in Psychology* 6 (2015): 970. https://doi.org/10.3389/fpsyg.2015.00970.

Sacks, Alexandra. "Reframing 'Mommy Brain,'" *New York Times*, May 11, 2018. https://www.nytimes.com/2018/05/11/well/family/reframing-mommy-brain.html.

Sacks, Oliver. *The Mind's Eye*. New York: Vintage/Knopf, 2010.

Sacks, Oliver. "This Year, Change Your Mind," *New York Times*, December 31, 2010. https://www.nytimes.com/2011/01/01/opinion/01sacks.html.

Sullivan, Regina, Rosemarie Perry, Aliza Sloan, Karine Kleinhaus, and Nina Burtchen. "Infant Bonding and Attachment to the Caregiver: Insights from Basic and Clinical Science," *Clinics in Perinatology* 38, no. 4 (2011): 643–55. https://doi.org/10.1016/j.clp.2011.08.011.

## CHAPTER 12: FAMILY PLANNING

Bouchard, Thomas, Richard J. Fehring, and Mary Schneider. "Efficacy of a New Postpartum Transition Protocol for Avoiding Pregnancy," *Journal of the American Board of Family Medicine* 26, no. 1 (2013): 35–44. https://doi.org/10.3122/jabfm.2013.01.120126.

Conde-Agudelo, Agustin, Anyeli Rosas-Bermudez, and Maureen H. Norton. "Birth Spacing and Risk of Autism and Other Neurodevelopment Disabilities: A Systematic Review," *Pediatrics* 137, no. 5 (2016). https://doi.org/10.1542/peds.2015-3482.

Doucleff, Michaeleen. "Secrets of a Maya Supermom: What Parenting Books Don't Tell You," NPR, May 11, 2018. https://www.npr.org/sections/goatsandsoda/2018/05/11/603315432/the-best-mothers-day-gift-get-mom-out-of-the-box.

Henrich, Joseph, Steven J. Heine, and Ara Norenzayan. "The Weirdest People in the World?," *Behavioral and Brain Sciences* 33 (2010): 61–135. https://doi.org/10.1017/S0140525X0999152X.

King, Janet C. "The Risk of Maternal Nutrition Depletion and Poor Outcomes Increases in Early or Closely Spaced Pregnancies," *Journal of Nutrition* 133, no. 5 (2003). https://doi.org/10.1093/jn/133.5.1732S.

Perel, Esther. *Mating in Captivity: Unlocking Erotic Intelligence*. New York: HarperCollins, 2006.

Schummers, Laura, Jennifer A. Hutcheon, Sonia Hernandez-Diaz, et al. "Association of Short Interpregnancy Interval with Pregnancy Outcomes According to Maternal Age," *JAMA Internal Medicine* 178, no. 12 (2018): 1661–70. https://doi.org/10.1001/jamainternmed.2018.4696.

World Health Organization. "Report of a WHO Technical Consultation on Birth Spacing," World Health Organization, Department of Reproductive Health and Research, 2007.

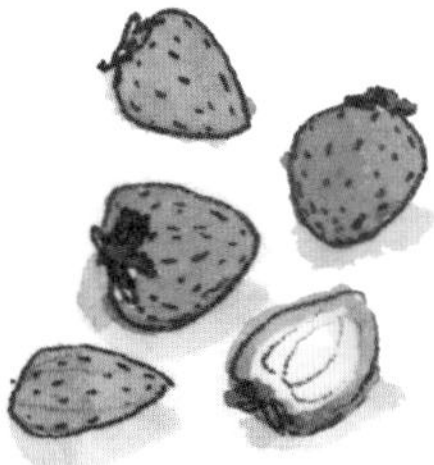

# Index

# About the Author

Amy J. Hammer is a writer whose work focuses on reproductive health, real food, movement, and the environment. She is fascinated by ecology, and her writing explores the relationships between humans and their environments and the impact of this relationship on overall health. She is a registered nurse and also has degrees in journalism and environmental studies and is pursuing a master's degree as a family nurse practitioner. Amy lives in the Great Basin Desert with her family, including one husband, two children, one brother named Bob, two cats, and eight chickens. In this arid landscape, they cultivate a thriving garden and forge meaningful connections to the land and their community. When she's not writing, Amy enjoys doing all the things she writes about: moving her body, gardening, making food, playing outside with her family, and living life with deep pleasure and, always, a sense of humor.

# About the Illustrator

Michelle Lassaline is an artist based in the Pacific Northwest. In addition to painting and drawing, her interdisciplinary art practice includes sewing and textiles, papier-mâché sculpture, and performance art. Michelle's work is in the collections of the City of Reno, the Oats Park Art Center in Fallon, Nevada, and Isle Royale National Park, where she was an artist-in-residence in 2016. She has been awarded grants from the City of Seattle, Artist Trust, 4Culture, and the Nevada Arts Council, and she is currently pursuing her Master of Fine Arts degree at the Maine College of Art.

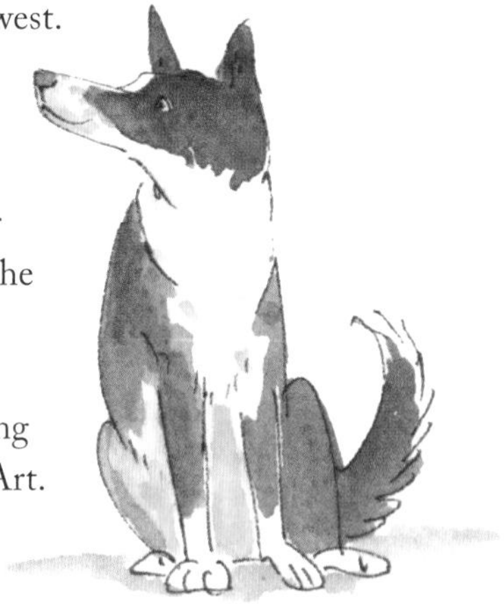